MINDFULNESS-BASED COGNITIVE THERAPY FOR BIPOLAR DISORDER

Mindfulness-Based Cognitive Therapy for Bipolar Disorder

Thilo Deckersbach
Britta Hölzel
Lori Eisner
Sara W. Lazar
Andrew A. Nierenberg

THE GUILFORD PRESS
New York   London

© 2014 The Guilford Press
A Division of Guilford Publications, Inc.
72 Spring Street, New York, NY 10012
www.guilford.com

Printed in the United States of America

This book is printed on acid-free paper.

Last digit is print number: 9   8   7   6   5   4   3   2   1

The authors have checked with sources believed to be reliable in their efforts to provide
information that is complete and generally in accord with the standards of practice that
are accepted at the time of publication. However, in view of the possibility of human error
or changes in behavioral, mental health, or medical sciences, neither the authors, nor the
editor and publisher, nor any other party who has been involved in the preparation or
publication of this work warrants that the information contained herein is in every respect
accurate or complete, and they are not responsible for any errors or omissions or the
results obtained from the use of such information. Readers are encouraged to confirm the
information contained in this book with other sources.

Library of Congress Cataloging-in-Publication data is available from the publisher.

ISBN 978-1-4625-1406-9

Illustrations by Steve A. McKinley, based on the work of Alexandra Rodman.

About the Authors

Thilo Deckersbach, PhD, is Associate Professor of Psychology at Harvard Medical School. He serves as Director of Psychology in the Bipolar Clinic and Research Program and as Director of Research in the Division of Neurotherapeutics at the Massachusetts General Hospital in Boston. Dr. Deckersbach's research has been supported by the National Institute of Mental Health, NARSAD, the Tourette Syndrome Association, the International OCD Foundation, and the Depressive and Bipolar Alternative Treatment Foundation. He has published over 95 peer-reviewed papers and book chapters. His clinical research concentrates on the development of cognitive-behavioral and mindfulness-based treatments for bipolar disorder; his functional neuroimaging research focuses on the interaction of cognitive and emotional processes in bipolar disorder. Dr. Deckersbach has been a dedicated meditation practitioner since 2008.

Britta Hölzel, PhD, is Research Fellow at the Institute for Medical Psychology at Charité in Berlin, Germany. She was previously Research Fellow in the Psychiatric Neuroscience Division at the Massachusetts General Hospital and Harvard Medical School. Dr. Hölzel is a mindfulness-based stress reduction instructor and a certified yoga teacher (Sivananda Organization), and has been a dedicated yoga and meditation practitioner since 1997. Dr. Hölzel's work has been supported by a Marie Curie International Outgoing Fellowship within the 7th European Community Framework Program, a Positive Neuroscience Award from the John Templeton Foundation, Varela grants from the Mind and Life Institute, and the Kusala Foundation. Her magnetic resonance imaging research focuses on the effects of mindfulness practice on the functional neuroanatomy of emotion regulation as well as on structural changes in the brain.

Lori Eisner, PhD, is Assistant in Psychology at the Massachusetts General Hospital's Bipolar Clinic and Research Program and Instructor at Harvard Medical School. Her work has been funded by the Harvard Medical School Kaplan Fellowship and the Clinical Research and Training Program. Her research has focused on the development and implementation of treatments to improve emotion regulation in people with bipolar disorder. She has examined the feasibility of a group treatment for emotion regulation that teaches mindfulness, emotion regulation, and distress tolerance skills adapted from dialectical behavior therapy. Dr. Eisner has coauthored four book chapters and has published in numerous peer-reviewed journals, including *Behavior Therapy, Clinical Psychology: Science and Practice, Journal of Psychiatric Practice,* and the *Journal of Abnormal Psychology.* She has been an avid yoga practitioner since 2003.

Sara W. Lazar, PhD, is Associate Researcher in the Psychiatry Department at the Massachusetts General Hospital and Assistant Professor in Psychology at Harvard Medical School. She is a board member of the Institute for Meditation and Psychotherapy and a contributing author to the book *Mindfulness and Psychotherapy.* The focus of Dr. Lazar's research is the elucidation of the neural mechanisms underlying the beneficial effects of yoga and meditation, both in clinical settings and in healthy individuals. Her research has been covered by numerous news outlets, including *The New York Times, USA Today, Time,* CNN, National Public Radio, WebMD, and *The Huffington Post.* She has been practicing yoga and mindfulness meditation since 1994.

Andrew A. Nierenberg, MD, is Professor of Psychiatry at Harvard Medical School. He serves as Director of the Bipolar Clinic and Research Program and as Associate Director of the Depression Clinical and Research Program at the Massachusetts General Hospital. He has been listed among the Best Doctors in North America for the treatment of mood and anxiety disorders since 1994, has received the National Depression and Manic Depressive Association Gerald L. Klerman Young Investigator Award, and was elected as a member of the American College of Neuropsychopharmacology. Dr. Nierenberg's research focuses on comparative effectiveness of existing treatments and the development of new treatments for mood disorders. He has published over 350 papers and 30 chapters and reviews and is a member of the editorial boards of over 15 journals.

Preface

This book describes the development and implementation of mindfulness-based cognitive therapy (MBCT) for individuals with bipolar disorder. It consists of 12 120-minute group treatment sessions conducted weekly over 3 months with concurrent individual therapy sessions, held every other week. It is grounded in MBCT for depression, developed by Zindel Segal and colleagues, as well as established cognitive-behavioral approaches for bipolar disorder and dialectical behavior therapy. The idea for this treatment originated at a time when the initial excitement about psychosocial treatments for bipolar disorder had begun to wane. Cognitive-behavioral therapy, for example, initially seemed to help prevent relapse in individuals with bipolar disorder above and beyond other types of therapy, but as it now stands, its utility in this regard is somewhat limited. Likewise, intensive psychotherapy for acute depression appears to add value only for patients who are in the earlier stages of bipolar disorder but not for those who are chronic. Therefore, we felt that additional therapeutic avenues for individuals with bipolar disorder were needed. MBCT for recurrent depression had moved beyond the stage of initial research, and its efficacy had become more established. Therefore, we thought MBCT might be a valuable option for patients with bipolar disorder, in particular for those with a multitude of mood episodes, co-occurring psychiatric problems, and cognitive difficulties. Because individuals with bipolar disorder face unique challenges, we modified MBCT for depression and supplemented it with treatment elements we felt would be beneficial for individuals with bipolar disorder. Specifically, we shortened the duration of meditations and yoga/movement exercises, added mood monitoring and mindfulness for preventing mania relapse, and included exercises in transferring mindfulness into daily life. The absence of depression (or depression symptoms) does not automatically translate into the presence of well-being for individuals with bipolar disorder. Therefore, we included self-compassion and loving-kindness in this treatment. Similar to dialectical behavior therapy, our treatment combines group sessions with individual therapy sessions. This serves to personalize MBCT treatment, helps patients who miss group sessions to stay up to speed, and provides additional support in crisis situations. The result of our efforts is the MBCT treatment for individuals with bipolar disorder described in Part II of this book.

For this manual, we have created audio recordings of the mindfulness practice exercises in the book, which can be streamed directly from the web or downloaded in MP3 format. Most participants find it helpful to use these audio recordings in their home practice. The audio tracks are available in two different locations: (1) on the instructor website, together with the reproducible handouts (*www.guilford.com/deckersbach-groupleaders*), and (2) on a website developed specifically for course participants (*www.guilford.com/deckersbach-audio*). You can direct your course participants to *www.guilford.com/deckersbach-audio* to access the recordings on their own. Alternately, you may wish to download the audio tracks yourself and burn them onto CDs or copy them to USB flash drives to distribute to participants at the first session.

Numerous individuals besides the authors have contributed to this book. We acknowledge their contributions with deep gratitude. We would like to thank Zindel Segal for his encouragement and ongoing thoughtful advice about our efforts to modify MBCT for individuals with bipolar disorder. Guidance on how to implement mindfulness for individuals with bipolar disorder also came from instructors at the Center for Mindfulness in Medicine, Health Care, and Society at the University of Massachusetts Medical School, as well as from other meditation teachers, among them Zayda Vallejo, Carole Legro, and Ruth Nelson. In this book you will meet patients who participated in the MBCT program at the Bipolar Clinic and Research Program at the Massachusetts General Hospital. We would like to thank them for letting us learn about their experiences, hopes, successes, and struggles as we joined them on their journey through this program, bringing mindfulness to their often chaotic inner lives. We have learned as much from them as we hope they learned from working with us. The people described in this book are real patients, but in order to protect their privacy we changed their identities, stories, and experiences so that they cannot be recognized.

Every book goes through multiple stages of writing and editing. Special thanks to Barbara Watkins and Jim Nageotte of The Guilford Press for their invaluable feedback on earlier versions of this book. For countless hours of proofreading we would like to thank Amanda Arulpragasam, Andrew Corse, Emily Bernstein, Stephanie Salcedo, Leah Shesler, and Elizabeth Greiter. Thank you to Steve McKinley and Alexandra Rodman for the drawings depicting the yoga/movement exercises and to Lynn Koerbel for her guidance on the meditation exercises and recording the scripts. This work was supported by a Career Development Award (K23MH074895) from the National Institute of Mental Health to the first author.

Contents

Part III. Reproducible Handouts

Purchasers can download audio files and larger versions of the handouts
at *www.guilford.com/deckersbach-groupleaders*
or *www.guilford.com/deckersbach-audio*; see page viii for details.

PART I

An Introduction to MBCT for Bipolar Disorder

CHAPTER 1

Bipolar Disorder and Mindfulness

Bipolar disorder is a mood disorder characterized by periods of hypomania or mania, and most often includes episodes of depression, interspersed with times of recovery. In its various forms bipolar disorder affects approximately 5.7 million Americans (Kessler, Chiu, Demler, Merikangas, & Walters, 2005; U.S. Census Bureau, 2005) and takes a huge toll on the affected individuals, as well as their families and friends. As most people who suffer from bipolar disorder will tell you, bipolar disorder is a recurrent, chronic, and often debilitating illness. Despite taking "mood-stabilizing" medications, people with bipolar disorder typically experience many recurrences and are rarely symptom-free. They have trouble succeeding in school, holding jobs, maintaining relationships, and getting along with others. Psychological treatments for bipolar disorder such as cognitive-behavioral therapy, family therapy, or interpersonal and social rhythm therapy may help to ease the burden. With one or more of these treatments, patients can delay the onset of new mood episodes and shorten their duration. These therapies, adjunctive to medications, can help patients function better and improve their quality of life. Yet, despite these advances, many patients continue to struggle in all areas of life.

This book describes a mindfulness-based cognitive therapy (MBCT) for people with bipolar disorder. The 12-session group program coupled with individual therapy sessions is designed to treat those who have experienced many mood episodes; have struggled with chronic, pervasive depressive and manic residual symptoms; and who may also have concurrent disorders such as anxiety disorders. We felt mindfulness would be a meaningful addition to the menu of therapeutic choices available to individuals with bipolar disorder adjunctive to medication.

The practice of mindfulness has been reported to produce beneficial effects for a number of psychiatric, functional somatic, and stress-related symptoms, and therefore has been increasingly incorporated into psychotherapeutic programs (Baer, 2003; Grossman, Niemann, Schmidt, & Walach, 2004). "Mindfulness" refers to paying nonjudgmental attention to experiences in the present moment (Kabat-Zinn, 1990). It has been conceptualized as comprising two components. The first is regulating attention in order to maintain focus on the immediate experience. The second involves approaching one's experience with curiosity, openness, and acceptance toward the encountered experiences, regardless of their valence and desirability (Bishop et al., 2004). Much of the emphasis of established psychosocial treatments for bipolar disorder adjunctive to medication is on "doing." Patients learn to monitor their moods, adjust their lives, acquire skills that help them to take medication regularly, adjust their rhythms, and learn to communicate and problem-solve more effectively. Nonetheless, many patients continue to experience days with depression, mood elevation, anxiety, irritability, worry, and rumination. Mindfulness involves learning to relate to these experiences differently—being rather than doing, mindfully. As we will see, changing the way of "being" with unpleasant and upsetting experiences, as well as pleasant experiences, can have a profound impact on how these experiences unfold for a person who has bipolar disorder. That said, the purpose of this treatment program is not simply to learn to "get used to" unpleasant experiences, or to compete with well-established treatment approaches that have been successfully used by people with bipolar disorder. Rather, our approach integrates three areas of expertise: (1) clinical knowledge about bipolar disorder, (2) therapeutic knowledge in established treatments for bipolar disorder, and (3) experience in mindfulness. We look at mindfulness as an additional therapeutic avenue that supplements the options that are already available for individuals with bipolar disorder. For this reason, our treatment incorporates and adopts many tools that have already been developed and successfully used in the treatment for bipolar disorder, and combines them with mindfulness.

WHO IS THIS BOOK FOR?

This book is for clinicians who already have experience in treating patients with bipolar disorder using other treatment modalities, such as cognitive-behavioral therapy (CBT), family-focused therapy (FFT), interpersonal and social rhythm therapy (IPSRT), or dialectical behavior therapy (DBT), and who are familiar with bipolar disorder and would like to expand their repertoire of therapeutic avenues to mindfulness. This book is also for experienced mindfulness teachers who would like to treat people with bipolar disorder. This book provides information about bipolar disorder, as well as guidance on how to adapt mindfulness to the signs and symptoms of bipolar disorder. The book also describes how to incorporate established cognitive-behavioral treatment strategies that we consider essential into the treatment of bipolar disorder.

THE ORGANIZATION OF THIS BOOK

We start this book by reviewing the most important clinical aspects of bipolar disorder. What are the symptoms of bipolar disorder? What are the different forms of bipolar disorder and how common are they? Clinicians also want to develop an appreciation for bipolar disorder as a recurring, chronic disorder, which despite interspersed periods of "recovery," often dramatically impacts people's functioning and quality of life. As mood-stabilizing medications remain the first line of treatment, we cover the most common medications and pharmacological treatment approaches, as well as their challenges. Our mindfulness-based program adopts treatment elements from other, already established treatments for bipolar disorder, and blends those with elements of mindfulness. Therefore, we also briefly describe the most commonly available adjunctive psychotherapies for bipolar disorder, their techniques, and what is known about their efficacy. This leads us to our rationale that mindfulness may be a meaningful addition to the portfolio of approaches to bipolar disorder. In this context we will review already established mindfulness-based treatments (mindfulness-based stress reduction, mindfulness-based cognitive therapy for depression), and what we know about the benefits of regular mindfulness practice (e.g., increased concentration abilities, more mood stability). We also review pilot studies that have been done in groups of people with bipolar disorder, including our own pilot studies at the Bipolar Clinic and Research Program at Massachusetts General Hospital in Boston. This MBCT program is designed to treat people with bipolar disorder who have experienced many mood episodes; have struggled with chronic, pervasive depressive and manic residual symptoms; and who may also have concurrent disorders such as anxiety disorders. As described in more detail in Chapter 2, it is a 12-session group program coupled with individual sessions. In Chapter 3, we provide helpful information about how to diagnose bipolar disorder and its associated problems. Chapter 4 covers the format and content of individual sessions supplementing group meetings. The remainder of the book includes a session-by-session description on how to implement the group part of this program and the handouts. This includes treatment elements such as how to conduct mood monitoring (Session 1), detect warning signs for mood episodes (Session 2), and design behavioral emergency plans for mood elevation (Session 3). Instructors will also learn how to teach yoga exercises (Sessions 1 and 2), sitting meditations, and body scans (Sessions 2–8), as well as how to transfer mindfulness into daily life (Sessions 1 and forward) and how to apply mindfulness to symptoms of depression or mania when they arise (Session 3 and forward). Increasing self-compassion, well-being, and mindfulness toward pleasurable experiences becomes a topic midtreatment, once basic mindfulness exercises have been introduced (Session 9 and forward). Instructors will also learn how to implement loving-kindness meditations and translate those into participants' daily lives. Group sessions are coupled with regular individual sessions (see Chapter 4) that are used to tailor mindfulness to participants' special needs and to provide help with crisis situations that often occur over the course of the treatment. In this book we have included scripts for the guided meditations we use in this treatment. Most participants find it helpful to have audio recordings of these meditation instructions to use in their home practice. We have created recordings of these instructions that can be downloaded for participants (see p. viii for details).

BIPOLAR DISORDER: THE BASICS

Symptoms

In this book, we concentrate on two of the most common forms of bipolar disorder: bipolar I disorder and bipolar II disorder (for a full list of bipolar disorders, see DSM-5, the latest edition of the *Diagnostic and Statistical Manual of Mental Disorders*). Both forms of bipolar disorder require a period of abnormally elevated or irritable mood (American Psychiatric Association, 2013). This includes symptoms such as elevated, expansive, or irritable mood coupled with being overconfident and more talkative than usual, having grandiose ideas, thoughts being more fluent and speeded, as well as being distractible, experiencing flight of ideas and decreased need for sleep associated with increased levels of activity often involving pleasurable and/or risky activities (e.g., overspending or gambling). The critical distinction between bipolar I and II disorder is the duration and severity of the mood elevation episode. People who experience expansive or irritable mood and the associated symptoms for at least 4 days, but not severe enough so that they markedly impair functioning (e.g., at work, in relationships), have a hypomanic episode (not a manic episode). If they have also experienced one or more episodes of major depression (see below), they meet criteria for bipolar II disorder.

Grandiose ideas and paranoia coupled with a lack of recognition of how unrealistic those ideas are (lack of insight) are examples of mood-congruent psychotic features consistent with a manic episode, provided mood elevation and the associated mania symptoms have lasted for at least a week. The presence of psychotic symptoms can easily be mistaken as signs of a non-mood psychotic disorder (Meyer & Meyer, 2009). As a sign of mania, psychotic features need to be congruent with the mood (e.g., grandiose) and only occur during the manic episode. The manic episode cannot be drug-induced or due to any other medical factors; otherwise it would yield a diagnosis of substance/medication-induced bipolar disorder (American Psychiatric Association, 2013). The presence of a manic episode leads to a diagnosis of bipolar I disorder. A history of depression is not a requirement for a diagnosis of bipolar I disorder, unlike bipolar II disorder. An episode of a major depression consists of depressed mood, and/or loss of interest or pleasure for most days over 2 weeks. Symptoms may include loss of energy, oversleeping, difficulties concentrating, being slow, lack of activity, and feeling completely worthless. The experience of depression may vary over time—for example, symptoms include becoming more anxious and irritable, ruminating, feeling restless, having difficulties falling and staying asleep, concentration difficulties, lack of appetite, and contemplation of suicide. When both manic and depressive symptoms are present at the same time, a person experiences what is called a mixed state. Mixed features (the simultaneous presence of symptoms of both depression and mania) are quite common. Also, full-blown mania and depression typically do not appear suddenly. Usually, there is a ramping up in symptom severity (called "prodromal signs") that can be used as warning signs that foreshadow the onset or worsening of hypomanic or depressive symptoms (Carlson & Goodwin, 1973). As we will later see, these warning signs, particularly for mood elevation, open a small window of time where one can intervene both medically and behaviorally in order to prevent their spiraling into hypomania or mania.

Prevalence and Course

Together, bipolar I and II disorder affect 2.1% of the U.S. population (Merikangas, Akiskal, et al., 2007). One percent of Americans have bipolar I disorder and 1.1% have bipolar II disorder. Another 2.4% of Americans suffer from less severe forms of bipolar disorder characterized by subthreshold hypomania with major depressive episodes, or recurrent hypomanic or subthreshold hypomanic episodes without major depression (Merikangas, Akiskal, et al., 2007). Bipolar disorder affects men and women equally. Most individuals (50–67%) experience their first episode before the age of

18 (Perlis et al., 2004). Between 15 and 28% develop the disorder before the age of 13 (Perlis et al., 2004). Bipolar disorder rarely occurs by itself. Ninety-eight percent of individuals with bipolar disorder have another lifetime psychiatric disorder that warrants treatment (Merikangas, Ames, et al., 2007). The most common include lifetime alcohol and substance dependence (60%) and anxiety disorders (50%) (Simon et al., 2004).

Nearly everyone experiences multiple episodes of mania and depression over their lifetime, but depression and ongoing chronic, pervasive depressive symptoms are the most difficult aspects of bipolar disorder to treat. The Collaborative Depression Study, a study that followed patients with unipolar and bipolar disorder, found that patients with bipolar disorder changed their symptom status an average of six times per year (Judd et al., 2002). Over the 13-year follow-up period, patients with bipolar disorder spent almost half of their time symptomatic, and depression accounted for three times as many weeks as mania or hypomania (Judd et al., 2002).

Findings from clinical and large-scale epidemiological studies also challenge the traditional view of bipolar disorder as an illness where mood episodes are interspersed with periods of full symptomatic and functional recovery (Judd et al., 2002; Kessler et al., 2006; Trede et al., 2005). Problems at work and with social and family functioning occur in 90% of individuals with bipolar disorder (Merikangas, Ames, et al., 2007). Tohen and colleagues (Tohen et al., 2003) followed people with bipolar disorder who had been hospitalized with their first manic episode for 2 years after discharge from the McLean Hospital near Boston. While nearly all of them (98%) reached a point during those 2 years when they did not meet criteria for mania anymore, only 72% reached a level where they had few or no symptoms. Only 43% within those 2 years returned to their level of functioning as it was the year before their manic episode. Similar results were reported by Keck et al. (1998) who found that in the 12 months following hospitalization for a manic or mixed episode, only 24% of patients were able to go back to work and socialize at their pre-episode levels of functioning (Keck et al., 1998).

Work-performing difficulties are common in individuals with bipolar disorder. In the National Comorbidity Survey Replication (NCS-R) study, a large nationwide epidemiological study of 9,282 people, individuals with bipolar disorder on average missed the equivalent of 65 days at work in a year (Kessler et al., 2006). This translates into the equivalent of 1 week of work missed every month. Depressive symptoms greatly contribute to people's ongoing functioning difficulties. In the NCS-R study, the number of workdays missed doubled for people who had a depressive episode in the past 12 months (Kessler et al., 2006). In the Collaborative Depression Study, when followed over time, functioning was worst when people were depressed (Judd et al., 2005). Changes in functioning over time mirrored changes in depressive severity (Judd et al., 2005), but people's functioning remained impaired even when patients remitted from a previous mood episode (Judd et al., 2008). At times, patients achieved restored levels of functioning in most areas (relationships, etc.), with the exception of work performance, where patients remained impaired a significant percentage of the time (Judd et al., 2005, 2008). With recurrent episodes and poor interepisode functioning, many patients with bipolar disorder have difficulties holding onto a job. In the Systematic Treatment Enhancement Program for Bipolar Disorder (STEP-BD), a large, multisite study funded by the National Institute of Mental Health and conducted at medical centers and universities in the United States, 15% of patients were disabled and 20% were unemployed (Kogan et al., 2004). Similar results have been obtained by the Stanley Foundation network: of 253 patients with bipolar I or II disorder, only one in three worked full time outside the home. More than half were unable to work or worked only in sheltered settings (Suppes et al., 2001).

Treatment

Medications

Bipolar disorder presents unique challenges for medication treatment, one of which is how to treat the multiple phases of the disorder: acute mania or hypomania, acute depression, maintenance preventative treatment, and the management of subsyndromal symptoms and comorbid conditions (Bersudsky & Belmaker, 2009). Few patients respond to monotherapy, and most require multiple medications to relieve their symptoms and distress (Ghaemi et al., 2006).

The overarching principle of pharmacological treatment of bipolar disorder considers multiple spheres of dysregulation including mood, energy, sleep, anxiety, and cognition, each of which can change depending on episode status, and each of which can be the target of pharmacotherapy. Acute manic and hypomanic episodes are the hallmark of bipolar disorder and are usually responsive to available treatments (Bersudsky & Belmaker, 2009). Broadly, the categories of medications effective for these episodes include the classic "mood stabilizers": lithium, valproate, carbamazepine, and the antipsychotics (first and second generation, including haloperidol, perphenazine, risperidone, aripiprazole, olanzapine, quetiapine, ziprasidone, asenapine, and lurasidone), either alone or in combination. Lamotrigine, a repurposed anticonvulsant (as are valproate and carbamazepine), appears to have unique preventative antidepressant properties, but weaker acute antidepressant effectiveness and maintenance antimanic effects (Geddes, Calabrese, & Goodwin, 2009).

Acute bipolar depressive episodes and depressive symptoms present the biggest challenge for patients with the fewest options (Belmaker, 2007). Treatments approved by the U.S. Food and Drug Administration (FDA) include the combination of olanzapine and fluoxetine and quetiapine monotherapy. Antidepressants have not been shown to be effective for bipolar depression in rigorous studies (Nierenberg, 2010), although the field continues to struggle with the discrepancy between the research data and practice. Clinicians prescribe antidepressants along with antimanic agents as the most common response to bipolar depression (Frye, 2011). A key randomized placebo-controlled trial from the STEP-BD study failed to find an advantage of antidepressants over placebo when added to a mood stabilizer (Sachs et al., 2007). Nonrandomized observational data from the same study found no difference between those who had a bipolar depressive episode and subsyndromal hypomanic symptoms and those who were or were not treated with antidepressants (Goldberg et al., 2007). Lamotrigine monotherapy showed acute antidepressant efficacy in a key trial in 1999, but subsequent studies failed to replicate this finding (Calabrese et al., 1999). A meta-analysis of all randomized studies of lamotrigine monotherapy found that, in aggregate, the studies found a modest effect of lamotrigine monotherapy (Geddes et al., 2009). But a key study of lamotrigine or placebo added to lithium found a statistically and clinically significant effect for lamotrigine (van der Loos et al., 2009). Thus, even though lamotrigine is approved by the FDA for the prevention of mood episodes, based on innovative prevention studies, many clinicians prescribe lamotrigine for the management of acute bipolar depressive episodes.

Even with state-of-the-art guideline concordant treatment, the outcomes of many bipolar patients remain suboptimal. Anxiety occurs frequently, and although some secondary analyses have found that medications such as quetiapine can have a beneficial effect on anxiety, no targeted studies have examined this important question. Many clinicians turn to benzodiazepines to help. Fatigue, too, persists in many and can either be a symptom or a side effect from other medications. Stimulants such as methylphenidate and awake-promoting agents such as modafinil are frequently prescribed, although with a risk, albeit uncertain, of exacerbating mania. Insomnia can also persist and cause problems with the rhythms of daily living and predispose bipolar patients to become manic. No specific pharmacological treatments have been studied, but hypnotics (e.g., zolpidem, eszopiclone, or benzodiazepines such as lorazepam) are used for insomnia. Finally, cognitive and executive dysfunction impairs bipolar patients even when they are outside of acute episodes, although there are no FDA-approved medications for cognitive impairments in bipolar disorder.

Despite pharmacotherapy, most patients will experience recurrence of mood episodes (Gitlin, Swendsen, Heller, & Hammen, 1995). Further complicating the picture, less than half of the patients who are prescribed medications are fully adherent to their medication regimen (Colom, Veita, Tacchi, Sanchez-Moreno, & Scott, 2005). Within 1 year after being hospitalized for a mixed or manic episode, up to 60% of patients discontinue their medications or do not take them regularly (Keck et al., 1998). A large community study found that the average length of adherence to mood-stabilizing medication was a little over 2 months (Johnson & McFarland, 1996). Not taking prescribed medications, or only taking them irregularly, dramatically increases the risk for relapse and rehospitalization (Keck et al., 1998; Scott & Pope, 2002).

Psychotherapies

Among other issues, psychological treatments have addressed the reasons for patient nonadherence to their medications. In the first study of CBT for bipolar disorder, Susan Cochran, at the University of California, Los Angeles, worked with bipolar patients for 6 weeks to address reasons for medication nonadherence (Cochran, 1984). Medications are disliked for multiple reasons, with medication side effects (sedation, weight gain, etc.) being just one of many. Not surprisingly, if side effects are experienced as intolerable, patients often do not take the medications for very long. However, in a Europe-wide survey of patients, side effects were ranked low (3%) on a list of reasons why patients felt bothered by taking medication (Morselli & Elgie, 2003). If severe side effects are not the reason, why then do patients discontinue medications? Reasons include the lack of insight into the chronic nature of bipolar disorder, lack of understanding of the need for medication treatment (Peralta & Cuesta, 1998), denial of the severity of the disorder, and fear of dependence (Morselli & Elgie, 2003). People are also ashamed about the need to take psychiatric medications, may see medications as unnatural, and don't want their feelings controlled by the medications. Others believe that if they just try hard, they can control mood without medications (Scott & Tacchi, 2002). Discontinuing medication can also be a prodromal sign of mood elevation (Keck et al., 1998), leading patients to believe that they do not need medication. Addressing these issues can increase patient medication adherence. At the end of the treatment (as well as at the 6-month follow-up) in Susan Cochran's 1984 study, patients were taking their medication (in this case lithium) more regularly, discontinued it less against medical advice, and had fewer mood episodes caused by nonadherence than patients who had received regular clinical care (Cochran, 1984).

Enhancing medication adherence was not the only reason why psychological treatments for bipolar disorder began to gain traction. Monitoring and detecting prodromal signs, especially those signaling mania, provides a window for early intervention (e.g., boosting or changing medication). It had also become increasingly clear that for many people psychosocial stress greatly increases the risk of recurrence of mood episodes (Ellicott, Hammen, Gitlin, Brown, & Jamison, 1990). Psychosocial treatment researchers felt that if they could work with people with bipolar disorder to learn more about their illness, monitor symptoms, help them to become more adherent, and adjust their behavior and their environment in ways that would minimize risk factors (irregular medication adherence, lack of sleep, alcohol and substance abuse, family criticism, stress) and maximize protective factors (regular schedules, etc.), that this would have beneficial effects on the course of the illness and ultimately improve people's quality of life (Miklowitz & Johnson, 2006). To date, psychological treatments have utilized an array of interventions. These include psychoeducation about bipolar disorder, mood monitoring and relapse prevention, communication and problem-solving training, cognitive restructuring (a technique to challenge maladaptive thoughts), activity scheduling, social rhythm adjustments, and interpersonal techniques. These have been combined in various forms in individual, group, or family treatments that were implemented at different stages of this illness (acutely ill, stable, etc.).

Free-standing psychoeducation programs for remitted, stable patients with bipolar disorder in conjunction with medication have been shown to lower the rate of manic recurrences (Perry, Tarrier, Morriss, McCarthy, & Limb, 1999) or both manic and depressive recurrences (Colom et al., 2009). Other treatment programs have combined psychoeducation with additional treatment modules (Bauer et al., 2006a, 2006b; Frank et al., 2005; Lam, Hayward, Watkins, Wright, & Sham, 2005; Lam et al., 2003; Miklowitz, George, Richards, Simoneau, & Suddath, 2003; Miklowitz et al., 2007; Simon et al., 2006). For example, Lam et al. (2003, 2005), who investigated a cognitive-behavioral approach for preventing relapse, combined psychoeducation with active mood monitoring, relapse prevention, modification of behaviors that could trigger mood symptoms (prodromes), and emphasis on regular routines and sleep (Lam et al., 2005; Lam et al., 2003). Lam et al. (2003, 2005), who compared their CBT relapse prevention program against treatment as usual, found that within the first year participants had fewer mood episodes, and within the first 2 years of follow-up experienced shorter mood episodes, fewer overall mood symptoms, better coping with prodromal manic symptoms, and fewer admissions to the hospital (Lam et al., 2005; Lam et al., 2003). In the two largest randomized studies conducted to date, Bauer et al. (2006a, 2006b) and Simon et al. (2006) combined group psychoeducation (recognizing triggers for episodes, monitoring warning signs, developing relapse prevention strategies, and increasing medication adherence) with sessions that focused on increasing functioning through achieving goals in life (Bauer et al., 2006a, 2006b; Simon et al., 2006). Patients were also assigned a nurse coordinator who would facilitate access, coordinate care, and reach out to patients (e.g., when they missed appointments, a sign that things may not be well). Both programs observed beneficial effects for shortening manic episodes (Bauer et al., 2006a; Simon et al., 2006) and lowering risk of manic episodes (Simon et al., 2006), although there were no effects on depression severity, weeks depressed, or depressive recurrences (Simon et al., 2006), confirming a growing realization that depression for people with bipolar disorder is more difficult to treat than mania.

David Miklowitz's (2008b) FFT for bipolar disorder educates families about the elements of bipolar disorder and teaches them to communicate more effectively and problem-solve together around the issues bipolar disorder creates for them. Miklowitz and colleagues who tested this program found that FFT participants had fewer relapses than patients who just received psychoeducation (Miklowitz et al., 2003; Rea et al., 2003). The role of interpersonal factors as well as that of the regularity of one's daily schedule (social rhythms) on the course of bipolar disorder have also been highlighted by Ellen Frank (Frank, Hlastala, Ritenour, & Houck, 1997; Frank et al., 2005). IPSRT was developed as both an acute and maintenance treatment for bipolar disorder to target nonadherence to medications, stressful life events, and disruptions in routines and social rhythms. IPSRT combines interpersonal psychotherapy with the social zeitgeber hypothesis. The social zeitgeber hypothesis states that disruption in daily routines can lead to instability of circadian rhythms, which, in vulnerable individuals, can lead to mood episodes (Frank et al., 2005). The treatment addresses the importance of maintaining regular routines and managing potential disruptions in that routine. Interpersonal aspects are drawn from interpersonal psychotherapy and focus on unresolved grief, interpersonal disputes, role transitions, and interpersonal deficits (Frank, Swartz, & Kupfer, 2000). In addition, the treatment addresses "grief for the lost healthy self," assisting the patient in mourning the life the patient may have lost because of the diagnosis and its accompanying limitations. IPSRT has helped individuals with bipolar disorder regulate their daily routines and sleep–wake cycles (Frank et al., 1997). Maintenance IPSRT, in combination with medications, also helps individuals maintain mood stability (Frank, 1999).

Overall, IPSRT may be most helpful when patients are experiencing acute episodes and is not recommended for individuals with bipolar disorder and comorbid anxiety disorders or high medical burden (Miklowitz, 2008a).

Finally, in the STEP-BD study, psychosocial researchers also turned their attention to treating acute depressive episodes. Depressed patients with bipolar disorder were randomized to either IPSRT, FFT, or CBT (consisting of mood monitoring, relapse prevention, and Beckian style CBT) (Miklowitz et al., 2007). All three treatments were equally successful in decreasing the length of the depressive episodes over the course of a year, compared to a low-level treatment condition that provided patients with a workbook with information about bipolar disorder and the opportunity to meet with a professional up to three times. Not only did the three treatments decrease the length of the depressive episode, but they also translated into more days well over the study year, and improved relationship functioning and life satisfaction (Miklowitz et al., 2007). With this array of impressive accomplishments of the existing psychotherapies for bipolar disorder, why was there a need for incorporating mindfulness?

MBCT FOR MAJOR DEPRESSION

When we started to think about additional therapeutic options for the patients in our clinic, mindfulness-based cognitive therapy for people with recurrent depressive episodes had already gained empirical support and had received much publicity. As they described it in their book *Mindfulness-Based Cognitive Therapy for Depression*, Zindel Segal, Mark Williams, and John Teasdale had looked for a psychological treatment that could help prevent future major depressive episodes in people with recurrent major depression (Segal, Williams, & Teasdale, 2002, 2013). They and many others had found that depressed people experience high levels of negative, self-critical thinking. Once recovered, however, negative thinking would normalize such that it could not be distinguished from that of never-depressed people. Likewise, decreased activity levels also tend to return to the normal range when people are no longer depressed. This removed pivotal targets for CBT as a treatment for the prevention of major depressive episodes.

Segal et al. (2002, 2013) were also aware of research done by Robert Post at the National Institute of Mental Health who had found that while life events often play a role early in the occurrence of major depressive episodes, they tend to lose their importance as precipitants as patients continue to experience major depressive episodes (Post, 1992). With unbiased thoughts, normal activity levels, and no life events to alter, Segal and colleagues turned their attention to mindfulness as a way to prevent the recurrence of major depressive episodes. They hypothesized that relapse, at a time of sad or lowering mood, involves the automatic reactivation of negative thinking, similar to the thought patterns that were active during people's previous episodes of depression (Segal et al., 2002, 2013). The more episodes of depression someone has experienced, the more the brain would be "trained" in this mode of responding, and the more automatic this mode of responding to sad or lowering mood would become (thereby also increasing the risk of future depressive episodes). More broadly, any thoughts and feelings associated with stored memories of depressed mood could serve as an internal context (a retrieval cue) that automatically reactivates depressed mood and its associated patterns of thinking and feeling (Segal et al., 2002, 2013; Williams, Teasdale, Segal, & Kabat-Zinn, 2007).

Part of this automatic pattern is a tendency to ruminate in response to negative affect (Johnson, McKenzie, & McMurrich, 2008). Rumination refers to behaviors and thoughts that focus one's attention on one's depressive symptoms and on the implications of those symptoms (Nolen-Hoeksema, 1991). This appears to create an automatic self-perpetuating cycle of ruminative, negative thinking; loss of positive affect; coupled with reduced motivation and goal-directed behavior leading back into depressive episodes. Segal et al. (2002, 2013) looked for a treatment that could help people to disengage from mind states characterized by self-perpetuating patterns of ruminative, negative thought. They turned to a treatment called mindfulness-based stress reduction (MBSR), developed by Jon Kabat-Zinn in the late 1970s (Kabat-Zinn, 1990). MBSR is typically taught to mixed groups of patients that present with a wide variety of problems ranging from stress-related health issues to chronic pain. This program is designed as an 8-week course for groups. The capacity for mindfulness is developed through multiple mindfulness meditation exercises, such as sitting meditation, walking meditation, mindful yoga, and the body scan. Participants are also taught to practice mindfulness in everyday activities, such as eating, cleaning the dishes, or taking a shower in order to facilitate the integration of mindfulness into daily life. Segal and colleagues adapted many of these exercises (e.g., body scans, sitting meditations) and coupled them with education about depression, mood, and thoughts (Segal et al., 2002, 2013). They tested the efficacy of their mindfulness-based cognitive therapy program in several clinical trials (Segal et al., 2010; Teasdale, Segal, & Williams, 1995; Teasdale et al., 2000). It turned out that for patients who had three or more episodes of major depression, MBCT reduced the recurrence of future episodes compared to people who had had only two or fewer major depressive episodes (Teasdale et al., 2000). More recently, Segal et al. (2010) found that among patients with unstable remission, MBCT substantially reduced the risk of occurrence, but there was no difference between MBCT and placebo for patients with stable remission (Segal et al., 2010).

MBCT FOR BIPOLAR DISORDER?

"Unstable remission"? Intermittent days, with lowered mood and negative self-critical thinking? This sounded familiar to us. As Michael, one of the bipolar patients who participated in our program described, "I may have a few good days, but then one morning I wake up and feel down, blah, just not right, with no energy. Or, there would be those days when I could not do anything right, no matter what I tried. Just a lot of self-critical, negative thinking, and being very irritable." Like Michael, even those patients with bipolar disorder who have infrequent recurrences experience ongoing, mostly depressive mood symptoms in between major mood episodes (Judd et al., 2002). In the STEP-BD program, most patients who were recovered at the time when they joined the study still experienced noticeable mood symptoms, among them difficulties sleeping, concentration issues, low energy, and self-critical thinking (Rodman et al., 2011). For patients who recovered in their first 2 years of the STEP-BD program, residual depressive or manic symptoms at recovery and proportion of days depressed or anxious in the preceding year shortened the time to depressive recurrence. Residual manic symptoms at recovery and proportion of days of elevated mood in the preceding year significantly shortened the time to manic, hypomanic, or mixed episode recurrence (Perlis et al., 2006). To us, these findings emphasized the need to treat ongoing depressive and manic mood symptoms.

Besides unstable remission and residual symptoms, people with bipolar disorder also seemed to share a tendency to ruminate about negative feelings and events (Kim, Yu, Lee, & Kim, 2012). Unlike people with major depression, however, people with bipolar disorder seemed to have a vulnerability to also ruminate about positive feelings (Johnson et al., 2008), suggesting self-perpetuating, ruminative responses as a potential avenue not only into depression, but also into mania. In healthy individuals mindfulness meditation decreases negative mood states (Jha, Stanley, Kiyonaga, Wong, & Gelfand, 2010) and reduces distractive and ruminative thoughts (Jain et al., 2007). Therefore, we could not help but wonder whether the practice of mindfulness could help people with bipolar disorder to treat their thoughts and feelings as transient mental events rather than reflections of reality, and whether this could help prevent the escalation of negative or positive ruminative patterns into depression or mania.

Mindfulness in Other Treatment Programs

Besides being effective in preventing depressive recurrences and rumination (Hofmann, Sawyer, Witt, & Oh; Segal et al., 2002, 2013), mindfulness has also been an integral part of other treatment programs. Among them, DBT for borderline personality disorder, a program for patients with intense emotions and severe emotion dysregulation difficulties (Linehan, 1993; Neacsiu, Rizvi, & Linehan, 2010), mindfulness-based relapse prevention for addictive behaviors (Bowen et al., 2006; Marlatt & Gordon, 2007), and mindfulness- and acceptance-based behavioral therapy for anxiety (Hofmann, Sawyer, Witt, & Oh, 2010; Roemer & Orsillo, 2009; Roemer, Orsillo, & Salters-Pedneault, 2008). Fifty percent of patients with bipolar disorder have a lifetime anxiety disorder (Simon et al., 2004). "Worry is a daily part of my life," said Holly, one of our patients, in a first meeting at the Bipolar Clinic. "It is particularly hard when I am depressed, but it still does not go away when things are better." Other people with bipolar disorder experience panic attacks and worry about their occurrence; yet other patients fear and/or avoid social situations or experience anxiety-provoking memories about traumatic events.

During mindfulness, practitioners expose themselves to whatever is present in the field of awareness, including thoughts, body sensations, and emotional experiences. They let themselves be affected by the experience, refrain from taking countermeasures, and instead bring an attitude of acceptance to bodily and affective responses (Hart, 1987). Practitioners are instructed to meet unpleasant emotions (such as fear, sadness, anger, aversion) by "turning towards them, rather than turning away" (Santorelli, 2000). Although this may be counterintuitive, novice practitioners soon discover that the unpleasant emotions pass away and a sense of safety or well-being can be experienced in their place—a process that is called "extinction," which underlies the highly effective exposure-based treatment for anxiety disorders (Chambless & Ollendick, 2001). Mark Williams and colleagues (2008) who employed the Segal et al. (2002, 2013) MBCT treatment in remitted patients with bipolar disorder, with a focus on in-between episode anxiety and depression symptoms, found that compared to a waiting-list group (no treatment), patients with bipolar disorder following 8 weeks of MBCT indeed showed reduced anxiety as well as depression symptoms (Williams et al., 2008).

Other Benefits of MBCT

Mindfulness also seems to have a beneficial effect on people's abilities to regulate strong emotions (Linehan, 1993; Neacsiu et al., 2010). "Don't tell me you know what I feel," Daniel, another participant in our program, complained. "I hate when people do this. I absolutely, absolutely hate it. When someone does this, I get so angry that I can barely think anymore," he says as he describes one of his many situations where strong emotional reactions get in the way of his getting along with others. Meditation training has been shown to lead to decreased emotional reactivity (the tendency to react strongly) and facilitates a return to emotional baseline (Goleman & Schwartz, 1976; Zeidler, 2007). Experimental work has shown that mindfulness training leads to a reduction in emotional interference (as assessed by the delay in reaction time after being presented with affective as compared to neutral pictures) (Ortner, Kilner, & Zelazo, 2007).

Another area that benefits from mindfulness practice is cognitive functioning. Once thought of as being a part of mood episodes, it has been recognized that for many individuals with bipolar disorder, cognitive problems persist even when they are not in mood episodes (Altshuler, 1993). Difficulties with attention (concentration), memory, and the organization of behaviors (often called executive functioning) extending beyond mood episodes affect approximately 30–40% of individuals with bipolar disorder (Cavanagh, Van Beck, Muir, & Blackwood, 2002; Clark, Iversen, & Goodwin, 2002; Deckersbach et al., 2004; Martinez-Aran et al., 2004). The reasons for this are likely multifaceted and may include medications, lack of sleep, and other factors. These difficulties can greatly impair one's ability to function in the workplace and at home (Altshuler, Bearden, Green, van Gorp, & Mintz, 2008; Atre-Vaidya et al., 1998; Dickerson et al., 2004; Dittmann et al., 2007; Gildengers et al., 2007; Harvey, Twamley, Vella, Patterson, & Heaton, 2010; Jaeger, Berns, Loftus, Gonzalez, & Czobor, 2007; Martinez-Aran et al., 2004, 2007). Regular meditators have enhanced attentional performance (Jha, Krompinger, & Baime, 2007; Slagter et al., 2007; Valentine & Sweet, 1999; van den Hurk, Giommi, Gielen, Speckens, & Barendregt, 2010) and mindfulness practice has been shown to positively impact attention, or conflict monitoring, such as the ability to disregard distractions in order to maintain an attentional focus (Chan & Woollacott, 2007; Jha et al., 2007; Moore & Malinowski, 2009; van den Hurk et al., 2010). Even brief meditation interventions can lead to improvements on attention tasks (Tang et al., 2007; Wenk-Sormaz, 2005) and increased activation in brain regions involved in the regulation of attentional processes in the brain.

Psychotherapy for Relapse Prevention and Acute Depression Revisited

Finally, some recent data from a clinical trial looking at relapse prevention for patients with bipolar disorder also encouraged us to look for an additional psychological treatment for patients with bipolar disorder. Jan Scott from the University of Newcastle had conducted a clinical trial in which she compared the effectiveness of cognitive behavior therapy with treatment as usual (TAU) for preventing the recurrence of mood episodes. Unlike other studies (Lam et al., 2003, 2005), she did not find any overall advantage of CBT over TAU in the ability to prevent recurrence. However, in a post-hoc analysis she discovered something interesting. For patients with 12 lifetime mood episodes, CBT and TAU were roughly equally effective in preventing relapse. For patients with fewer than 12 lifetime mood episodes CBT was more effective, whereas patients with more than 12 lifetime mood episodes, TAU seemed to be the better option. In fact, this effect became much more pronounced for patients with 20 or 30 lifetime mood episodes, suggesting that CBT may not be the best treatment for people with particularly severe and recurrent bipolar disorder.

We also wondered whether the beneficial effect of psychotherapy for recovery from acute depression in the STEP-BD program was dependent on the chronicity of bipolar disorder, and we looked at the number of lifetime depressive mood episodes as a potential moderator (Peters et al., in press). We found that psychotherapy (CBT, FFT, IPSRT), compared to three sessions of education about bipolar disorder (called "collaborative care") had its biggest impact on recovery rates for patients with 10–20 lifetime depressive episodes (psychotherapy: 79%; collaborative care: 27%), whereas it did not make a difference for patients with 1–9 lifetime depressive episodes (psychotherapy: 76%; collaborative care: 73%) or for patients with more than 20 lifetime episodes (psychotherapy: 63%; collaborative care: 52%) (Peters et al., in press).

Taken together, these findings suggested that MBCT might be a treatment option particularly for more chronic patients with bipolar disorder, who experience other concurrent psychiatric disorders (e.g., anxiety disorders) and deal with emotion regulation issues, and cognitive problems. In the next chapter we discuss why we decided to modify MBCT for depression.

CHAPTER 2

An Overview of MBCT for Bipolar Disorder

HOW WE MODIFIED MBCT FOR BIPOLAR DISORDER

We were not the first to modify MBCT for depression as the basis for treating patients with bipolar disorder. Some of our modifications were influenced by previous modifications. The first to modify the Segal et al. (2002, 2013) program for people with bipolar disorder were David Miklowitz then at the University of Colorado, and Guy Goodwin and Mark Williams, at the University of Oxford (Miklowitz et al., 2009). They included two additional treatment elements that were specific to participants with bipolar disorder: education about mood changes and its provoking factors (e.g., interpersonal conflict, sleep–wake cycle disruptions) and learning to observe one's mood, thinking, or behavior nonjudgmentally during periods of mood escalation (Miklowitz et al., 2009). Thus, the same strategies that were used to help participants manage their depressive states were now also applied to managing hypomania and mania. Using this modified MBCT protocol, Miklowitz and colleagues observed small-to-medium effects for decreases in depression and anxiety in remitted participants with bipolar disorder in an open trial (Miklowitz et al., 2009; Segal et al., 2002, 2013). Participants would identify their prodromal (warning) changes in mood symptoms and apply mindfulness when they observed these symptoms recurring. They would also identify specific action steps that could be implemented to respond effectively to these periods of increased risk (Miklowitz et al., 2009). We also felt that mood monitoring and the early detection of warning signs foreshadowing mood elevation were important additions for bipolar participants to prevent recurrence of manic episodes.

When becoming hypomanic, patients typically engage in behaviors that increase mood elevation, leading them into hypomania or mania. Lack of sleep, increased talking, increase in goal-directed activities, particularly pleasurable ones, as well as frequent shifts of attention when patients constantly switch among multiple tasks would fuel mood elevation, creating a spiral upward into mania. Conversely, however, not engaging in these activities with increasing mood elevation would make patients feel uncomfortable. As Elizabeth, one of the participants, pointed out in the program early on, "This is what my body wants at that time. It wants to talk and do multiple things all at once. It wants to accomplish things. What do I do with this excess energy if I don't engage?" We felt that mood monitoring, identifying warning signs, and bringing mindfulness to changes in mood, especially early in the process, could be ways to prevent manic mood escalation.

Besides teaching about mood changes, we also felt participants would benefit from a better understanding about the automatic vicious cycles involved in ruminative depressive or hypomanic thinking, mood elevation, anxiety, and irritability. Addressing the role of psychosocial triggers for mood episodes was another important element that other programs for bipolar disorder had already implemented (Bauer et al., 2006a, 2006b; Simon et al., 2006) and that should not be missing from ours. Finding a balance between omitting or modifying triggers (e.g., interpersonal conflict) that could increase the risk for mood episodes and bringing mindfulness to those that could not be avoided or modified would help participants to live more stable lives and avoid mood escalation.

In terms of formal practice, we felt that some of the exercises included in the MBCT program (at least initially) would be too difficult for participants with cognitive difficulties, who have problems sustaining their attention for longer periods of time. For example, the first Body-Scan Exercise (an exercise in which attention is moved through the body in a sequential fashion) in the Segal et al. (2002, 2013) MBCT program spans 45 minutes. For participants with bipolar disorder, we felt a more stepwise approach that would gradually increase the length of these exercises might be helpful to prevent participant frustration and disengagement from the program. We also added emotion-focused meditation exercises that would help participants practice to become more mindful with their strong feelings. Likewise, after discussion with MBSR teachers and Zindel Segal, we also opted to include Mindful Yoga Exercises into our program (an MBSR component omitted in MBCT), as mindful movement exercises would provide a grounding and focusing experience that would help participants who have struggles with concentration and are easily distractible. This choice also contributed to our decision to extend our program to 12 sessions (compared to the eight used in MBSR).

As commonly done in MBSR and MBCT, we also wanted participants to build mindfulness in their everyday lives. Yet, given our participants' often disorganized and chaotic lives, and their memory difficulties, we were not quite convinced that this result would really materialize if we did not add some more concrete help in terms of "how to" actually inject more everyday mindfulness into their lives. Therefore, we employed cognitive-behavioral strategies to increase the frequency and consistency of participants engaging in mindfulness in daily life (e.g., systematic use of reminder cues for implementing mindfulness) (Deckersbach et al., 2010). We also felt that, similar to dialectical behavior therapy (Linehan, 1993), participants would benefit from semiregular individual meetings with the mindfulness instructor to help them overcome obstacles on their way to incorporating mindfulness into their lives. From our experience with working with bipolar participants, having a forum and hands-on help for problem solving around concrete life issues would be a welcome help to keep them on track and address crises that would periodically occur throughout their participation in the program. Finally, there were some other elements that caught our attention that we felt deserved recognition. As Segal et al. (2002, p. 55) had pointed out, learning to "decenter from negative thoughts and unpleasant feelings" (mindful observance) was essential but not enough. Rather, MBCT and MBSR instructors would guide participants to adopt a kind and welcoming attitude toward difficult experiences.

In our own training, we had noticed that instructors increasingly emphasized not only the ability to be accepting but also the ability to be compassionate with ourselves when dealing with difficult or unpleasant experiences. This recognition was also beginning to resonate among researchers. As shown in a study by Van Dam and colleagues, self-compassion (independently from mindfulness) predicted decreases in symptom severity and increases in quality of life in a large group of people from the community who completed a mindfulness-based self-help book for problems with anxiety (Van Dam, Sheppard, Forsyth, & Earleywine, 2011). We had also learned that the absence of negatives did not mean the presence of positives. That is, many of our participants even when they were not terribly depressed or overly self-critical felt unmotivated and complained about their lack of joy and well-being. "I just did not feel happy," Michelle noted as she looked back to the time before she started our mindfulness program. "I was not really depressed, but I just felt blah. I did not look forward to things. It was as if someone had taken the life out of me." Indeed, negative affect and positive affect had already been recognized as independent constructs (Watson, Clark, & Tellegen, 1988; Watson & Tellegen, 1985). The decrease or absence of depression (or depression symptoms) does not seem to automatically translate into the presence of positive affect or well-being (Fava, Rafanelli, Cazzaro, Conti, & Grandi, 1998; Ryff & Singer, 1996).

Perhaps self-compassion could be an important component, especially for positive mental states (Germer, 2009). We hoped that participants would learn not only to become more mindful (observant, accepting) of negative and self-deprecating self-evaluations and difficult feelings, but also to begin to become more gentle and compassionate with themselves (Neff, 2003). Loving-kindness meditations became the vehicle with which we introduced this idea into our program. However, we did not want participants simply to replace negative and ruminative thoughts with positive and self-compassionate ones. Therefore, loving-kindness meditations became part of the second half of our 12-session program, after participants had already worked on mindful-accepting types of meditation exercises in the first half of the program. As in the first half, we coupled those formal loving-kindness meditations with exercises transferring loving-kindness and self-compassion into daily lives. We worked with participants to include self-soothing activities in their daily lives and bring mindfulness to joyful and pleasurable experiences as they arose.

THE MBCT FOR BIPOLAR DISORDER PROGRAM

MBCT for bipolar disorder consists of twelve 120-minute group treatment sessions conducted weekly over 3 months with concurrent individual sessions held every other week.

Assessment

At the beginning of this MBCT treatment is an assessment of prospective participants by the instructor in an individual meeting (see Chapter 3). This involves determining the bipolar disorder and the ongoing risk for mania or depression. What kind of symptoms and difficulties functioning are present? What co-occurring psychiatric or medical conditions does a participant have? This information will help to tailor the program to the specific needs of each individual participant. Likewise, we would like to know whether a participant's expectations for the program are realistic and whether his or her life situation is such that participation in this program makes sense at this time.

Group Sessions

The topic of the first two sessions is becoming aware of the present moment by learning to observe the sensations of movement brought on by simple yoga exercises leading into short Body Scans. In Body Scan exercises, attention is directed to different parts of the body. The concept of mindfulness ("mindfulness is paying attention in a particular way, on purpose, in the present moment and nonjudgmentally"; Kabat-Zinn, 1994, p. 4) is introduced by the raisin exercise, in which participants explore the raw attributes of a raisin (e.g., texture, color, scent; Session 1). All these exercises are designed to ground participants, make them aware of the present moment, and begin to teach them the process of observing what is present. As we would like participants to transfer this newly experienced observant awareness into daily life, in Session 1, a short Breathing Exercise (Introduction to the Breathing Space) is introduced and participants are asked to engage in this exercise whenever they switch from one activity to the next in order to become aware of what is present in that very moment. Growing awareness in this program will be directed to mood symptoms and in order to intervene before participants become manic or fully depressed. Therefore, in Session 1, mood monitoring is introduced as a way of keeping track of mood symptoms. Participants keep a Mood Diary in which they record mood symptoms daily. Instructors and participants review these Mood Diaries at the start of every subsequent session.

Starting in Session 2, we broaden mood monitoring by introducing the concept of becoming aware of warning signs (i.e., mood symptoms, thoughts, feelings, and behaviors that signal the worsening of mood). Warning signs and mood symptoms are then monitored daily using a Mood Diary for the remainder of the program. In Session 2, mindfulness to routine activities is introduced as another way of being present in the moment. In terms of formal practice, participants transition to practicing a short body scan without movement-induced sensations providing an anchor for attention. At the beginning, all formal meditation exercises are deliberately short (e.g., about 15 minutes) to accommodate those participants with difficulties focusing and sustaining attention. As all meditation exercises (e.g., yoga, body scans, sitting meditations) are practiced during the week as homework, we encourage participants to gradually stretch the practice longer as they become more proficient. In addition, the first 3 sessions include guidance about strategies (e.g., placing reminder cues or preplanning exercises) to work with obstacles to practice in daily life.

In Session 3, we begin to design action plans for what participants could do when warning signs of worsening mood arise. We also move beyond warning signs, and begin to direct attention to triggers. The term "triggers" refers to all factors that increase the likelihood of occurrence of warning signs. This can range from bad sleep habits, to overly high expectations a participant has regarding him- or herself, or difficulties saying "No" to assignments and feeling overwhelmed with work. Becoming aware of triggers will be a process that continues for the remainder of the program. In Session 3, participants begin to practice an expanded version of the Breathing Space (the 3-Minute Breathing Space). This version not only involves becoming present in the moment, but then also centers participants on the breath and grounds them, before widening the attentional focus again, beginning a process of decentering. In all these exercises, acceptance of "whatever is" is implicitly woven into the instructions. In terms of formal exercises, starting in Session 3, participants begin to explore mindful observing of different aspects of their inner landscape, down the road leading to an increased ability to holding all those aspects in a wider, accepting awareness.

This involves mindful observance of breathing (Session 3), mindfulness of breath and body (Session 4), mindful sitting with of sounds and thoughts (Session 5), and being mindful with strong feelings (Emotion-Focused Meditations; Session 5). As being mindful with strong feelings tends to be challenging for most participants, Emotion-Focused Meditations are practiced for several weeks (Sessions 5–9) before moving on to an Open Awareness Meditation (Session 9) in which participants begin to hold thoughts, feelings, sensations, and sounds in a wider, decentered accepting awareness. Starting in Session 4, participants will begin to work with triggers they have identified. This involves eliminating triggers where possible, or becoming more mindful with those that cannot be avoided. The expanded version of the Breathing Space (the 3-Minute Breathing Space) is now brought into those moments when participants are triggered in order to help them decenter from difficult thoughts and unpleasant feelings. Then participants begin to problem-solve how to best respond to those triggers going forward. This process continues for the remainder of the program.

In Session 5, participants begin to learn more about the interaction of thoughts, feelings, and behaviors that unfold when they find themselves becoming more depressed, manic, angry, or anxious. This involves beginning to recognize automatic negative, hyperpositive, or catastrophic thoughts, and learning more about mood-congruent information processing and behaviors that intensify the self-perpetuating cycle of thoughts and feelings rather than slowing them down. As these vicious cycles tend to be highly overlearned and unfold quite automatically, we call them "autopilots." Accepting awareness will now be explicitly emphasized as part of the instructions. Going forward, participants begin to initiate the expanded 3-Minute Breathing Space with Acceptance whenever they encounter triggers and an autopilot begins to unfold in daily life. The end of the Breathing Space is a choice point for the participant to learn how to move forward in a given situation. How can I respond most mindfully to what I am experiencing right now?

To provide guidance, we amend action plans for depression and mania by guiding participants in exploring ways of how to bring mindful acceptance into those moments and how to respond to these moments most skillfully. In addition, we create plans that include options about how to be more mindful with anger and anxiety. These modes of responding will be practiced for the remainder of the program. The discussion of autopilots and action plans will focus on depression first (Session 5), as this is the most pervasive problem for most participants with bipolar disorder. Next we focus on mania (Session 6), as the consequences of manic episodes can be devastating. Anger can be part of both depression and mania, hence the anger autopilot is discussed in Session 7 before addressing the autopilot associated with anxiety disorders (Session 8), which are often co-occurring with bipolar disorder.

With Session 9, formal emotion-focused meditations as part of the practice in the group are coming to an end and we introduce open awareness: the practice of holding thoughts, feelings, and sensations or sounds in a wide, open, spacious awareness without getting involved or tangled up in them. Session 9 is also the beginning of compassionate coaching and loving-kindness (Sessions 9–12). Up to this point, compassion was implicitly woven into the instructions and the discussions with group participants. Starting in Session 9, how to become more compassionate with oneself will be an explicit topic. This involves a formal loving-kindness meditation (Session 9) and participants beginning to act as their own kind and compassionate coaches in dealing with difficult thoughts and feelings, as well as life issues going forward (Session 10). We also ask participants to treat themselves well by systematically engaging in self-soothing and enjoyable activities (Session 10) and practicing actively to send loving-kindness to others, as well as to themselves (Sessions 10 and 11). As the program comes to an end, the last session (session 12) serves as a review of the skills participants have learned and a discussion of how participants can continue with mindfulness as they are moving on, before saying good-bye.

Individual Sessions

Group sessions are coupled with semiregular individual therapy sessions every other week or, if needed, more often. These individual therapy sessions serve several purposes (see Part I: Individual Sessions). First, in our experience, only a minority of participants will come to all 12 group sessions. Therefore, participants who miss one or more group sessions may fall behind. Falling behind and feeling one is not keeping up with group is one of the reasons participants may quit. Individual sessions, while not intended to fully replace group sessions, are an avenue to help participants catch up and stay with the program.

Second, individual sessions are used to support participants in crisis situations. Many of the elements built into the group sessions are meant for practicing and skill building, but group sessions usually do not provide a lot of time for the instructor to work with participants individually, and help the participant to problem-solve when crisis situations arise. Yet crises situations are often those times during the program when participants call in that they cannot come to group or just don't show up.

Third, individual sessions provide a forum in which to individualize mindfulness exercises, discuss particular challenges a participant may have with these exercises, and address obstacles to practicing. They also serve to deepen action plans for depression and mania, and to deepen knowledge about warning signs and triggers. When depression and mania strike, individual sessions are used to bring in treatment elements that ordinarily would be introduced later in the MBCT program. For example, when participants are slipping into depression, behavioral activation and self-soothing activities are implemented at that time, rather than waiting until Session 9. Likewise, for participants who are becoming hypomanic, action plans may need to be initiated before Session 3 and some mindfulness skills (e.g., 3-Minute Breathing Space) may be part of that action plan even though participants have not had much (or no) time to practice this before. Furthermore, participants who have become hypomanic need to be monitored more closely clinically than a once-a-week group session permits. Finally, individual sessions can be used as a forum to discuss participants' concerns regarding medications (e.g., wanting to change or discontinue them).

Homework

This program asks participants to practice meditation exercises in their daily lives in between sessions. In many ways, adopting mindfulness involves learning new skills. This works best with repeated practice. Therefore, we ask participants to practice yoga and meditation exercises at home. To facilitate this process, we provide recordings of the instructions participants receive in class as well as handouts (see Part III). Recordings can be downloaded (see p. viii for details). At the end of each session, we specify which exercise should be practiced at home, including the name of the track, and give out the handouts pertaining to the homework. Practicing meditation (or yoga) exercises at home using these recordings is a good start. Once a participant feels comfortable, he or she can transition to a self-guided practice without recordings. In our experience, adhering to a formal meditation practice is difficult for many individuals with bipolar disorder. Not only are their lives often chaotic, but attention and memory difficulties may impede practice. However, rather than barring interested and willing participants from this program for these reasons, we opted for taking this as a challenge that comes with the disorder. Therefore, this book includes instructions on how to implement short, more informal, meditation exercises (Breathing Spaces) in daily life and how to be reminded about it.

HOW WELL DOES MBCT FOR BIPOLAR DISORDER WORK?

After 2 years of discussion, consultations, designing and redesigning our program, we were ready to start our first MBCT groups in the spring of 2009. First, we wanted to see whether we could successfully implement what had been designed in countless hours of discussion. Therefore, despite its methodological limitations, we initially opted for conducting an open trial in which participants were aware that they were treated with MBCT for bipolar disorder (Deckersbach et al., 2012). From the Bipolar Clinic and Research Program at Massachusetts General Hospital, we recruited a small group of 12 patients with bipolar I or II disorder who had experienced residual depression or decreased interest at least 3 days every week during the month preceding the study, but did not have full depression. We also did not want participants to be hypomanic or manic at the time they entered the study. Thus, we limited the degree of permitted residual mood elevation symptoms (a score of <12 in the Young Mania Rating Scale; Young, Biggs, Ziegler, & Meyer, 1978). Most participants were taking mood-stabilizing medications. The group followed a pretreatment assessment that included measures of mindfulness, depression, mania, rumination, and worry, as well as attention difficulties, positive affect, well-being, and overall psychosocial functioning. Participants then completed 12 sessions of this MBCT for bipolar disorder followed by a posttreatment assessment at the end of treatment (after Session 12), and a 3-month follow-up assessment. MBCT for bipolar disorder consisted of twelve, 120-minute group treatment sessions conducted weekly over 3 months but without the concurrent individual sessions yet (a modification we made after this initial study).

In terms of feasibility, two of our participants dropped out after the initial screening visit with no further visits. Ten participants completed treatment (8 females). One participant who completed the treatment moved out of the area and could not be reached for the follow-up. All but two participants had more than a total of 12 lifetime mood episodes. Overall, participants attended an average of 8.5 sessions.

The results are encouraging. On the Five Facet Mindfulness Scale (our measure of mindfulness) participants significantly improved their ability to observe thoughts and feelings, and became less judgmental and less reactive to difficult thoughts and feelings. They also experienced less depression (as measured by the Hamilton Depression Rating Inventory), and there was no change in the degree of residual manic symptoms. We also found that at the end of our treatment, participants ruminated less, had better concentration abilities, were less emotionally reactive, and reported better cognitive and overall functioning (Stange et al., 2011). These effects held up when we only looked at participants with bipolar I disorder and participants with concurrent anxiety disorders. They also remained when we only looked at those participants with more than 12 lifetime mood episodes. In fact, numerically, the effects became stronger, as the two participants with fewer episodes of all the participants had the smallest amount of gains. However, we recognize that larger randomized clinical trials are needed to establish the overall efficacy of this program.

PROGRAM ISSUES

Who Is Qualified to Conduct MBCT for Bipolar Disorder?

Two types of clinicians are qualified to conduct MBCT for bipolar disorder: (1) clinicians with experience in treating participants with bipolar disorder using other types of treatments (e.g., CBT, FFT, IPSRT, or DBT) and who would like to include mindfulness in their repertoire of therapeutic avenues; and (2) experienced mindfulness teachers who are familiar with bipolar disorder and would like to treat people with bipolar disorder. Clinicians experienced in teaching mindfulness will recognize the adaptation of many mindfulness-based stress reduction exercises. For this group, we describe in detail (see Part II) how to incorporate the established CBT strategies that are built into this program (e.g., mood monitoring). For clinicians with experience in CBT, FFT, IPSRT, or DBT, a critical question is, How much experience in mindfulness and meditation is needed?

Mindfulness Experience

We embarked on developing this program after completing several MBSR classes (T. D.) and becoming a licensed MBSR instructor (B. H.). Overall, we consider the therapist's active embodiment of mindfulness one of the most important ingredients of a successful intervention. There are several aspects to this:

1. With the degree of the therapist's own mindfulness practice, mindfulness instructions will become richer. Having paid close attention to the sensations of breathing in the abdomen oneself, or having encountered the impermanence of emotions, thoughts, and body sensations in one's own experience, the therapist will have better access to rich and multifaceted descriptions, pointing the participants to every new aspect of these seemingly boring practices.

2. Explanations will flow most naturally and most logically when taught out of one's own experience. Participants will come up with a vast number of questions and doubts about the practice. Giving standard-type responses that one has learned out of a manual won't satisfy participants, but will instead bore them, and comes along with the danger of making the mindfulness practices seem dead. Only when the participants can feel that the therapist has in-depth, personal experiences, and brings in his or her own curiosity about experience, fascination with the practice, and honest and open receptivity to the question, will they be able to really open up for it.

An important dimension of learning mindfulness practice is experiencing the therapist as a role model who embodies the practice with the way he or she interacts with the participants, faces his or her own emotions, and takes a posture in the class. (Mindfulness can be contagious.) Mindfulness facilitators will have to be able to stay centered within themselves in the midst of difficult emotional turbulences from group participants. Bipolar participants will come into class with very high or very low mood and energy levels. Mindfulness practice will help the therapist acquire a position from where he or she is able to intimately relate to the participant's experience, while at the same time staying centered within his or her own experience. Having trained to stay centered in the midst of his or her own internal conflicting emotional experiences during his or her own practice, he or she will be able to respond from a position where he or she is holding both of these in awareness within the same space. This will support participants by making them feel fully "seen/heard" and accepted the way they are, while at the same time pointing in a direction of more calmness and safety. The therapist will thus convey a message of "You are perfect the way you are *and* there is room for improvement."

Mindfulness teachers will also have to be able to pause in the midst of difficult group interactions. Participants with bipolar disorder can have a tendency to involve the group in conversations that take off in completely different directions than intended by the facilitator. Within such potentially unstable/inherently unstable dynamics in the class, choosing to act out of a place of mindful awareness of the entire situation and one's own internal reactions to it, will bring the therapist into a position to respond more adequately and skillfully.

More generally, having an active mindfulness practice will help therapists to connect to the difficult and challenging aspects within their own experiences. It will thereby enable them to engage participants with humility and connectedness, with a perspective that life is difficult and challenging for all of us: "within this human life, we are all somewhat in the same boat." Rather than discouraging therapists with no mindfulness practice from learning this program, we would like to encourage them to take up a regular mindfulness practice and to step into this fascinating encounter. More specifically, if you have never meditated and would like to incorporate mindfulness in your work with participants, we recommend taking at least one or more MBSR classes, and establishing your own regular meditation practice. We also recommend participating in a silent retreat, as this also has a profound impact on the experience and teaching of mindfulness. Finally, we recommend arranging for supervision through experienced MBSR and MBCT instructors when you embark on your first MBCT treatment group. With this level of experience and additional supervision, this treatment manual provides the tools to successfully implement MBCT for individuals with bipolar disorder.

Which Patients Should Try This MBCT for Bipolar Disorder?

Although with a limited empirical basis it is challenging to make recommendations, we also recognize clinicians' need for guidance for whom MBCT may be helpful. Most of the patients who participated in our studies (or have received MBCT clinically in the Bipolar Clinic and Research Program) fit what Scott et al. (2006) termed "severe, recurrent bipolar disorder." Our participants have lived with bipolar disorder for over a decade and have experienced well over 20 lifetime mood episodes. While medication adherence waxed and waned, these participants have learned that mood-stabilizing medications are the cornerstone of their treatment. Almost all of them also had concurrent psychiatric disorders, mostly anxiety disorders (panic disorder, generalized anxiety disorder [GAD], obsessive–compulsive disorder [OCD], social phobia, and posttraumatic stress disorder [PTSD]). All of them were struggling with ongoing depressive symptoms, difficulties organizing their days, or overall functioning. Some of them met criteria for major depression when they started the program. These are the participants who have benefited from our treatment as it is described in this manual.

Therefore, based on the available data, we recommend the MBCT for bipolar disorder described in this book for patients with pervasive recurrent depressive symptoms. Since the initial pilot trial, patients with major depression have also successfully completed this MBCT program. Therefore, we also recommend this program for patients who experience full major depression at the time when they start the program. We recommend this treatment for patients with co-occurring anxiety disorders and with past substance abuse or dependence. Finally, we recommend this program for patients with residual or intermittent increases in mood elevation. In this program, these patients will learn how to recognize the early signs of mood elevation and how to prevent escalation using mindfulness (among other established antimania behavioral techniques). However, for patients who are already hypomanic or manic, this is not the time to start this program. We also recommend this treatment for individuals with bipolar disorder who struggle with intense emotional reactions, as many of our exercises are designed to help patients to disengage and decenter from strong feelings and thoughts. This program is for clients who already take mood-stabilizing medications. We recommend taking mood-stabilizing medications for at least two reasons: (1) medications reduce the likelihood of a mania relapse and (2) they may buffer the severity of mood swings. This makes it easier for clients to learn and implement the MBCT skills they are taught.

Individuals who actively and frequently use drugs should consider a detoxification program followed by a drug rehabilitation program. For example, for drug and substance abuse as the primary problem, the program developed by Bowen and colleagues (Bowen, Chawla, & Marlatt, 2011) can be considered. What about younger patients, who were just diagnosed with bipolar disorder, struggling to make sense of the diagnosis, dealing with the aftermath of their first mood episodes? Mindfulness is a skill that seems to have beneficial effects for many areas of health. We feel this treatment could be helpful for patients in the early phases of their illness, provided they are open, interested, and motivated to practice and cultivate mindfulness. Often, however, the needs of patients coming out of their first episode or those in the early stages of the illness differ from those who have experience with bipolar disorder for 10 or 20 years. Younger patients may need more comprehensive psychoeducation than this program offers in order to help them accept the illness. Those with beliefs and thoughts that interfere with medication adherence (not just forgetting to take their medications) may also need to focus on psychosocial treatments early on, helping them to make the necessary life-style adjustments, which this program does only to some extent. For families, Miklowitz's FFT program clearly is the first choice and has received solid empirical support. Nonetheless, in our experience, clients who participated in our program who had spouses have successfully embraced many of the exercises together.

Group Size, Composition, Setting

Group Size

We recommend a group size of six to ten participants: six participants as the lower bound, because, at any given time, some participants will not come to group. With one or two participants not coming in any given week, it is still possible to work with participants as a group with four or more participants present. Ten participants is the upper limit, so that each participant still has a chance to provide input and share his or her experience as part of the group discussions.

Participant Composition

Participant groups can be mixed in terms of diagnosis (bipolar I and II), mood status (residual depression or mania, fully depressed), comorbid conditions (e.g., anxiety disorders), and chronicity and functioning (e.g., number of previous mood episodes; employed or unemployed). In our experience, having a diverse group greatly enriched the experience participants had in group.

Number of Instructors

The group can be run by one instructor. However, whenever possible, we recommend including a second clinician (or trainee) as a coleader. This facilitates the process of checking Mood Diaries at the beginning of each group session. This will also be helpful when crisis situations come up and a participant needs to be attended to individually at the time of group.

Room

As the first two sessions involve movement/yoga exercises and body scans, the room should be big enough that participants have sufficient space to move their arms and legs without getting into each other's space. A white board (or chalkboard) is helpful to visualize content for the group (e.g., autopilots in Sessions 5–8), although working with handouts and regular paper is acceptable.

Clothing and Material

Participants should bring comfortable clothes. This is particularly important for the yoga and movement exercises especially in the first two sessions. They may also want to buy a yoga mat and a meditation cushion if this is not provided as part of the setting. For sitting meditations, regular chairs can also be used. Participants should have an MP3 player and arrange for Internet access so that they can download recordings for homework practice.

In Chapter 3 we review the assessment and orientation session that takes place with each prospective participant before he or she is invited to join the MBCT program.

CHAPTER 3

Assessment and Orientation
for Prospective Participants

Before the first MBCT group, we schedule one individual session with each potential participant. This session serves two main purposes: (1) for us to determine whether a participant is a good candidate for the group and (2) for the potential participant to determine whether his or her hopes and goals for the program match what the program has to offer. At the end of this chapter, we provide instructors with a checklist of the most important points to consider when meeting with a prospective participant. In this assessment meeting, we cover the following topics:

- Diagnosis of bipolar disorder
- Current mood status, mood patterns, triggers, and habitual coping
- Co-occurring psychiatric disorders
- Co-occurring medical conditions
- Hopes and expectations for MBCT
- MBCT for bipolar disorder: The roadmap
- Mindfulness and medication

DIAGNOSIS OF BIPOLAR DISORDER

For determining whether a participant has bipolar disorder, we use structured clinical interviews such as the Mini-International Neuropsychiatric Interview (M.I.N.I.; Sheehan et al., 1998) or the Structured Clinical Interview for DSM-IV (SCID; First, Spitzer, Gibbon, & Williams, 1995; Sheehan et al., 1998). These interviews use the diagnostic criteria described in the DSM and determine a participant's subtype of bipolar disorder. Why is this important? Because it provides information about the risk for and the severity of hypomanic or manic episodes. As the instructor, you would like to know how frequent and severe episodes of mood elevation have been. Did your participant have full-blown manic episodes or only hypomania? Did manic episodes involve psychotic thinking (i.e., grandiosity, paranoia, or religious delusions)? Were high-risk activities such as excessively spending money, gambling, taking drugs, or risky sexual behaviors involved? During the program you will encounter decision-making points where this information will be helpful to guide the decisions you and the participant will make. For example, on the one hand, if you know that excess energy and speeded thinking have never escalated into full-blown mania for a given participant, usually decrease without intervention, and are not associated with high-risk behaviors, you and the participant may decide to work on those periods using mindfulness skills. On the other hand, if you already know that even some mood elevation tends to escalate into full-blown mania quickly, then time is of the essence. Not contacting the treating psychiatrist or increasing (or adding) mood stabilizing and/or antipsychotic medications would be a risky course of action. In these moments, your participant's safety comes first and immediate action may be required. Mindfulness skills can support this process in helping the participant become more aware of the need for supportive medical care, and can guide him or her in making skillful choices and taking care of him- or herself in a more active way.

You also want to be aware of ongoing suicidal ideation, previous suicide attempts, whether the participant currently has a plan, and what his or her contingencies are (i.e., Under which circumstances would the participant shift from having a plan to having a plan and intent?). Experience has taught us that participants, despite their and our best efforts, may become fully depressed during the program, or painfully suffer through periods of mixed depressive and manic symptoms. These times tend to indicate the biggest risk for suicide, and it is therefore good to be aware of any suicidal ideation, plan, or intent.

CURRENT MOOD STATUS, MOOD PATTERNS, TRIGGERS, AND HABITUAL COPING

The M.I.N.I. or SCID will also help you determine the participant's current mood status (i.e., Does your participant currently meet criteria for depression, hypomania, or mania?). Questionnaires such as the Beck Depression Inventory (BDI-II; Beck, Steer, & Brown, 1996) and the Quick Inventory of Depressive Symptomatology Self-Report (Quids-SR; Rush et al., 2003) or clinical rating scales such as the Hamilton Rating Scale for Depression (HRSD; Hamilton, 1960) and the Montgomery–Asberg Depression Rating Scale (MADRS; Montgomery & Asberg, 1979) can also help to guide the exploration. A good starting point for the program occurs when participants are experiencing intermittent or ongoing residual depressive or residual manic symptoms. We have also included participants who met full criteria for depression. However, if you have a difficult time getting a word in, your participant seems to be overconfident about the program, or shifts topics of conversations frequently and you find yourself having a hard time following him or her, this participant may be experiencing significant mood elevation (hypomania or mania). This is not a good starting point for learning mindfulness skills.

As described earlier, many participants experience ongoing, fluctuating, and chronic residual depressive and manic symptoms, which increase the likelihood that they may spiral into full-blown depression or mania. Thus, you want to learn more about a participant's pattern of ongoing residual symptoms. For example, with respect to depression, participants may describe their underlying mood as "low" and state that they "have a hard time motivating themselves," although they do not experience all the associated signs of full depression, such as sleep or appetite problems. Other participants may report that they are feeling "OK" for a while, but then there are days when "it hits them." This can happen when something sets them off without any predictive event. Remember, with repeated episodes of depression or mania, it appears that the brain switches into ruminative modes easier, without identifiable triggers. This state may only last for a day or a few days before the participant seems to "switch out of it," but it can also culminate in full-blown depression. As you monitor your participant throughout the group, this information will help you to guide clinically meaningful decisions in your participant's best interest. Also, knowing more about your participant's inner experience during these periods will help you to facilitate him or her in becoming more mindful.

The same questions should be asked with respect to interepisode manic symptoms. Which ones do participants have? Are they ongoing? Are they intermittent? Participants may notice that they have a little too much energy and get easily excited about projects or activities. They may also notice that they start feeling more activated and confident intermittently at times of achievements, which may increase their risk for hypomania or mania. Overconfident thinking and excitement about projects, plans, or ideas can be a leftover symptom from a recent hypomanic or manic episode that puts a participant at risk for increasing activities and potentially risky behaviors.

We tend to go through all the depression and mania symptoms listed in the DSM and inquire about their presence, duration, and frequency. We get a better sense of events, feelings, thoughts, and behaviors that may trigger or increase a participant's depressive or manic symptoms so that we can recognize their triggers more easily when they come up during the group phase. We also like to get a better sense of what topics send participants into a tailspin of depressive (or manic) rumination, like worrying that things may not work out, feeling lonely or unloved, or seeing yourself as an underachiever. Also, for example, the potential of achievements can create excitement and positive rumination. "Relationships are a big one for me," as Holly in our first meeting described one of her recent tailspins into several days of feeling depressed. "If a guy does not call me back after a date, I spend hours and hours figuring out what I did wrong. I end up talking to all my friends, to my therapist, just finding out what I did wrong. I am a nice person!" Sean, on the other hand, who started the group at the tail end of a 6-month manic episode, found it difficult to stop thinking about what he had learned about dating in a dating class he had taken while manic. "With all this new knowledge, I want to get back into dating and I can't help thinking about how great this will be."

We also like to get a better sense of the intensity of participants' emotional reactions and emotion regulation strategies when they are faced with painful, depressive, irritable, or positive ruminative thinking and experiences. For example, are they trying to shift their thoughts away from painful experiences or do they ruminate about them? In the case of Holly, she goes into fixing mode, doing everything she can to prove to herself that she is worthy of a relationship. Or do they try to avoid anxiety-provoking situations? Several questionnaires have been designed to assess the intensity of emotional reactions and participants' ways of emotion regulation more formally. These include the Emotion Reactivity Scale (ERS; Nock, Wedig, Holmberg, & Hooley, 2008) and the Difficulties in Emotion Regulation Scale (Gratz & Roemer, 2004). That said, the purpose of this session is not to collect an exhaustive set of triggers and assess all habitual coping strategies at this point in time. Also, many participants do not recognize their triggers and are not able to verbalize their inner experiences. Nonetheless, for the instructor, it offers a glimpse into the triggers that may affect a participant. The session also may help to better the participant's journey into mindfulness and signal some obstacles that could lie ahead.

CO-OCCURRING PSYCHIATRIC DISORDERS

Almost all participants with bipolar disorder have co-occurring psychiatric conditions, most commonly anxiety disorders (panic disorder, GAD, social phobia, and somewhat less often PTSD and OCD), substance abuse or dependence, and attention-deficit/hyperactivity disorder (ADHD). Based on the M.I.N.I., we assess whether participants currently meet the criteria for any of these or other comorbid conditions. This will help you tailor some of the mindfulness exercises toward your participant's needs. For example, anxiety is a common experience for many participants with bipolar disorder. Anxiety and the corresponding associated emotion-focused meditation are covered in Session 8. However, participants for whom anxiety is a major issue can, and should, start emotion-focused meditations geared toward anxiety as early as Session 5 when emotion-focused meditations ("Working with Difficult Feelings") are introduced. Knowledge about co-occurring disorders also provides information about participants' inner landscape when doing mindfulness exercises.

For example, for a participant with panic disorder, noticing physical symptoms (e.g., heart beat) while engaging in yoga or sitting meditations may trigger catastrophic thoughts ("What if I get a panic attack?"), anxiety, and increased physical symptoms due to anxiety, possibly leading into a panic attack. This does not mean that such a participant should not do mindfulness exercises. Rather, the instructor may decide to provide further education about the vicious cycle of panic attacks early on. This may provide the participant with some critical knowledge that will put him or her in a better position to do these exercises and gradually increase mindfulness toward anxiety-related feelings and thoughts. It will also prompt the instructor to inquire about catastrophic thinking that may have occurred during a mindfulness exercise and how the participant experienced and dealt with it.

Participants with GAD may find themselves engaging in worry and rumination about everyday topics ("Will my boss be fine with my work?," "Is this the right decision?") and having a hard time disengaging, whereas for a participant with social phobia, the idea of being in a group with other people may be a terrifying idea. This will all be part of the participants' experiences to which they will increasingly bring mindfulness. Also, for the instructor, it is knowledge critical to creating a careful balance between providing safety cues and facilitating mindfulness so that participants can adopt a more mindful stance toward anxious experiences over the course of the program. For participants with anxiety disorders, it can be helpful to utilize questionnaires that provide information about feared internal sensations (e.g., the Anxiety Sensitivity Index [ASI]; Peterson & Reiss, 1992) and catastrophic cognitions (Chambless, Caputo, Bright, & Gallagher, 1984).

More than half of all participants with bipolar disorder meet criteria for substance abuse or dependence at some point during their lives. If a participant frequently uses drugs or alcohol and this appears to be the primary problem, the participant is not a good candidate for this program. However, we did not exclude participants with a history of substance abuse. As part of the initial meeting, we review what drugs have been involved and the pattern of use. From the perspective of a mindfulness program, learned, or conditioned, cravings are central to drug and alcohol abuse and dependence and increase the risk that a participant may use drugs or alcohol again. These triggers can be not only times of the day and places, but also difficult emotional states for which alcohol and drugs have served as coping mechanisms. As part of the program, participants want to become more aware of these cues and gradually bring mindfulness into these moments. Participants with a long-standing history of drug and alcohol abuse may also suffer from cognitive problems such as difficulties remembering, focusing, concentrating, and getting organized.

Similar issues are faced by participants with comorbid ADHD or cognitive problems associated with bipolar disorder. Subjective cognitive problems can be assessed using rating scales such as the ADHD Self-Report Scale (Kessler, Adler, et al., 2005), the Frontal Systems Behavior Rating Scale (FrSBe; Grace & Malloy, 2001), and the Behavior Rating Inventory of Executive Function (BRIEF; Roth, Isquith, & Gioia, 2005). For participants with memory problems and difficulties focusing over longer periods of time and getting organized, emphasis was placed on using reminder cues for doing mindfulness exercises. Likewise we focused on raising awareness when bad judgment could derail a participant from doing his or her exercises. Mindfulness exercises (e.g., Body Scans, sitting meditations) are short at the beginning and can gradually be lengthened by participants themselves. We recognize the value of longer mindfulness exercises, even at the beginning of a mindfulness program. However, if participants feel that the practice is too difficult early on, they will disengage.

CO-OCCURRING MEDICAL CONDITIONS

Many participants with bipolar disorder have medical issues. While co-occurring medical issues do not preclude participation in a mindfulness program, they warrant extra and possible ongoing attention. You should pay attention to medical issues for two main reasons. First, some of the symptoms participants may experience may be due to a medical condition. The purpose of becoming more mindful is to become more aware of and to change the way participants relate to any uncomfortable and challenging experience. However, from a health perspective, this goal refers to experiences that cannot be treated medically. Acute appendicitis should be treated by surgery, not mindfulness, although mindfulness may help to cope with the pain before or after surgery. A participant with bipolar disorder who feels tired all the time and has little energy or motivation may have hypothyrodism. Weight loss, rapid heart beat, anxiety or irritability, and sweating can be signs of hyperthyrodism. Both conditions should be treated medically.

Second, medical conditions necessitate adjusting some of the program's exercises. Let's consider participants who are overweight or have musculoskeletal issues. We may simplify some of the movement exercises. The purpose of movement exercises is to make participants become more in tune with their bodies, not to increase their physical fitness. This goal can be achieved by simple movements and by paying attention to bodily sensations, without including more challenging motions like bending over. For participants with blood pressure issues, we also advise caution with respect to some of the exercises that involve bending over.

HOPES AND EXPECTATIONS FOR MBCT

Everyone who considers participation in a MBCT program for bipolar disorder has a wish list of what he or she would like to accomplish, such as to have fewer mood episodes, get a quieter mind, free the self from strong feelings, stop being pushed around by emotions, stop ruminating, have more control over thoughts, just feel normal, not feel anything, or simply find peace. False expectations can lead to disappointment and dropout. On account of this problem, we inquire about and discuss these hopes and expectations for MBCT before the start of the program. Our review of the MBCT program (see below) can help to debunk some myths about meditation and mindfulness and serves to adjust overly high or false expectations. At the end of the session, participants are provided with Handout 1, which summarizes the most common misconceptions about mindfulness. Common misconceptions about MBCT, meditation, and mindfulness are described below.

1. *With meditation, I will have no more mood episodes.* This is unlikely. As part of the MBCT program, participants will learn to recognize warning signs for depression, hypomania, and mania and bring mindfulness to them. This response will help to prevent symptoms from spiraling into full-blown depression, hypomania, or mania. With these new skills, there is a good chance that they may have fewer mood episodes, but it is unlikely that they will all be fully prevented.

2. *I will be able to "treat" my depression and mania with only mindfulness.* Mindfulness will become part of the treatment, but is unlikely to be the only component. Among other things, participants will learn to bring mindfulness to the experiences that come with depression, hypomania, or mania. One hopes this will shorten periods of depression, hypomania,

or mania and make them less severe. However, especially for mania, not addressing symptoms with medication is a risky course of action (see below).

3. *Meditation will help to quiet my mind.* Sometimes when people meditate, they encounter moments with few or no thoughts. However, this is not the goal of or the reason for practicing meditation. Meditation involves learning to become more aware of thoughts and to pay attention to thoughts in a different, nonjudgmental way. This helps interrupt ruminative patterns of thinking that often worsen mood symptoms in depression, hypomania, and mania.

4. *Meditation stops rumination.* Though true, this does not mean meditation can block out thoughts. Rather, mindfulness involves learning to recognize maladaptive thought patterns and to bring observant, nonjudgmental attention to them, instead of engaging in endless loops of rumination.

5. *Meditation stops depressive and manic thoughts.* Meditation involves learning how to pay attention to and disengage from these thought patterns in a novel, nonjudgmental way. This skill will not necessarily stop the depressive and manic thoughts.

6. *Meditation relaxes, calms, and evens out strong feelings.* Though this can happen, this is not the purpose for practicing meditation. Rather, mindfulness involves a different, observant, and nonjudgmental way of being with thoughts and feelings. In fact, as many meditation teachers have pointed out, being mindful is especially important when feelings are strong.

7. *Meditation can help to control strong feelings.* Meditation can help to control strong feelings in a different way than most people think. Mindfulness is not about trying to relax when strong feelings are present. In this program, participants learn to create a "wider space" within themselves from which they can observe, notice, and be with strong feelings and thoughts without getting tangled up in them.

8. *Meditation involves music and mentally going to peaceful places.* This is true for some meditation exercises, but not for those used in this program.

MBCT FOR BIPOLAR DISORDER: THE ROADMAP

False hopes and expectations can be addressed by giving participants a brief overview of the program (see Handout 2). The overview can help participants determine whether this program is what they are looking for and whether it is a good time for them to start participating. The purpose of the roadmap is not to provide an exhaustive description of the program, but rather to highlight the most salient aspects.

1. Overall, mindfulness is about developing skills to decenter from strong feelings and thoughts that come with depression, hypomania, and mania. Participants learn to create a wider space within themselves from which they can observe, notice, and be with strong feelings and thoughts without getting tangled up in them.

2. Mood episodes (depression, hypomania, mania) usually do not occur out of the blue, although it may seem that way. Typically there are warning signs, indicating that the mood is getting worse (e.g., becoming depressed or hypomanic). For example, depression may be foreshadowed by an increased frequency of negative thoughts, more rumination, and feeling less motivated, while initial signs of hypomania or mania may involve increased energy, confidence, and motivation, or increased irritability. As part of the program, participants will learn to bring awareness to the presence of these warning signs and begin to implement mindfulness as they arise.

3. Participants also learn to direct awareness and bring mindfulness to thoughts, feelings, behaviors, and situations that may lead to warning signs. For example, exercising before bedtime may cause lack of sleep, which leads to warning signs for hypomania like speeded thoughts and increased energy. Likewise, not finishing a work assignment may make someone feel like a failure, leading to rumination about being inadequate, which can be a warning sign for depression. The program strives to increase awareness of such situations, and their associated thoughts and feelings. Participants should aim to find balance by reducing exposure to such situations when possible, bringing mindfulness to thoughts and feelings if exposure is unavoidable, and applying problem-solving strategies in a mindful way (like responding rather than reacting).

4. We also employ mindfulness during periods of depression, hypomania, and, if possible, mania. Mindfulness will still likely be one aspect of a broader intervention that involves cognitive and behavioral strategies and medication. (For the discussion of medication, see below.) For instance, if a hypomanic participant notices increased energy and motivation, develops new plans and ideas on the spur, and feels talkative, an intervention may involve taking a mindful stance toward the exciting thoughts and ideas, as well as reducing stimulation (e.g., staying home), preventing risky activities (e.g., buying, gambling), limiting conversations, increasing medication, and bringing further mindfulness to the uncomfortable feeling of not spending the excess energy or following the urge to talk.

5. Finally, in the second part of the program, participants work on becoming their own kind and compassionate coaches for dealing most effectively with the challenges of bipolar disorder. This involves learning to take better care of their own needs, treating themselves with kindness, and bringing in soothing and pleasurable activities to help them buffer the stress of daily life.

These goals are accomplished through practice. Over the course of the program, participants learn to create a wider space within themselves from which they can observe, notice, and be with strong feelings and thoughts without getting tangled up in them. This process involves practicing mindfulness exercises. Mindfulness is a skill that can be acquired. It will be taught in 2-hour group sessions each week. The acquisition of this skill, like any other skill, requires practice. A skill that is only practiced once a week will take a long time to grow; therefore, practice during the week is highly encouraged. Practice comes in two forms. The first includes mindfulness exercises for which participants are asked to set aside blocks of time to practice on a daily basis, if possible. This may include formal practice, which comprises movement exercises and sitting meditations. In addition, there will be informal practice, in which mindfulness exercises are built into a participant's daily life. For example, we may ask a participant to practice checking in with him- or herself about what is going on in a particular moment or to begin observing more consciously which thoughts, feelings, and bodily sensations are present in a given moment. This way, one can incorporate moments of mindfulness into daily life. Over time, the frequency of those moments will increase. For example, one can become mindful about being in the subway, sitting in a chair, eating a meal, or feeling frustrated, angry, and irritated. Group sessions will be complemented by biweekly individual sessions that provide the participant with additional support, help tailor mindfulness practices, and help solve life issues that may interfere with participation in the MBCT program (see Chapter 4).

A summary of the roadmap is provided in Handout 2, given to participants at the end of the session. Participants will vary considerably in their ability to implement formal mindfulness practices. However, if a participant feels that working on increasing daily mindfulness would be too great of burden for him or her, some caution is advised for enrolling this person. Do not be surprised if after this initial overview few participants are deterred by the time and effort the program requires. Once the programs' demands begin, prior underestimation of time and effort can make participants more likely to drop out. Therefore, learning more about a participant's personal life can be helpful for an instructor in assessing whether his or her participation in the MBCT program is a good choice.

MINDFULNESS AND MEDICATION

Medications almost always become a topic of discussion at some point. Not only do they tie into participants' hopes and expectations for the MBCT program, but also at times during the program there may be a need to boost or change medications if participants experience clinically severe worsening of symptoms, particularly if they are at risk of becoming hypomanic or manic. Consequently, we review medication and related concerns with the participant before the program starts. We also like to have a jointly agreed-upon course of action should symptoms of mania or depression increase in severity.

Should a participant take medication when participating in the program? In general, we recommend MBCT for bipolar disorder in addition to pharmacotherapy. Specific medication needs will depend on the person, his or her diagnosis, and his or her clinical course of bipolar disorder. On the one hand, not taking mood-stabilizing medications or antipsychotic medications is a risky decision for a participant with bipolar I disorder who had a recent manic episode and has a history of previous manic episodes with psychotic symptoms. On the other hand, for a participant with a long-standing history of depression and intermittent hypomanic episodes that have never impaired functioning, medication options may be more variable, especially given the undetermined efficacy of many antidepressant medications for bipolar disorder. Reviewing medications involves getting a sense of what, if any, medications the participant takes. If the participant has a psychiatrist, it is helpful to get permission to communicate with him or her, as establishing this communication tends to be more difficult when the participant is already hypomanic or manic. We also inquire about concerns regarding medications, as they may influence participants' adherence to medication regimens. If there is reason to believe that a participant is taking medications that seem inadequate or inconsistent with the recommendations of the practice guidelines for bipolar disorder, we may recommend an independent medication consultation. Sometimes, a participant's primary care physician prescribes his or her medications. In this case, we recommend that he or she find a psychiatrist prior to starting this program. As described earlier, despite adequate pharmacotherapy, it is common for participants to continue to experience residual, pervasive mood symptoms and episodes of depression, hypomania, or mania—hence the need for this program.

Some participants envision that with the help of MBCT they may achieve greater control over their mood to a degree that they will be able to discontinue medication altogether. While this belief provides a great source of motivation, it can also be a reason for profound disappointment. Most participants we have worked with have been able to achieve greater mood stability and some have even lowered their medication doses following the completion of our program. However, if discontinuing medication is a participant's goal, clarifying the potential effects of mindfulness on evening out mood and emotional control may help to adjust unrealistic expectations regarding posttreatment mood stability and the need for continued medication.

Some participants who inquire about the program will be medication-free. Should they start the MBCT program? It depends. If a participant recently discontinued medication, it is possible that this occurred in the context of the beginning of a hypomanic or manic episode when the participant felt increasingly confident about his or her ability to manage bipolar disorder without medication. Unless that participant is willing to restart his or her medications before enrolling in the program, we do not recommend participation. In the context of noticeable or reported symptoms of mood elevation, reassurance from the participant that he or she is "feeling fine," "doing well," or "handling this" may indicate lack of insight, that is, this participant is underestimating the degree of mood elevation that has already unfolded. In this case, we alert the participant to the symptoms of mood elevation that we notice, including overconfidence, and recommend discussing these symptoms with his or her psychiatrist and family, if possible, to get a second opinion about his or her mood and possible need for medication. Other nonmedicated participants may have reportedly done well for a while, but demonstrate signs of alcohol or drug abuse. For those participants, we also recommend restarting medication prior to beginning an MBCT program. For some participants a drug detoxification program may be the appropriate treatment plan.

Other nonmedicated participants may not yet have had a recurrence of depression or mania since discontinuing medications. These participants may be reluctant to restart medications because they had purported success managing bipolar symptoms without medications. We discuss the risks they take, especially if they have had manic episodes in the past. If such a participant otherwise seems like a good fit for the MBCT program, but continues to be reluctant to consider medication on a regular basis, our next course of action is to negotiate rescue medication. That is, we offer participation in the program contingent on the participant's willingness to take rescue medication should symptoms of mania arise. If the participant agrees, we work out a plan with the participant and his or her psychiatrist under which circumstances rescue medication should be started. This plan identifies the warning signs that initiate the rescue plan. In general, instructors should expect that negotiations around medications take place throughout the program. This involves negotiations about when to boost or change medication and for how long. We address concerns about boosting or changing medications before or after group sessions and also in individual meetings with the participant, as there is often not enough time to address such concerns during group sessions.

PREPARING FOR THE FIRST GROUP SESSION

Participants with bipolar disorder often come across as bright and very functional, masking how severely functioning may be impaired. One individual who had intended to participate in the group got lost on his way to the group's meeting location. He was so dismayed by his inability to simply find a building that he never came back to start the group. On the day of the first group, some participants simply forgot about the meeting. For others, something "urgent" came up and they could not make group. These experiences taught us to prepare participants for the first day of group. First, we discuss these potential obstacles to attendance openly with participants in the assessment session. Participants may or may not think that forgetfulness or poor judgment applies to them, but most are willing to grant us permission to implement our support system. This includes identifying support people, like spouses, to support participants' attendance. They can also remind participants to come to group. In addition, we place reminder calls a couple of days before and on the day of group sessions. Reminder e-mails can serve the same function. On the day of group meetings, we have participants' cell phone numbers as well as their psychiatrists' and support persons' cell phone numbers on hand so that we are able to call if a participant is not on time.

Before we proceed in outlining the first group session, let us review the rationale, content, and structure of the individual therapy sessions designed to complement group sessions (Chapter 4).

Instructor Checklist: Do You Know Your Participant?

- Bipolar subtype? Bipolar I, II, or NOS?
- Current mood status:
  - Depressed?
  - Hypomanic?
  - Manic?
  - Ongoing depressive and/or manic symptoms?
  - Ongoing mood symptoms: Which ones? Frequency? Duration? Intensity?
    - Pattern: Ongoing? Intermittent?
    - Known triggers for mood symptoms? Sleep? Achievements? Anxiety?
    - Which types of emotion-regulation strategies?
- Co-occurring disorders: Anxiety disorders? Alcohol or drug abuse? ADHD?
- Co-occurring medical issues?
- MBCT hopes and expectations: Are they realistic enough?
- Time and effort: Can the participant meet the demand?
- MBCT and medication:
  - Does the participant have a psychiatrist?
  - Do you have the phone number/contact info?
  - Is medication adequate?
  - If nonmedicated: Is the participant willing to consider rescue medication?
- Preparing for the first session: Is a support person identified? Do you have participant's and support person's phone number?

CHAPTER 4

Individual Sessions

MBCT group sessions are coupled with semiregular individual therapy sessions, during which the instructor meets with each participant every other week or as needed. These individual therapy sessions serve several purposes:

- Problem solving for crisis situations
- Review of previous sessions, including:
  - Individualizing or adjusting mindfulness exercises
  - Refining action plans for depression and mania
  - Deepening knowledge about warning signs and triggers
  - Problem solving for obstacles to practicing
- Dealing with mania
- Dealing with depression
- Discussing medication and raising insight

PROBLEM SOLVING FOR CRISIS SITUATIONS

A day before the second group session, Christina called and left a message saying that she could no longer participate in the program. When the instructor called her back, she explained that her son, who was battling drug addiction, had just been admitted to another detoxification program. He was more or less living on the street and doing drugs, leaving his mother constantly worried about his well-being. Usually things would calm down for a while and then it would start all over again. Needless to say, Christina was worried about her son, felt completely overwhelmed, and did not do any of the exercises that had been assigned in the first session. "I just can't do this. It's too much," she said apologetically, explaining why she needed to drop out of the program. Situations like this are more common than you might think. About one-third to one-half of the participants in our program encountered crisis situations that felt overwhelming and led to their considering dropping out of the program. During group sessions, there was hardly ever enough time to sufficiently address these situations. We found ourselves talking to participants individually on the phone or in person, helping them to work through the situation that had unfolded. Implicitly, we had adopted a model that dialectical behavior therapy (DBT) has employed for years: skills training as part of the group treatment and helping participants to apply these skills in an individual-session format. Therefore, we started to offer semiregular individual sessions as part of the program.

What does problem solving for crisis situations mean? Let's use Christina's experience as an example. When she learned of her son's situation, Christina's mind immediately went to catastrophic thoughts—first she thought he would die, he would be homeless, or she would have to take him in, which would make her life chaotic. She thought, "Please, not again," and "Why can't he get his act together?" Her mind was a stream of mixed catastrophic thoughts and attempts to find a solution. Getting more anxious and overwhelmed as there did not seem to be any good solution to this problem, she tried to get more information about housing and drug treatment centers so that she could provide her son with some options. Between trying mentally to fix things and attempting to get more information, Christina ended up having a full-blown panic attack. Somewhat reluctantly, she agreed to come in and meet with the instructor. "What should I do?," she repeatedly asked as she was describing the situation. Indeed, how can you become mindful with this kind of situation and also problem-solve? No matter how far the group has advanced, we always use the 3-Minute Breathing Space as a way to ground oneself and begin the process of stepping out of automatic pilot (see Session 3). After listening to Christina explain the situation and how she felt, as the first part of the Breathing Space, the instructor asked her to come into the present and notice what she was feeling right then and there. In the second part of the Breathing Space, the instructor guided her to focus on her breathing, and to follow her in-breath and her out-breath. That day, Christina spent several minutes just following and returning to the breath as a way of grounding herself. She could then widen her attentional focus to re-include her whole body as the third part of the Breathing Space. She continued in "noticing and being mode," returning to the breath whenever needed.

Situations like this often come with only imperfect solutions. All solutions Christina had entertained in her mind came with emotional drawbacks. Thinking about taking her son in caused anxiety because she was afraid of his "chaos" and what it would do to her life. Not taking him in "made her a bad mother" and caused huge feelings and thoughts of guilt. There did not seem to be a good or even acceptable solution. Thus, her mind kept going back and forth between the various alternatives. Just observing the mind's attempt to find an acceptable or perhaps even perfect solution can be quite revealing to participants. "It really looks like I don't have a good way out here, no matter where I turn," Christina acknowledged. For Christina, becoming aware of her "need to fix" and the "fixing" routine of the mind also helped her when turning to the practical side of problem solving.

Mindful problem solving after completing the Breathing Space considers the various alternatives that one has available to respond to a situation. The emphasis is on mindful responding to a situation, rather than reacting with intense feelings and thoughts. With Christina, we considered her various options. Should she let her son live with her again? Should she look for a drug treatment program? Were there any other resources that could be available to her son and herself? As we looked into these options, which all came with disadvantages, the instructor continued to ask Christina to check in with herself and to notice what thoughts and feelings she observed as she considered what to do. This check-in also involved accepting the fact that there were no solutions without drawbacks. At various times, when she noticed the feeling of becoming overwhelmed, Christina grounded herself by attending to the breath before opening up again. That day Christina decided that talking to a social worker and finding out what resources may be available to her son felt like the best option.

When difficult situations do not have painless solutions the mind continues to worry and ruminate, looking for a way out. Mindfulness involves gradually becoming more aware of this desire for a painless solution that keeps the mind running, and bringing acceptance to what cannot be fixed. When it comes to problem solving in the context of crisis situations and mindfulness, we follow these general steps: (1) the Breathing Space (see Session 3) and (2) mindful consideration of the various options to respond to the situation. During this second phase, it is particularly important for the instructor not to fall into the trap of trying to hunt for a painless solution. Rather, we use this practical phase to guide the participant to accept the mind's and body's reactions when painful or unwanted alternatives are considered, as well as the tendency to continue to search for palatable solutions that come with little or no disadvantages. Responding involves making a more mindful, reflective choice, rather than reacting to the mind's grooves. This could result in choosing to delay a response.

At the beginning of this process, Christina concentrated more on her body and on noticing the sensations she felt, because it was often too painful for her to directly pay attention to her thoughts. She and her instructor talked about noticing and being with what unfolded in her body without trying to fix it and bringing gentleness to her own pain as she was considering the various options available to her. As the program continued, she gradually realized more and more the pattern her mind was going through: cycling between considering solutions, rejecting them, revisiting solutions she had rejected before, and striving for one solution that came without feeling anxious or guilty. She became more and more aware of her need to make things right, and gradually learned to become "less tangled up" in attempts to fix a situation with no acceptable solution. She also gradually realized that she needed to take care of herself while taking care of her son, which helped her to make some difficult decisions along the way and "to be" with some difficult decisions; this manifested as not letting her son move in with her, but rather helping him find housing after completing a drug rehab program. In crisis situations like Christina's, instructors should also be flexible. For example, for Christina, not feeling obligated to engage in formal exercises was a big relief. Based on the individual session she had with her instructor, she felt comfortable practicing and using the Breathing Space going forward. Interestingly, she started practicing the Movement Exercise right after her first individual session and it became one of her favorite ways of grounding herself in moments when her mind was taking off.

REVIEW OF PREVIOUS SESSIONS

When there is no crisis to address, instructors and participants can simply focus on reviewing the previous group sessions. For instructors, this is a valuable opportunity to learn more about a participant's experience of the group session and exercises. We also discuss any additional questions a participant may have, clarify misconceptions, deepen the participant's understanding of the material, help to remove obstacles, and help participants to include mindfulness in their daily lives. For example, for the first sessions, this agenda can involve clarifying why movement exercises and being present in the moment, even for mundane activities such as eating or brushing teeth, are relevant for when negative thoughts or unpleasant feelings arise. This involves deepening their understanding of how warning signs for depression and mania are related to negative thoughts and unpleasant feelings and what kind of triggers the participant has noticed in the past (see Session 3). We also refine action plans for when mania strikes or intermittent depressive symptoms spiral into depressive episodes (see Session 3). Mindful problem solving often addresses difficulties implementing the exercises and adjusting them to a participant's needs. Some commonly discussed issues include forgetting to practice, procrastination, and misconceptions about the mindfulness exercises.

Forgetting

Not completing the exercises is sometimes just a matter of not remembering to do them. As described earlier, some participants with bipolar disorder have memory difficulties. This involves forgetting to do exercises one had planned on doing at a particular time. How do you increase the likelihood that participants will remember? As described in the first group session, one way of forming habits is to engage in repetition. Always doing the same activity at a given time will associate this particular activity with this specific time. To help participants remember, we tend to place reminder cues to do the exercise. This can be a Post-it note, a phone alarm, or a reminder by a spouse that it is time to do the exercise. It also helps to attach the mindfulness exercises to specific activities or times. For example, do the Movement Exercise before dinner. Over time and with repetition, participants will find that they independently remember that it is time to do the exercise. That is, one has moved from relying on external reminder cues to internal reminder cues.

Procrastination

Even when participants remember that they should do an exercise at a given time, more often than not you will hear participants say, "I knew that I was supposed to do my exercise, but I just could not bring myself to do it." This is a common experience. In this case, it is not an issue of forgetting or not having time. Rather, the thought of doing the exercise is unpleasant, and doing something other than the practice seems more attractive. Once you start paying attention to this pattern, you will be amazed by how often it plays out even for the most mundane activities, like making a phone call, writing an e-mail, or paying a bill. The first step in addressing procrastination is becoming aware of it. Mindfulness is the perfect tool for this. When participants report that they found themselves procrastinating, we simply ask them to switch into "mindful observation mode" the next time. What better opportunity is there to become more aware of feelings, sensations, or thoughts than a situation where a "I should do X, but do not want to do X" is present? The participant should take notice of the sensation at this moment and where the feeling is located. What thoughts lead us to not engage in the Movement Exercise, the Sitting Meditation, or the Body Scan we had scheduled for this particular time? Do you notice that the mind is engaging an excuse that makes us feel less guilty for not doing the exercise? Is this habitual? Do you recognize this playing out in other situations as well? Sometimes, perhaps surprisingly to participants, we ask them to continue in this observational mode for a while and just notice what unfolds in their minds and bodies at that particular time. Why? Because, from our perspective, the formal and informal exercises in this program are vehicles or tools to gradually adopt a more mindful way of being. The road a participant takes matters less than does nearing this goal. Therefore, we ask them to seize that moment when they become aware of procrastination unfolding and to begin the process of inquisitively observing the inner workings of their minds and bodies. We may also ask participants with increased awareness to initiate the scheduled mindfulness exercises despite the body and mind wanting to engage in something else. Curiously, we observe how this course of action changes the experience they are having at that particular moment.

Misconceptions about the Exercise

Participants will adopt their own ways of conducting these mindfulness exercises. The individual sessions offer additional opportunities for the participants to share their experiences. For the instructors, this may provide an opportunity to guide participants who have adopted ways of doing the exercises that may not be helpful. For example, soon after starting the Movement Exercise, Sara found that if she focused really hard on some of the sensations, they would lessen and then simply go away. "What a fabulous experience this is," she said. "I would have never thought that by doing this you can actually get rid of the pain." With a participant like Sara, the instructor has various choices. He or she can simply point out that the purpose of the exercise is to notice without making any active attempt or effort to change things as they happen. He or she could also help Sara to bring some curiosity to that moment when she experiences pain and the aversion it creates. After all, this is the reason why Sara shifts attention away. Alternatively, he or she could advise Sara to bring some gentle curiosity to the pain, explore how it feels (e.g., burning, stinging) and what unfolds if she does not attempt to alter the experience.

Courtney, on the other hand, found herself quickly returning to the breath when painful or unwanted experiences arose during the Body Scan. The instructor worked with her such that she would gradually allow herself to revisit the painful area and explore the pain sensation as best as she could, always with the option of going back to the breath as her anchor. In addition, the instructor worked with her to gradually realize the aversion that the pain caused and how it was a trigger for rumination, encouraging thoughts like "What if I will be stuck with the pain forever?"

Finally, Michael figured out that when he became aware of unwanted and painful thoughts, quickly moving his attention to the breath and filling his mind with the experience of breathing would make the painful thought go away. He had begun to use "mindfulness" as a way of stopping unwanted thoughts. Previously, he had engaged in endless rumination about painful thoughts, which usually made him feel very depressed. With education on mindfulness, he had realized that elaborating on these thoughts "just made it worse" and "did not change anything." Therefore, he would now decisively focus on the breath when those thoughts arose. Clearly, Michael had become proficient in the business of thought suppression. The instructor asked him how it would be to gradually reapproach the thought after focusing on the breath and, for as long as he felt capable, to gently include this thought in the field of awareness without trying to change it. Interestingly, in this case it also started to go away by itself, although initially it came with a moment of feeling pain, which Michael began to explore as well. In all of these instances, the individual sessions provided extra space and opportunity for exploration and guidance for the participants to progress on their way to becoming more mindful.

Personalizing the Exercises

We also individualize and adjust the mindfulness exercises depending on participants' needs. This can involve altering the length of the exercise and guidelines for how to be mindful with symptoms of depression, mania, anger, irritability, and anxiety. Most exercises in this program are initially kept brief and take about 15 to 20 minutes. This is particularly true for Body Scans and Sitting Meditations. Many participants with bipolar disorder have difficulties concentrating or sustaining attention for longer periods of time. The act of focusing and refocusing attention as part of these exercises can quickly become aversive. We recognize that learning to observe aversion and bring an accepting awareness to this experience is an integral part of any mindfulness program. However, if exercises are too aversive, participants may quit doing them. Therefore, our exercises (e.g., Body Scans, Sitting Meditations) are designed such that participants can gradually stretch them out as much as they feel able to. As Jennifer pointed out after completing the program, "At the beginning, 5 minutes of sitting meditation made me itchy. I just could not stand it. Giving me permission to exit at any time was great. This way I challenged myself a little bit more each time, and gradually got up to about 20 minutes. This is huge for me!" We alert participants early on that progress will not be linear. Intuitively, people tend to expect that with practice things get a little bit easier each time. Reality looks a bit more like a roller coaster, where ups and downs are part of the experience. But if one hangs in there, one can see how things are steadily looking better.

The instructor's guidelines for how to be mindful with symptoms of depression, mania, anger, irritability, and anxiety are provided in Sessions 5–8 (see also participant Handouts 15, 20, 25, 27). For each individual participant, the instructor works with these guidelines to help him or her find his or her own way of becoming mindful with these experiences. The qualities of aversion and attachment are noteworthy for bipolar disorder. Many experiences that participants encounter day in and day out, such as feeling depressed or anxious, are aversive. Participants do not like them, do not want them, and would much rather have them go away immediately. Part of what participants will learn in this program is to bring an accepting observance to those aversive experiences, rather than fixing them with rumination and worry, or trying to ignore or suppress them in some other way. Attachment comprises other experiences that are desirable. They feel good. The body wants more. Often, but not always, these are experiences associated with mood elevation. For example, once the urge to talk has set in, talking feels good and amplifies the urge to talk more. Likewise, if working on multiple tasks all at once or engaging in multiple activities makes one feel confident, the body wants more. Conversely, not talking more and not engaging in activities becomes aversive. Participants often encounter aversive frustrations first and then the urge to express the anger by telling someone off or yelling, for example, second. Individuals with bipolar disorder, in many moments, experience both aversion and attachment (desire). Participants are guided to not engage in those desired experiences that either risk mania or intensify mood elevation, but to bring accepting observance both to the desire and the aversion that arises when not engaging in something that mind and body want at that time. Each participant has his or her unique experiences of aversive and desired experiences to which he or she will learn to bring mindfulness.

DEALING WITH MANIA

"I am manic" Sara said, when the instructor returned her call after she had paged him on a Saturday morning. A more comprehensive assessment of the situation revealed that Sara had smoked weed the day before. Weed disrupted her sleep and that usually made her manic. Sara was talkative. "Isn't this a perfect situation to find out what mindfulness can do?," she asked, seemingly excited about the situation. "Now I can practice being mindful with mania." In addition to her obvious need to talk—it was hard to get a word in on the phone—her thoughts were fast and "jumpy." "My mind is coming up with all sorts of things I probably should not do," she said, "I want to go back on eBay." Through further inquiry, the instructor learned that she called from her boyfriend's apartment, that he was around, and that she was safe for the moment. "I guess it's time to initiate our mania action plan," the instructor said. Sara enthusiastically agreed. Lack of sleep, with or without smoking weed, had been one of the triggers for mania that Sara had identified. Her action plan had several components. First, make sure that she had a safe place where she could stay. Fortunately, her boyfriend's apartment was that place. Second, she called her psychiatrist, who, in accordance with the action plan, increased the dose of her antipsychotic medication. This made her tired, but also decreased her drive to engage in pleasurable activities like going on eBay. Next, with Sara's permission, her boyfriend changed the passwords to Sara's and his own computer, so that she could not get online. As negotiated before, Sara also gave up her credit cards for the time being.

For the next couple of days, she stayed in her boyfriend's apartment, keeping stimulation low, listening to music, watching TV, and at times talking to friends. Her psychologist checked in with her daily and worked with her to bring mindfulness to the experience of feeling manic. For guidelines of how to be mindful with mania, see Session 6 (Handout 20). Coming into the present, noting what is going on in the mind and in the body, and then refocusing attention on the breath is a way of anchoring and grounding oneself, before widening the space to include the whole body. Sara noticed the increased energy of wanting to be active and wanting to do things, mostly in her diaphragm and abdomen. As is common for mood elevation, not engaging in desired activity made her feel uncomfortable. Sara practiced allowing these sensations to be in her body, noticing the aversion, and, as best she could, bringing acceptance to these sensations and feelings. Her mind kept producing ideas of what she wanted to buy and sell on eBay, drawing her toward thinking and fantasizing about things she had long wanted. Sara practiced acknowledging these thoughts, labeling them as "manic thoughts," and then gently redirecting her attention back to the breath as her anchor, without pursuing or elaborating on them.

Behaviorally, she was guided to mindfully do only one activity at the time (see Mindfulness to Routine Activity). Mania often motivates people to multitask, which results in frequent task shifting, and tends to increase distractibility and speeded thoughts. Likewise, when she talked to her boyfriend, she also noticed that talking for a while increased the need to talk more. Therefore, when she noticed this urge to talk, she mindfully anchored herself on the breath and then included this feeling into her field of awareness while refraining from talking. That week Sara stayed home and managed to avoid unpleasant consequences, like spending money or hospitalization, which were typical during a manic episode. Symptoms of mood elevation, like increased energy or feeling talkative, continued to wax and wane for the better part of a week before things became calmer again.

When warning signs for mood elevation arise, or when participants become hypomanic, as instructors we tend to be directive in how to use mindfulness for the various experiences or symptoms of mania, and then adjust the approach based on the participant's feedback. Action plans, like Sara's, include behavioral (e.g., reduce stimulation, do only one activity at a time, do not log on to the computer), pharmacological (e.g., increase mood stabilizer or antipsychotic medication), and mindfulness elements tailored to the participant's needs. When a participant comes to group and warning signs are present, we assess whether the participant is capable of participating in the group with a Mood Diary check. If the participant is capable, we meet with him or her afterward to address the warning signs or hypomania that has unfolded. If the participant is not capable of participating in group because he or she may talk too much or would be too disruptive, the group coleader, if available, may leave with the participant to work through the situation with him or her individually. While individual sessions are usually scheduled every other week, the occurrence of mania may require talking to a participant more often, possibly every day, on the phone or in the office, as long as the participant and the situation can be safely managed on an outpatient basis.

DEALING WITH DEPRESSION

What if a participant is depressed at the time when he or she starts the MBCT program or gets depressed while participating? Fully depressed participants encounter negative thoughts more frequently and more intensely than participants with residual depressive symptoms, and it may take longer to quell them. This may involve more intense self-critical, angry, or anxious negative thoughts. Negative thoughts may also be more believable for depressed participants, and it may be more difficult for them to keep perspective. Depression also comes with reduced motivation, decreased interest, and lower activity levels.

Initially, we do not do anything different for depressed participants than for participants with residual depressive and manic symptoms. They complete the Movement and Body Scan exercises in Sessions 1 and 2. They also start practicing the Breathing Space at scheduled times in Sessions 2 and 3. Starting in Session 4, they will also apply the Breathing Space at times when they are feeling "down" or depressed. As described in Session 4, the end of the Breathing Space represents a choice point for participants to ask themselves what they may need for themselves at that point in time. This is an opportunity to begin mindfully engaging in activities that are soothing or pleasurable (for a list of suggested activities, see Session 9). In cognitive-behavioral therapy, activity scheduling has been found to be an effective intervention for depressed mood. Being actively involved in a task or an activity is also an effective tool against rumination. Therefore, in the individual sessions with depressed participants, we work with them to identify activities and behaviors that are pleasurable (or used to be pleasurable), and participants begin to work those activities into their schedules. This work will be continued in subsequent individual sessions, and participants will also gradually add mastery-based activities into their schedules. Because many depressed participants have lowered activity levels, we start activity scheduling as early as the second individual session.

Engaging in activities can have its own challenges for depressed participants. Michael described his "failed" attempt to hang out with some of his friends at a local bar, saying, "I know that I should have gone, but I just could not get myself to, although I really tried. I just could not get into the mood." Like Michael, many participants try to get themselves to feel "OK enough" to "get going." They try to motivate themselves to do things, but this feeling of "not wanting," "not being in the mood," and "heaviness" keeps them from engaging in whatever activity they had planned on doing. In this case, we have participants practice becoming more aware of the sensations and thoughts that come with these feelings. They notice and observe them mindfully, such as how the thoughts might predict that meeting friends at the pub will be no fun. Participants work on trying to not change the thoughts, just noticing where the feeling of not wanting is located in their bodies and bringing curiosity to how the raw experience of "not wanting," of "heaviness," or of "not being in the mood" is in their bodies. Then, and only then, after having noticed this feeling for a while, do we ask them to complete a Movement Exercise. In this case, it is the Movement Exercise of getting dressed and going out, in which they observe movement. When feeling depressed is associated with anxious or irritable features, we use the guidelines described in Sessions 7 (Handout 25) and 8 (Handout 27) to mindfully move forward after initiating the Breathing Space whenever they become aware of feeling irritable, angry, or anxious.

DISCUSSING MEDICATION AND INSIGHT

When a participant presents with warning signs for hypomania or mania, beyond bringing in mindfulness, it is often advisable to boost or possibly change medications to counteract the early symptoms. This can be a challenge for several reasons. First, participants may be reluctant to increase or change medication. Second, they may not be sufficiently aware that symptoms of mania have arisen. The suggestion to increase, change, or add medication may conflict with a participant's preference, as he or she is taking the mindfulness class in order to reduce medications and is now being asked to potentially increase them. Boosting medication often also comes with unwanted side effects, such as feeling more sedated, drowsy, or "knocked out," which are the most common ones in our experience. "And you don't think that we could get around this?," Michael asked after his instructor had noted in Michael's Mood Diary that his mood was elevated for most of the week before the second group session. Michael acknowledged that he had been feeling more talkative than usual and that the usual sluggishness in his thoughts had vanished. "And it's been sticking around for most of the week," he admitted, "not just a couple of days." He had welcomed it as a nice change because he usually was more on the "depressed side," although he was aware that his mood elevation could "get out of hand." Nonetheless, he was not enthusiastic about the idea of calling his psychiatrist, as he anticipated that this would result in a medication augmentation, which would make him feel sedated and knocked out.

How do you negotiate with participants to swallow this "bitter pill"? In these situations, we remind participants that if we miss this window of opportunity, the medication change that comes with treating full-blown hypomania or mania is often worse. The side effects now may be minor and temporary compared to those they may experience with a more substantial medication change. It also helps to refresh participants' memories about the aftermath that follows mania. Mania can be followed by a crash into depression or a period of substantial mood lability. This emotional roller coaster involves cycling between days with mood elevation, days with depression, or days with both. This can go on for weeks and is something that participants want to avoid. In helping participants reach a decision about whether or not to get in touch with their psychiatrist, it may be useful to acknowledge that at this moment they are caught between "a rock and a hard place." That is, they are trying to choose between two undesirable options: boosting medications and side effects now, or becoming manic and needing a bigger boost or medication change with potentially more side effects and mood lability later. We readily acknowledge that they would likely prefer to pick neither option. With this choice not available, it comes down to picking the "lesser of the two evils."

But what if a participant says, "I feel fine," although the instructor clearly picks up on some warning signs? The participant may be more talkative than usual and is more engaging in group, contrary to how he or she usually behaves. It is possible that the participant is aware of the change, but does not want to acknowledge it because he or she is feeling "better" and does not want risk medication "taking this away." Alternatively, he or she may not be aware of the change. Especially when participants have been on a roller coaster with their mood for years, it gets harder and harder to know what is a "normal mood," as the frame of reference gets lost. In terms of managing this situation, there is no magic trick. We simply tend to share our observations and ask the participant whether he or she, and possibly others, has noticed these changes as well. It can be easier to point out observable behaviors, rather than internal states. Our observations are framed as a question: Could the observed behavioral changes be a warning sign for mania? If the possibility cannot be denied, then the question becomes: What are the consequences if we ignore those signs? Again, the question guides the participants toward the "lesser of two evils." Nonetheless, sometimes the best that can be negotiated in a situation like this is for the participant and his support system to agree to continue to observe, be highly vigilant, and contact the instructor or psychiatrist if symptoms persist or get worse.

One may argue that the approach of early medication boosts or changes when warning signs for mania arise defeats the purpose of mindfulness— becoming more mindful with symptoms and thereby preventing the spiraling from negative or speeded thoughts into full-blown mood episodes. If participants learn at the beginning of the program that they need to shift or boost medication in order to deal with a change in symptoms, does that not reinforce the wrong message? We tend to remind participants that mindfulness is a skill that will improve over time. Like with learning how to play a musical instrument, practice makes perfect. Who goes on stage after playing the violin for just a week? Down the road, with more mindfulness practice under their belts, the point at which medication adjustments are made may change. With the review of the individual sessions completed, we are now ready to embark on the description of the 12 group sessions in Part II.

PART II
The Group Sessions

Welcome in the Moment

- Welcome
- Movement Exercise and Brief Sitting Meditation Practice
- Participant Introduction and Group Guidelines
- A First Taste of Mindfulness: The Raisin Exercise
- Relating the Raisin Exercise to the Goals of the Program
- Yoga Leading into a Short Body Scan
- Mood Diary
- Introduction to the Breathing Space
- Formal and Informal Practice
- Homework
  - Audio recordings (see p. viii for details)
  - Yoga–Body Scan—once a day (audio track 1)
  - Introduction to the Breathing Space—as often as possible (audio track 2)
  - Mood Diary (daily)

INSTRUCTOR MATERIAL FOR SESSION 1

- Script for Movement Exercise and Brief Sitting Meditation Practice and Movement Exercise Diagram (Box 1.1)
- Script for the Raisin Exercise (Box 1.2)
- Solutions for the Mindfulness Discussion Questions (see the section "Relating the Raisin Exercise to the Goals of the Program" in this chapter)
- Script for the Yoga–Body Scan (Box 1.3) and Handout 4: Yoga Exercise
- Script for the Introduction to the Breathing Space (Box 1.4)

PARTICIPANT HANDOUTS FOR SESSION 1

- Handout 3: Mindfulness Discussion Questions
- Handout 4: Yoga Exercise
- Handout 5: Mood Diary
- Handout 6: Planning Your Mindfulness Practice
- Handout 7: Homework Sheet

WELCOME

How do you arrive where you already are? After rushing through the evening commute, you may be wondering whether you will find the place, be on time, who you will meet, and what to expect. Or, perhaps, you are already where you are supposed to be, sitting in a room full of people, yet with your thoughts still at home or at work. As you may know, people are rarely in the present moment: their thoughts usually are focused on what is coming next, or still stuck in the past, on what happened today. Mindfulness, however, means coming into the present, into the *here* and *now*. Therefore, after a brief, yet warm welcome, we start the program with a movement and brief sitting meditation exercise that is meant to help the participants to arrive at where they are. Audio recordings for this session include the Yoga–Body Scan (audio track 1) and the Introduction to the Breathing Space (audio track 2).

Box 1.1. Movement Exercise and Brief Sitting Meditation Practice (15 Minutes)

Movement Exercise

Position numbers given below correspond to the illustrations on the movement exercise diagram. (Note for the instructor: Pause in between the sentences.)

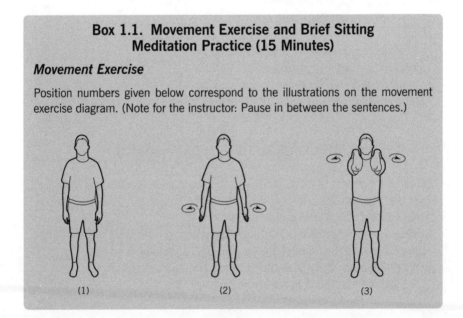

(1)   (2)   (3)

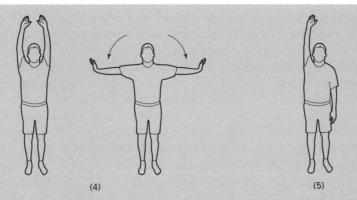

(4)   (5)

- Please come into a solid standing position with the feet about hip-width apart, the back straight, and your shoulders relaxed. You can always close your eyes if you feel comfortable doing so [Position 1].
- Wrist rotation: rotating the hands. Noticing what parts of the arms are involved. What movements can your wrists actually do? Stretching the fingers, finding out what movements of the fingers feel comfortable [Position 2].
- Shoulder rotation: placing the hands on the shoulders and bringing the elbows together in front of the chest. Now making big circles with the elbows, inhaling as you bring the elbows up in front of you, and now exhaling as you lower them back down to your back. After a while, change directions, doing it gently [Position 3].
- Reach up: in a standing position, stretching arms up (as you inhale), lengthening the arms and hands but relaxing the shoulders. Noticing where in the body you can feel this movement. Maybe noticing some tingling sensations as the arms return to the sides [Position 4].
- Side stretch: stretching the arms up (as you inhale), keeping them parallel and bending sideways. First, bending over to your right side, while noticing the stretching in the left side of the body. Becoming aware of the stretch in your whole side of the body from the fingers to the feet. Now, slowly coming back to center. Taking a moment here to notice any sensations in your body. Now, continuing on to the other side. Now, coming back to center and releasing the arms. Noticing the effects of this practice on the body and the breath [Position 5].

The movement exercise leads into a brief introspective sitting practice.

Seated Introspective Practice

- Please come sit on your chair. Sitting comfortably with a straight back and relaxed shoulders. If you feel comfortable closing your eyes, you can do so. You can also have your gaze focused on the ground in front of you.
- Bringing the feet in solid contact with the ground, becoming aware of the soles of the feet and noticing how the weight of the legs is distributed on the soles of the feet. Feeling into the legs, noticing the angle of the knees.

- Becoming aware of the regions where the thighs are in contact with the chair and allowing this region of contact to become a bit wider by letting the weight of the legs sink into the chair. Noticing the buttocks sinking into the chair.
- Also bringing awareness to the parts of the thighs that are not in contact with the chair, perhaps being aware of clothing touching, the skin, whatever sensations are present. Noticing how the weight of the arms rests on the thighs.
- Now bringing awareness to the stomach; noticing how your abdomen expands with each inhalation and how it falls back toward the spine with each exhalation. Noticing the movement of the chest with each breath.
- Allowing the shoulders to relax and to sink toward the ground.
- Bringing awareness to the face, allowing the jaws, eyes, and mouth to relax.
- Now bringing awareness to how the breath flows into the nose and how it leaves the body.
- And now taking a moment to bring awareness to the thoughts and feelings that may be occurring right now. There is nothing to be changed about them; just noticing what is happening.
- There might be some thoughts or feelings regarding the fact that we are beginning this class today. Maybe there are some expectations, hopes, or perhaps some fears or worries. . . .
- Just become aware of whatever you might encounter in the realm of thoughts and emotions.
- Now, I'd like to invite you to ask yourself the questions "What are my aims related to the class? What do I hope for?"
- And in case you have already found an answer, you could put it aside and once again ask yourself the questions "What do I want from this class? What brought me here?"
- Now, gently bringing awareness back to the body and back to the sensations related to sitting here on the chair, sitting in this room, becoming aware of the sounds surrounding you. Now slowly opening your eyes and bringing movement back into the body, wiggling the fingers and toes, moving your arms and legs, stretching or doing a movement that is good for you.

PARTICIPANT INTRODUCTION
AND GROUP GUIDELINES

Conducting this Movement and Sitting Exercise right at the beginning of the program helps participants to ground themselves and come into the present. Right from the outset, it also sets the stage for all coming sessions where learning will be experiential in many ways. That is, we introduce a shift toward noticing what is going on in the here and now and adopting an observant accepting stance toward whichever experiences are encountered at any given moment. Once they arrive in the present, participants are asked to introduce themselves to the group, and, if they choose to do so, share some of their goals and hopes for participating in the program. We also review the usual guidelines of confidentiality and privacy that apply to group treatments (e.g., not revealing the identity of group members to nongroup members, not talking to one member of the group about another person in the group). From the very beginning, the following ideas of self-care and self-compassion are implicitly woven into the instructions and conversations with participants: respecting physical restrictions and the boundaries of one's body during movement and yoga exercises, not "over-doing," and being "gentle" to one's self. Likewise, participants are asked to refrain from giving advice to other group members and to allow everybody the chance to experience and discover for themselves.

A FIRST TASTE OF MINDFULNESS: THE RAISIN EXERCISE

As mindfulness is best learned through experience, we, like most other programs of this kind, then introduce the concept of mindfulness experientially through the Raisin Exercise.

Box 1.2. Raisin Exercise (10 Minutes)

Note for the instructor: Pause at least 10 seconds between phrases, and deliver the instructions in a matter-of-fact way, at a slow but deliberate pace.

- I'm going to go around the class and give you each a few objects. (Raisins are handed out/passed around).
- Now, what I would like you to do is focus on one of the objects and just imagine that you have never seen anything like it before. Imagine you have just dropped in from Mars at this moment and you have never seen anything like it before in your life.
- Taking one of these objects and holding it in the palm of your hand or between your finger and thumb. (*Pause*)
- Paying attention to seeing it. (*Pause*)
- Looking at it carefully, as if you had never seen such a thing before. (*Pause*)
- Turning it over between your fingers. (*Pause*)
- Exploring its texture between your fingers. (*Pause*)
- Examining the highlights where the light shines . . . the darker hollows and folds. (*Pause*)

- Letting your eyes explore every part of it, as if you had never seen such a thing before. (*Pause*)
- And if, while you are doing this, any thoughts come to mind about "What a strange thing we are doing," "What is the point of this?," or "I don't like these," then just note them as thoughts and bring your awareness back to the object. (*Pause*)
- And now smelling the object, taking it and holding it beneath your nose, and with each inbreath, carefully noticing the smell of it. (*Pause*)
- And now taking another look at it. (*Pause*)
- And now slowly taking the object to your mouth, maybe noticing how your hand and arm know exactly where to put it, perhaps noticing your mouth watering as it comes up. (*Pause*)
- And then gently placing the object in the mouth, noticing how it is "received," without biting it, just exploring the sensations of having it in your mouth. (*Pause*)
- And when you are ready, very consciously taking a bite into it and noticing the taste that it releases. (*Pause*)
- Slowly chewing it, . . . noticing the saliva in the mouth, . . . the change in consistency of the object. (*Pause*)
- Then, when you feel ready to swallow, seeing if you can first detect the intention to swallow as it comes up, so that even this is experienced consciously before you actually swallow it. (*Pause*)
- Finally, seeing if you can follow the sensations of swallowing it, sensing it moving down to your stomach and also realizing that your body is not exactly one raisin heavier.

The Raisin Exercise provides an opportunity to begin the process of directly *observing*, which is an essential part of mindfulness. After all, we already know what a raisin looks like, don't we? We have memories of what a raisin typically looks like, its usual color, its texture, and, conceptually, we know it is a dried fruit, and we can eat it without any harm. But, what does *this* raisin look like, the very raisin each participant is holding in his or her hand? To guide this process of observant exploration, we begin the discussion with an open-ended question, "So, what have you noticed, looking at this raisin in this way?" As participants share their experiences, we follow up with additional questions, conveying a sense of inquisitive curiosity, perhaps some naiveté at times, wanting to know more about the nature of the experience and its details. "Can you tell me more about it?", "What else have you noticed?" To alert participants to the contrast with how they usually eat a raisin, we ask, "Have you noticed things about this raisin you have not noticed before?", "How is the experience of seeing/tasting/smelling a raisin in this way different from how you usually eat?" As Michael pointed out, "I never really noticed how rocky the raisin's surface is." Jennifer realized a "particular smell: sweet, rotten, and a bit alcoholic" that she had not consciously noticed before. The experience of tasting a raisin in this fashion is also often described as "less passing, richer, and sometimes more fulfilling compared to the usual way of eating raisins." "It felt a bit like time was standing still for a moment, and there was just this raisin, rather than a raisin and a million other things," Courtney recalled.

When describing the raisin experience often participants convey conceptual thinking and utilize comparisons. We try to steer their attention to the "raw" experience, rather than using comparisons and conceptual thinking. As Stephen pointed out, "Having it in my mouth feels a little bit like a rock," but when asked about saying more, he began to explain that he was noticing the raisin's surface being uneven, the curves and crevices his tongue was sensing. Why is it important to shift from conceptual thinking to the raw experience? Participants already label experiences in certain ways ("I am depressed"; "I am angry"; "I am anxious") rather than allowing themselves to experience the very sensation/feeling itself. Thus, the Raisin Exercise is a glimpse into practicing how to relate to the raw sensation, whether this refers to a raisin, or, down the road, to thoughts, feelings, and sensations associated with depression, mania, anger, or anxiety.

The Raisin Exercise also allows participants to experience and raise their awareness of the mind's reactions to exploring the raisin in this particular fashion—many of which participants may ordinarily not have noticed if they had eaten the raisin their usual way. These experiences include emotional reactions (pleasure, aversion), judgments, and mindwandering—all of which become the object of observation as participants progress in the program.

JUSTIN: This was not pleasant at all.

INSTRUCTOR: Would you like to describe this to us?

JUSTIN: I just wanted to move on, rather than spending so much time on exploring a raisin. This was very different to how I usually do things. . . .

INSTRUCTOR: Can you tell us more about this?

JUSTIN: I never pay that much attention to what I do because I usually do other things while I am eating, like being on the web or answering e-mails.

INSTRUCTOR: So, what did you notice?

JUSTIN: I noticed that I was becoming impatient, wanting to move on. I kept thinking to myself, "Come on, are you kidding me, spending that much time on a raisin?"

INSTRUCTOR: So you had thoughts like saying "wasting time"?

JUSTIN: Yes, and a pressure feeling in my stomach, just wanting to keep going. . . .

For Veronica, the Raisin Exercise made her aware of some aversions:

VERONICA: I also did not like it very much. Not so much because of impatience, but because I don't think I am that much of a fan of raisins.

INSTRUCTOR: What is it about the raisins that you did not like?

VERONICA: It's the taste. The alcoholic sweetness.

INSTRUCTOR: What did you notice going through your mind as you were holding the raisin in your mouth?

VERONICA: Just this sense of not liking it, not wanting to continue with it.

INSTRUCTOR: How did you notice this in your body?

For Michelle, tasting the raisin triggered associations, and brought back images from a vacation in Italy she and her husband had taken a while ago, whereas for Brian his mind wandered away from the exercise.

BRIAN: All of a sudden, I found myself thinking about other things.

INSTRUCTOR: Interesting. You think you are in the present tasting a raisin and all of a sudden you find yourself somewhere else. What did you notice?

BRIAN: I was thinking about family stuff, dinner when I get home later, bringing the kids to bed, but then what I still have to do for tomorrow morning at work. . . .

INSTRUCTOR: Interesting—while you are trying to focus in the present moment, your mind just wanders away by itself to completely unrelated topics taking away from your experience in the present moment.

Brian's experience can be used as an example that mindwandering is a perfectly normal process. It happens daily to everyone, and it is something the brain does without our being aware of it. In summary, (1) paying attention in this fashion makes participants aware of facets of a situation they would not have ordinarily noticed before, (2) paying attention changes the experience participants have in the moment, and (3) the mind has a tendency to wander away from the present.

RELATING THE RAISIN EXERCISE TO THE GOALS OF THE PROGRAM

How does the Raisin Exercise relate to mood and coping with bipolar disorder? To give participants an intuitive understanding, we discuss the relationship between mindwandering and happiness with the group (Handout 3). Psychologists Matthew Killingsworth and Daniel Gilbert (2010) conducted a survey to find the extent to which people's minds wander day to day. At random times people were asked to report via their smart phones what they were doing and whether they were thinking about something other than what they were currently doing. Results showed:

- People were not thinking about the present about half of the time they were awake (question 1; correct answer: b, 47%).
- Regardless of what people were doing in the moment, people were always happier when they were thinking about the present than when their minds had wandered away (question 2; correct answer: c, happier).
- Surprisingly, the mind wandering to pleasant topics did not lead to more happiness when compared to being in the moment (question 3; correct answer: b, false).
- People were also happier when they were in the moment than when their minds wandered to neutral or unpleasant topics (question 4; correct answer: a, true).

After completing the survey, we ask group participants about their answers and discuss them. The take-home point for the group is that people tend to be happier being in the present moment compared to when the mind drifts toward neutral and unpleasant topics. In addition, wandering away to pleasant topics does not make people feel happier than being in the present. As Killingsworth and Gilbert concluded, "A wandering mind is an unhappy mind" (2010, p. 932).

For participants with bipolar disorder, the mind has a tendency to wander away toward self-critical negative topics or go toward thoughts and feelings that can lead to mood elevation, anger, or anxiety. Therefore, catching the wandering mind early and remaining grounded in the present will help participants to disengage from thoughts and feelings that worsen their mood. In addition, being more in the present will help participants detect *warning signs* of worsening mood. In the same way as paying attention to the raisin can reveal characteristics previously undetected, paying attention to their thoughts will help participants discover changes in mood that foreshadow mood episodes. In fact, many participants can easily relate to this concept with respect to mania. Most of them have experienced states in which decreased sleep, increased speed of thoughts, or perhaps increased confidence, energy, or feeling more talkative, in hindsight, were preludes to hypomanic and manic episodes. Usually, these warning signs tend to wax and wane over time. Once present with a certain intensity and frequency, they seem to signal that things are taking a turn for the worst. These warning signs will become the objects of observation as part of the mood monitoring introduced later in this session.

YOGA LEADING INTO A SHORT BODY SCAN

Acquiring a particular way of paying attention (to the present moment, nonjudgmentally) and raising awareness will be a gradual process. The first step for participants is learning to come into the present moment, and just as in the Raisin Exercise paying direct attention to bodily sensations, relating to their bodies and their physical sensations in an observant, accepting way. The following Yoga–Body Scan (audio track 1) is designed for reaching these goals. Initially, this provides a focus for attention through movement-induced sensations that become the object of the observation, which then leads to observing physical sensations (or the lack thereof) while laying still on one's back (during the brief body scan portion of the exercise). The drawings of the different movements are provided in Handout 4. This handout will also be given to participants at the end of the session as a guide for practicing the Yoga–Body Scan as homework during the week.

Box 1.3. Yoga–Body Scan (25 Minutes)

Yoga

Position numbers given below correspond to the illustrations on Handout 4: Yoga Exercise.

- Please find a comfortable *standing position* [Position 1], standing either on a yoga mat or on the floor. If you haven't done so yet, taking off your shoes if that's comfortable for you.
- Standing with the feet about hip-width apart, the legs straight but knees soft, and bringing awareness to the body's position.

- Becoming aware of the contact of the soles of the feet on the floor.
- Noticing how the weight of the body is distributed on the soles of the feet.
- Now becoming aware of the position of the pelvis, feeling free to tilt the pelvis forward a bit, so that the lower back can straighten. You might imagine having sand in your back pockets, which can allow the lower back to release a little toward the floor.
- And now softening the belly and opening the chest to the front so that the breath can flow fully into the chest and belly without hindrance.
- Allowing the shoulders and neck to release and soften if that's possible right now, and having the arms and hands hang alongside the body.
- And now, becoming aware of the flow of the breath. Without modifying the breath in any way, just noticing its natural flow, becoming aware of the abdomen rising with the inhale and the abdomen falling back toward the spine on the exhale.
- During the whole yoga exercise, it is important that you honor your limitations and be gentle with yourself. Not trying to go beyond what you're capable of in any of the positions. Being respectful of your boundaries and recognizing your limitations. Always feel free to come out of a position if that feels appropriate. Your own expert knowing of your body and its capacities is more important than following the instructions precisely.
- Now we'll be beginning with a *stretching position* [Position 2]. While inhaling, bringing the arms out to the sides, and stretching the arms and hands toward the sky.
- Extending the arms, hands, and fingers, while continuing to breathe. Allowing the shoulders to release down, so the arms and hands are straight, but the shoulders are relaxed.
- Noticing this stretch in the arms and hands, as well as in the other parts of the body. And continuing to breathe.
- And now, slowly lowering the arms back down, by the sides, turning the palms down as you do so [Position 2].
- Noticing sensations in hands and arms as you are doing this.
- And now fully releasing and relaxing the arms, and noticing the effects of the stretch. How are the hands and arms and shoulders feeling after completing this stretch?
- Noticing sensations in the whole body.
- Now we'll be doing a *diagonal stretch* [Position 3]. So with the next inhalation, bringing the right arm up and stretching the right hand up and a bit to the right side.
- And now lifting the left leg straight out to the side just a little bit. Having the foot about 1 or 2 inches off the floor so that you have a good diagonal stretch from the right hand down into the left foot. Stretching the hand up. Breathing.
- Lifting the left leg higher, if that's possible. This is also a balancing posture. Being aware of the sensations in the arms, in the right arm in particular and in the left leg, as well as the right leg, which is stabilizing you.

- Slowly bringing the arm and leg back down, bringing the foot down to the ground, and releasing the hand and arm back down by your side. Taking a moment to notice the effect of the stretch.
- Now continuing to the other side. Bringing the left arm up, stretching the left hand to the left upper side, and slightly raising the right foot up so you have the diagonal stretch from the left hand down into the right foot.
- Stretching to the left, as if you were trying to pluck an apple from a tree, lifting the right leg away from you. Continuing breathing and being aware of the way this feels. Feeling how the muscles are engaged as you are doing this. Breathing.
- Now slowly lowering the arm and leg back down, releasing that position. Releasing this position. Noticing how the back, arms, legs, and whole body are feeling after this diagonal stretch.
- Now we're going to be doing *shoulder rotations, or shoulder rolls* [Position 4]. So standing with the feet about hip-width apart, and just moving the shoulders with the arms and hands resting at your sides. Begin by bringing the shoulders to the front and now raising them up toward the ears and then moving them back. Bringing the shoulder blades together and then lowering them. Continuing this rolling, rotating movement at your own pace. Exploring the movement possible here. Noticing any difference between the two shoulders. Letting the breath flow as it naturally flows. Exploring this rotation in a way that it might feel if you were giving yourself a good massage. Noticing where in the back this movement is noticeable.
- Doing this movement, at your own pace.
- You might be noticing the movement in the shoulders, shoulder blades, and perhaps even the lower back. Simply being attentive to wherever in the body you can feel this movement.
- Now, changing directions, and moving in the other direction. Pulling the shoulders back, now up toward the ears and lowering them down to the front.
- Again, choosing your own pace, and enjoying this movement like a massage.
- There is no need to bring any tension into the hands or face. Noticing what body parts can be released and softened.
- Now releasing and coming back to a straight and upright standing position. Staying in contact with the sensations in the shoulders. How are the shoulders feeling right now after you have done this movement? And where else in the body is this effect of the movement noticeable?
- Perhaps you do not notice any effects. Or the effects might be very small or subtle. This is fine. Just becoming aware of what you are actually feeling.
- Now, we will be moving into the *chair pose* [Position 5]. While inhaling, bringing the arms up to shoulder level. Stretching the arms out in front of you, parallel to the floor.
- While exhaling, bending the knees as if you were sitting back onto a chair. Continue breathing, and bring awareness to the thighs.

- The thighs are doing a strong job here, keeping you in the position. It is a strong pose. Breathing.
- This is an excellent pose to work with your boundaries and limitations.
- Honoring them, not pushing yourself in any way, being respectful to your body.
- Feeling free to come out of the pose when you feel you've had enough. But also noticing how far and how long you can actually go.
- And now when you are ready coming out of the pose, straightening the legs, and, while exhaling, lowering the arms back down.
- Noticing how it feels to release this pose.
- This is quite a challenging posture, and you might notice that the breathing rate has increased and the heart is beating a bit faster. You may feel warmth or tingling, or a sense of release in the legs.
- Simply noticing this and being aware of how the breathing and heart rate are slowly coming back to normal.
- Now let's move to a *cat and cow practice* [Position 6]. Making your way to the floor, supported on the hands and knees. Having the knees directly below the pelvis and the hands directly below the shoulders.
- If you are not comfortable getting on the knees, or if you have knee problems, you can do this practice while sitting in a chair. What is important is to be moving the spine.
- While inhaling, raising the head up and lowering the belly toward the floor. As you exhale, rounding the back like a scared cat, pushing the middle spine up toward the ceiling while dropping the head and tailbone down, toward the floor.
- Now coordinating the breath with the movement, including the whole spine into the movement. The whole spine should be moving in this practice.
- Repeating this movement at your own pace, at a tempo that feels right for you. This is excellent practice for keeping the spine flexible and healthy. You might choose to linger over areas of the spine that feel tight or numb. Enjoying the movement. Finding what works best for you.
- Using this as a way for letting go of tensions or fatigue in the back. Doing all of this with an intention of being good to yourself, doing something good for yourself, for the body, for the mind, for your whole being. And now releasing this practice, and coming down directly onto the belly, lying flat [Position 7].
- Resting the arms alongside the body. Turning the head to rest on one cheek or the other. If this position isn't comfortable, you can fold the hands underneath the forehead, with the neck in a neutral position.
- From this position, we'll be doing *leg raises*. While inhaling, bringing the right leg up just a few inches off the ground while keeping the leg straight. Raising it behind the body. Keeping it here for a few seconds. And while exhaling, lowering the leg.
- When you are ready, inhaling, lifting the other leg up, just a few inches, holding it for a brief moment. And when you are ready, exhaling and lowering the leg.

- Try this a few times at your own pace. Coordinating the breath with the movement. Raising one leg, holding it for a moment, bringing it down, and shifting to the other side. Noticing where in the back or anywhere else in the body you can feel these movements. And as you are ready releasing all effort here. Resting. Taking a moment to become aware of the effects of the practice. Breathing.
- Now, slowly and with awareness, rolling onto your back.

Body Scan

This exercise is done while lying on one's back, immediately following the yoga sequence. (Note for the instructor: [. . .] indicates a pause.)

- Now as you are lying on the back, perhaps setting an intention to rest in the present, letting go of the past and the future. Letting everything fade into the background but the body. Meeting whatever you find in the body with openness, curiosity, and acceptance.
- This practice is like taking a tour of the body—noticing what is here in this moment. No need to move any of the body parts. Simply noticing and experiencing them, one by one.
- Starting by bringing awareness to the flow of the breath in the abdomen. Becoming aware of the expansion of the abdomen with each inhalation, and the slight falling back with each exhalation. No need to change the flow of the breath in any way. Just being with its natural flow . . .
- Now moving awareness from the breath all the way down through the body and into both feet. Noticing the contact of the heels with the mat, pressure here, perhaps. Being aware of sensations in the toes, and moving to the bottoms of the feet, and the tops . . .
- Now, allowing the feet to fade from the field of awareness and moving attention up to the ankles. Noticing whatever sensations are present in the ankles . . .
- Now, letting go of the ankles, and moving to the calves, and up into the knees, and further up into the thighs . . . aware of the contact with the floor perhaps, clothing, or maybe the feel of the air along the skin . . . what sensations are here? . . . temperature maybe or tightness . . . what is here to be felt, to be known?
- Now moving awareness up into the pelvis. Aware perhaps of the pressure of the buttocks on the ground . . . sensations in the lower belly, aware perhaps of sensations at the level of the skin and also deeper in the body.
- Now slowing moving awareness up the back: the lower back, the middle back, and the upper back. And then shifting awareness to sensations in the front of the torso, the belly, and the chest . . . the movement of the ribcage with the breath . . .
- Now shifting awareness to the upper arms, to the area of the shoulders where the upper arms meet the torso, and then moving down from the upper arms

into the elbows, the lower arms, the wrists, the hands. Present to sensations in the palms and fingers . . . the thumbs, pulsations here or tingling, moisture or dryness . . .

- Now moving the focus of attention to the neck and shoulders. Noticing sensations in the throat, and in the head . . . Becoming aware of what is present in the face right now: the forehead, the eyebrows and eyes, the nose, cheeks, jaws, the mouth, lips, and tongue . . . exploring what can be felt here.
- And now slowly expanding the field of awareness to include the entire body. The body in its entirety from the top of the head down to the tips of the toes and the fingers . . . Being aware of the breath as it flows through the body . . .
- Right now, there is nothing to do, nowhere to go. Just being here, aware of the presence of this moment . . . Everything is complete as it is . . . Being aware of the wholesomeness of this awareness of just being, being in the present moment . . .

As with the Raisin Exercise, we invite participants to share their experiences during the Yoga–Body Scan. The following issues typically come up.

Thoughts and Judgments

When people take on a new task, they strive to get it right. The yoga exercise is no exception in this regard. Participants wonder whether they stretched enough, did the postures right, or were breathing the correct way (especially those who have prior yoga experience where ways of breathing are part of the instructions). Participants also talk about "how hard it was to get one or the other posture right." From the perspective of mindfulness, these experiences are used to illustrate a key concept: the yoga exercise just serves as a vehicle to learn to observe whatever experiences there are in the present moment.

> *Instructor*: "There is no right or wrong way of doing this exercise. Paradoxically, we are not trying to achieve a certain posture, even though we are showing you how to do this exercise. The exercise is just something we are doing in order to learn to observe whatever is present in this very moment. This can be bodily sensations induced by movement, or feeling the breath, but at the same time, there may be questions crossing our minds, or judgments like 'Am I doing this right?' In the spirit of the exercise, we can now practice to also notice and observe those questions or judgments as they arise without getting tangled up in them. In fact, now that you have become aware of it, next time this happens, just make a mental note—'*Am I doing this right?*' *judgment*—as you then continue with the exercise."

Similarly, during the body scan portion, participants feel they failed because they noticed their minds wandered away or thoughts kept crossing their minds that distracted them from the task at hand (noticing and observing bodily sensations).

> *Instructor*: "However, we are not trying to empty our minds, or prevent our thoughts from wandering away. In fact, I would like you to welcome these experiences as you become aware of them. As you may find out over the course of the program, our minds do wander all the time, as this is built into the very architecture of our brains, and therefore it is bound to happen. But what I would like you to do is to welcome this as an opportunity to become aware of it when it happens, note the experience, and then gently return to the Yoga–Body Scan, no matter where it has led you."

Feelings

A common expectation is that yoga should be relaxing. This is particular prominent for participants who have done relaxation exercises or experienced yoga before (especially afterward). So, what if participants could not relax? As these statements come up we invite participants (similar to the Raisin Exercise) to explore their experiences further, although we do point out that we are not trying to achieve a special state of relaxation: "Rather, now that you have noticed this, when you are doing the exercise, you may become more aware of these 'should' statements." As participants further explore their "cannot relax" experiences, they may discover that they were comparing how they were feeling while doing the exercise to some designated or desired state about how they should feel at this time ("relaxed"). Perhaps they were even scanning their body for certain signs of relaxation they could not detect, which was giving rise to the "I do not feel relaxed, but should feel relaxed" thought.

"I Got Anxious."

The yoga exercise induces physical sensations (both musculoskeletal and cardiovascular). Some of these sensations may trigger anxiety (e.g., "What if this triggers a panic attack?"), in particular for participants with a concurrent anxiety disorder (e.g., panic disorder). As Courtney pointed out, "I did not like this exercise at all. It made my heart beat so much harder, and this reminded me how it feels when I am about to get a panic attack. This really made me tense." For other participants, anxiety is triggered during the body scan, when there is no contextual justification (moving/exercising) for sensations they experience. It can be quite discouraging and frustrating for participants with anxiety disorders who had pinned their hope on meditation as the "magic bullet" for becoming more relaxed and less anxious to experience that yoga and meditation exercises at least initially can do the opposite. For these participants, it is often helpful to teach them that although the exercises initially may be somewhat more uncomfortable, with continued practice, this will get better over time. During the Yoga–Body Scan, we encourage participants to be particularly gentle with themselves and only do as much as they feel they are able to do. This way, participants usually keep sufficient safety cues/behaviors in place that they may allow themselves to notice and observe whichever bodily experiences (or catastrophic thoughts) come up without getting "tangled up in it." During both the yoga and the body scan parts of the exercise, we encourage participants to bring a gentle curiosity to the sensations they experience, especially to those that come with anxiety, and to notice the "raw" sensations they are experiencing ("What sensations are telling you that your heart is beating harder?", "What tells you that your chest is tied tight?"). On the other hand, we guide participants to go back to the breath as an anchor whenever they feel that it is becoming too difficult or too overwhelming, until they feel they are able to approach these sensations again. The same approach is also used for participants who tend to have more intense emotional reactions, whether this may be anxiety or any other emotional reaction (anger, etc.).

Sensations

When engaging in the yoga exercise, participants may encounter sensations of physical discomfort, even mild pain, when doing certain postures. In this case we tend to emphasize two things: (1) that participants should respect their own limits, be gentle to themselves, and listen to their bodies about how much they can do (self-compassion), but then (2) as much as they feel comfortable, be able to bring some curiosity to those sensations as they arise in their bodies. The general stance the instructors take is:

> *Instructor:* "Just allow yourself to notice whatever is in your body at any given moment. There is nothing you need to do about this. Notice, observe, and let it be there without getting tangled up in it or trying to control it. Whatever it is, it is OK for it to be there. Nothing needs to be done about it other than noticing and observing whatever is present at any given moment, whether these are sensations, feelings, thoughts, or judgments."

MOOD DIARY

The Mood Diary is used as a tool to help participants raise their awareness for the occurrence of warning signs that foreshadow the worsening of mood. Participants are provided with a copy of the Mood Diary (Handout 5). Early detection of warning signs provides a window of time during which participants can intervene by initiating action plans that may prevent the down-spiraling of mood symptoms into full mood episodes. Action plans will be worked out in session 3. Although the idea of mood charting often has intuitive appeal to instructors, they should not be surprised that this idea is not greeted with a warm welcome by all participants. In fact, many participants do not like monitoring their mood. This is understandable if one takes into account that directing attention toward one's own mood, especially if things are not going so well, may make mood symptoms more noticeable, elicit negative thoughts and self-evaluations, and trigger rumination. As Michelle, one our participants, pointed out quite candidly, "I don't like this idea. I think I am just doing better not paying this much attention to my mood, because overfocusing just seems to make it worse." We found it helpful to explain to participants that, for this very reason, the mood charting itself is kept relatively brief and won't keep participants focused on the mood for very long. But also, part of the class is about bringing this new type of attention (observing and noticing nonjudgmentally) to warning signs, triggers, associated negative thoughts, and ruminative old grooves and that this may change their experience with those.

At first glance, the Mood Diary, with its columns and rows, may appear complicated. However, it can be filled out in as little as 10–20 seconds on a given day (for another approach, see Otto et al., 2009). Each column represents a day of the month (column one = day 1). Each day, participants just complete one column. We advise participants to keep the Mood Diary on their nightstand or right next to their bed, as moving it around increases the chance that it will get lost. At the beginning of the day, we ask participants to note the number of hours of sleep that they got. At the end of the day, right before they go to bed, participants check the boxes that correspond to the moods they experienced during the day. If they experienced neither elevated nor depressed mood during the day, they should check the box marked "normal." The upper rows are reserved for mood elevation, and the lower rows for depressed mood. In addition, participants rate how anxious and irritable they were during the day and whether they took their medication (which should be listed on the bottom of the diary). In order to start the process of identifying triggers, participants can make notes about any stressful or positive events that occurred during the day.

This way, the Mood Diary not only serves as a tool for raising awareness, but, with continued use, it also allows the participant to see the course of depression and/or mood elevation symptoms at one glance over a month. Since the first session often takes place at night, the participants fill out the Mood Diary for that day. This also gives the instructor the chance to check with every participant for relevant symptoms of hypomania or depression (i.e., the instructor should go around and take a look at each participant's Mood Diary). Should this Mood Diary check reveal significant symptoms of hypomania/mania for a participant, the instructor should meet with this participant after the session to determine the best course of action (guidelines for how to deal with hypomania/mania are provided in Chapter 4 and Session 6). Likewise, the guidelines for dealing with depression are provided in Chapter 4 and Session 5.

INTRODUCTION TO THE BREATHING SPACE

Following the instructions for the Mood Diary, we introduce participants to the first part of the 3-Minute Breathing Space Exercise. The full 3-Minute Breathing Space Exercise will be introduced in Session 3. This brief exercise is meant to give participants the opportunity to step out of whatever they are doing at a given moment and check in with themselves about what is going on. Observe and notice for a few moments before moving on with the next activity (see informal practice below). It is modeled after the first part of the 3-Minute Breathing Space Exercise designed by Segal et al. (2002, 2013) to help implement mindfulness in participants' daily lives. This is practiced with the group once before discussing aspects of formal and informal practice.

Box 1.4. Introduction to the Breathing Space

- This is a practice of coming into the moment wherever you are.
- Whether you are standing, sitting, or lying down, taking a definite posture, letting the body express a sense of being present and awake. Closing the eyes, if this feels comfortable to you.
- Now, becoming aware of what is going on with you right now.
- Becoming aware of what is going through the mind. What thoughts are around? As best as you can just noting the thoughts as mental events.
- And also becoming aware of any feelings that are around at this moment . . . allowing any sense of discomfort or unpleasant feelings to be with you, rather than pushing them away or shutting them out. Just acknowledging them.

- Similarly, becoming aware of sensations in the body. Are there sensations of tension? And again, just allowing yourself to be aware of them. Simply noting them.
- Whatever it is you are noticing right now, thoughts, feelings, or sensations, simply allowing yourself to just notice what is going on right now.

Adapted in part from Segal et al. (2002, 2013). Copyright 2003, 2013 by The Guilford Press. Adapted by permission.

FORMAL AND INFORMAL PRACTICE

This program, like all other programs of this type, asks participants to engage in regular homework and practice. Mindfulness relies on participants' ability to learn. The type of learning mindfulness draws upon requires repetitive practice of the same exercise. One meeting a week accounts for only a fraction of time spent practicing in a given week. How can we expect to see changes if we do not practice what has been learned in session and apply it in real life? Traditionally, there have been two types of practices in mindfulness-based programs: formal and informal. Formal practice involves activities that require participants to set aside a dedicated period of time every day for practicing yoga and other exercises that are taught as part of this program. Informal practice involves bringing mindful attention to internal and external experiences as participants go about their daily lives (Orsillo & Roemer, 2011, p. 99). Like a violinist who has regular rehearsal hours but then also takes the instrument at other times to practice, both types of practices help to develop mindfulness skills. To some extent, this program blurs this distinction as we ask participants to conduct many brief "informal" daily mindfulness practices (such as the Breathing Space Exercise), but we work with participants on strategies to increase the frequency of these "informal" exercises as much as possible.

Guidelines for scheduling times for mindfulness practice are provided in Handout 6. Scheduling time for formal practices is often challenging for participants with bipolar disorder. People with bipolar disorder often have disorganized and chaotic lives, and they usually get derailed despite their best intentions. Memory difficulties also pose a challenge for participants remembering to do these exercises and what they actually looked like. This may not happen during the first week, when everything is new, fresh, and perhaps exciting, but these obstacles tend to be encountered later. Let's use the Yoga–Body Scan as an example for how to address these obstacles. We find it helpful to pair up participants and have them engage in concrete planning (see Handout 6 for guidelines on how to plan). When and where do they want to do the exercise? What obstacles could come their way? And what could they do when they find that they are reasoning with themselves about whether they should do the exercise now or at a later point? After participants have identified a particular time and place, we like them to mentally walk through what they usually do at that time of the day in order to anticipate obstacles that may come up. Numerous things can interfere with practicing, such as running late in the morning, an unanticipated phone call, a meeting going longer, needing to pick up the kids, or simply not feeling like doing the exercise after a long stressful day. Some of these obstacles can be overcome by planning in advance: if you anticipate not doing the exercising because you may not have comfortable clothes available in that particular moment, place them there in advance. If the exercise requires you to move furniture, or to create space, do so in advance, or consider a different place. In fact, it is often the simple additional things that need to be done before one can do the exercise (move furniture, etc.) that can get participants derailed; one should not underestimate the power of such obstacles. If after the "mental walk-through" a day and time seems unrealistic, participants should pick a different time and place and repeat the mental walk-through. That said, there will not be a perfect time, just one when interferences are less probable or can be circumvented more easily. Once a time and place are identified, participants should ask themselves how they can remind themselves to do the exercise. Some participants with bipolar disorder have memory difficulties and may not remember to do the exercise despite their best intentions. Scheduling reminders using phones, putting the practice in the schedule book, or placing colored postings as reminders can be helpful to increase the likelihood that participants will remember the time for the exercise. Often, it is helpful to schedule the practice after doing something someone always does on a daily basis. For example, Michelle ended up doing the Yoga–Body Scan after reading the newspaper in the morning and before going grocery shopping. The newspaper was a daily routine for her. Likewise, some participants may find it helpful to enlist their spouse or significant other as a support person. This person can simply remind the participants about doing the yoga exercise, free up time with their help, or, for some participants, actually join in and do the exercises. For example, Justin and his wife determined that the time before dinner was an ideal time for him to practice. Usually they would prepare dinner together, but she was perfectly fine with his practicing the Yoga–Body Scan during this time. In addition, with dinner-time approaching, his wife would remind him about doing the exercise. We also ask participants to pay attention to their mind finding excuses not to practice ("I am too tired," "Not in the mood," "Just too much"). In fact, we not only anticipate this to happen, we ask participants to switch into their observant mode and then still to do the practice, rather than debating and arguing with themselves.

Informal Practice

We should not underestimate the power of informal practice. In fact, many of the exercises, as the program unfolds, will take place in daily life. As we have learned, formal exercise, despite our best efforts as instructors, often does not materialize. That is not meant to discourage or deemphasize formal practice, but it raises awareness for maximizing informal practices in order to achieve our goals. Our first informal practice is the first part of the 3-Minute Breathing Space (Box 1.4, Introduction to the Breathing Space). We would like participants to complete this exercise as many times during the day as possible. In its shortest form, the exercise does not take more than a minute to complete. Imagine if we could get someone to do this 10 or 20 times each day—they would have a total of 10 or 20 minutes of practice every day when he or she totals the minutes. This feels like a lot, but think about how many times during the day you are not doing anything in particular other than waiting for something or bridging time in between other, more "important" activities. Some examples include waiting for the subway in the morning, the minute before starting your car, standing at a traffic light, before getting out of your car, being in the elevator, walking into your office, before switching on the computer, the minute after getting a coffee before starting your next task, the minute before going to lunch, or coming back after lunch.

> *Instructor*: "Here is how I would like you to start thinking about what you do, day in, day out. Everything you do consists of small 'chunks' of activities [Duhigg, 2012]. Think about making coffee. You place the filter in the machine, you add the coffee and the water, and then you click the power button. I bet that this is one of those moments, when most of the time we do not really pay much attention anymore, because, this is the 'coffee-making routine'—it is so overlearned and ingrained that it does not require much conscious attention. In fact, it looks like the brain stores the coffee-making routine as one chunk of motor behaviors that are being executed once you decide to make coffee. A lot of what we do, day in and day out, is executing these kinds of chunks, like making coffee, sending an e-mail, placing phone calls, and so forth. When a chunk of behavior is set in motion, the program runs pretty automatically, and often we do not need to pay attention anymore. But, at the end of that chunk, that is often a moment of pausing, a moment of orientation, which, for the Breathing Space,

gives us a great chance to utilize it right in the middle between two chunks: before taking the coffee and going back to the desk to write the next e-mail. After finishing an e-mail and going on to the next one, or before or after making a phone call—this is what I would like you to do with the Breathing Space Exercise. Start to plug it in at the end of one small activity you do, before you start the next [Duhigg, 2012]."

Next, as with the formal practice we ask participants to mentally walk through their day and identify transition points in their behaviors when they could do the Introduction to the Breathing Space. As with the formal practice, this can be done by mentally walking through the day and identifying the beginning and end of small chunks of activities where the Breathing Space can be brought in before or after. Common examples include:

- After getting into the car, before starting the engine
- After stopping at a red traffic light
- After parking your car
- After sitting down in a bus or subway
- After writing an e-mail
- Before opening an e-mail one received
- Before starting a meal
- After finishing a meal

Participants should place additional reminders using their phones for random times, so that they are reminded about paying attention to the beginning and end of activities, and initiating the Breathing Space as often as possible.

Instructor: "This is one of the most important take-home points for today. Perhaps the biggest gift you can give yourself going forward from here is to bring awareness to the present moment. This can be done, for example, by plugging in the Breathing Space between different things that you do. For example, when you leave here, you will leave the clinic, go to the elevator, and then press the button for the elevator to come. This moment—waiting for the elevator—is a chance for you to take a Breathing Space. Or perhaps you may decide to take a Breathing Space in the elevator. Then, when you walk to your car, before you open the door, you could do a Breathing Space. You could do a Breathing Space before you start the engine. If you start thinking about your behavior in these units, you may find lots of opportunities to do Breathing Spaces every day. The nice thing about this is that the more often you do this, the time being in the present accumulates, and all of a sudden you may find yourself in the present all the time!"

HOMEWORK

We ask participants to practice the Yoga–Body Scan (audio track 1) and fill out their Mood Diary (Handout 5) once a day, and do the Introduction to the Breathing Space as many times as they like (audio track 2). Handout 4, which depicts the positions and movements of the Yoga–Body Scan, is designed to help participants remember the positions and movements. Participants are encouraged to first practice the Breathing Space by listening to the recording a number of times (audio track 2). Once they feel comfortable, they should implement the Breathing Space without listening to the recording when they shift activities. Handout 6 provides participants with guidelines on how to set up their mindfulness practice. Before the session ends, we also like to remind people, that while the practice, hopefully, is fun and enjoyable, experience tells us that it may not be. Sometimes, it may feel like just another chore participants need to do. It may also heighten their awareness of tension and anxiety, which makes people shy away from it. Nonetheless, we encourage participants as best as we can to start up the practice. We ask participants to make notes about their practice throughout the week using Handout 7. The session ends with scheduling individual meetings with the instructor.

Welcome Back to the Present

OVERVIEW

- About This Session
- Welcome Back and Mood Diary Check
- The Mindfulness Paradox
- Yoga–Body Scan
- Obstacles to Practicing
- Awakening: The Breathing Space
- Mindfulness to Routine Activities
- Mood Diary and Warning Signs
- Body Scan
- Responding versus Reacting
- Homework
  - Body Scan (audio track 3)
  - Introduction to the Breathing Space (audio track 2)
  - Mindfulness to routine activities
  - Mood Diary and attention to warning signs

INSTRUCTOR MATERIAL FOR SESSION 2

- Script for the Yoga–Body Scan (Box 1.3) and Handout 4: Yoga Exercise
- Script for the Body Scan (Box 2.1)

- Handout 5: Mood Diary (in case a participant forgot to bring his or hers)
- Handout 7: Homework Sheet
- Handout 8: Worksheet for Warning Signs and Action Plans

ABOUT THIS SESSION

In this session we deepen the practice of the Yoga–Body Scan, leading toward a Body Scan in which participants move their attention through different body parts without inducing movement. This Body Scan exercise can be practiced as homework using the Body Scan recording (audio track 3). As many participants will readily acknowledge after the first week, making time for practice may have been more difficult than initially thought. Therefore, we problem-solve around obstacles for practicing. Coming into the present continues to be an ongoing process. Breathing Spaces are meant to support it. In this session this process is broadened and deepened by deliberately bringing mindfulness to activities that normally do not receive much attention (routine activities), such as brushing teeth, eating, or washing dishes. Participants' increased awareness will be directed to the presence of warning signs that signal the worsening of their mood (in order to develop action plans down the road). Finally, we also begin to address some of the paradoxes that center around mindfulness: changes in participants' experiences arise from deliberately adopting an observant stance toward sensations, feelings, and thoughts, without trying to change them. Yet, at the same time, mindfulness does not mean passive endurance: it involves learning to respond more skillfully to experiences and aspects of one's life that may deserve change.

WELCOME BACK AND MOOD DIARY CHECK

As participants return after their first week, before the start of the group, we briefly check each participant's Mood Diary individually, and inquire how things are going. When we welcome people back to group we simply ask whether we may take a quick "peek" at their Mood Diary. This will become an established routine that will be part of participants' return to group. If a participant has not filled it out or forgot to bring the diary, we provide him or her with a new sheet and ask him or her to fill it out retrospectively. This sets the expectation that the Mood Diary will always be checked. At the beginning of the group, instructors want to be aware of any significant mood changes that may have taken place over the course of the week. This is particularly important for detecting early signs of hypomania/mania, as addressing these symptoms is often time-sensitive in order to prevent the spiraling of these symptoms into full-blown mania. That being said, some fluctuations in mood symptoms (symptoms associated with both depression and mania) are common. In order to determine the significance of any mood shift, we ask participants how intense and interfering the symptoms are/were, and whether this is a substantial deviation from the typical waxing and waning of mood. Likewise, we inquire whether, in their experiences, this shift foreshadows taking a turn for the worse (note that the warning signs are a topic discussed later in this session as part of mood monitoring). If not, the participants' experiences can be shared in class and folded into the exercises conducted in class and during homework. But what should the instructor do if a participant returns to group feeling energized, keyed up, with speeded thoughts, or being more talkative? First, if symptoms have become severe, immediate action may need to be taken (e.g., call or page the psychiatrist, send a participant over to a psychiatric emergency room). If noticeable, yet a participant could still participate in class, then we may give this participant instructions about how to be mindful with these experiences during class (see Session 6 and Handout 20 for guidelines about how to be mindful with symptoms of mania).

For example, when Michael returned to the second group session with some mood elevation, it turned out that his mood elevation was mild enough that he could participate in the program that day (see also the individual session "Negotiating Medication and Insight"). However, we gave him some guidelines concerning what to do with his increased feeling of energy and his urge to talk and be witty. Specifically, we asked Michael to be extra gentle with himself, rather than trying to spend extra energy during the yoga exercise. We directed him to attend to his urge to talk, or allow himself to observe the "impulse to say something and wanting to be funny," rather than following it. Michael's task became to note and observe where the urge to talk was located in his body, how it felt, what sensations it came with, as well as being with uncomfortable sensations or feelings, which might arise with him not acting on that urge. Michael also agreed to "switch" into this "mindful mode" whenever the instructor would give him a sign by raising his or her eyebrows. Several times during the session, when Michael got carried away talking, the instructor signaled him, and Michael used this cue to switch into observant mode. After the session, he and the instructor met, contacted his psychiatrist, and went over the guidelines about how to be mindful with the symptoms of mania that had arisen (see Session 6 and Handout 20). With symptoms of mania present that are either severe enough or foreshadowing a spiraling down into mania, we recommend getting in touch with the psychiatrist. The purpose of this communication is to ask the psychiatrist to boost medication or temporarily add medication to counteract the symptoms of mania. As this may not be the participant's preference, some negotiation may be needed (see Chapter 4 for guidelines about negotiating medication changes).

THE MINDFULNESS PARADOX

What motivates participants to come to a 2-hour class once a week, attend individual sessions, and shoulder the burden of homework? Ultimately, it is the hope for change for the better. "I just hoped that this mindfulness would be something that could get my mood more stable," Justin recalls. "Even these minor ups and downs were draining, and no matter what I would do, there would not be a week or sometimes even a day without getting set off. It was as if bipolar was always lingering in the back, always ready to give me a hard time, and no matter how hard I would work, once it hits the ground, it's running. I just wanted things to be peaceful and quiet." Other participants have described similar hopes and expectations to us: "getting my head less busy," "getting better control over my feelings," "stopping cascades of mood spiraling up or down," and "learning to cope with anxiety or anger."

What stood out to us from most of these pregroup interviews were two things: first, with few exceptions, many people who participated in our program had painfully realized that taking medication was not enough for them to stabilize their mood and treat all the other problems that often come with bipolar disorder (e.g., anxiety, anger). Second, all of them were willing and highly motivated to work hard to make things better. It is this commitment to work hard in order to change things that sets forth the dialectic that becomes a recurring theme throughout the program.

Mindfulness is not about learning how to switch off thoughts or how to keep strong feelings at bay, nor how to not feel down, anxious, or angry. These experiences are unavoidable. Mindfulness is about learning to relate to these experiences in a different way: seeing them as events in our minds and our bodies, or streams of thoughts, feelings, and sensations that will pass, followed by other thoughts, feelings, and sensations. One of the core skills in mindfulness practice is to adopt an observant, accepting stance toward these experiences in each and every moment. This attitude facilitates disengagement from impulses, strategies, and habits of the mind trying to fix things, change the experience, make it better, less aversive, or more palatable. Paradoxically, it is this very practice of purposefully not trying to fix or change things that often transforms that very experience that participants would like to change. For the instructor, this means weaving this thread into both formal instructions and conversations: Comments like "being with whatever is," and "noticing whatever is in this very moment," and "allowing things to be as they are," convey a sense that nothing needs to be changed or fixed in this very moment, encouraging participants to notice and observe whatever is whenever it happens.

Naming the "paradox" of this principle as such can be helpful for participants in order to understand the idea. Often, participants will ask what they are supposed to "do" with these experiences. "How should I deal with this?" "What can I do about uncomfortable or painful sensations?" "What if this makes me feel awkward or anxious?" The answer may surprise, because of its simplicity "Do nothing, absolutely nothing, other than noting and observing what unfolds in the body and in the mind at any moment." This is true for all formal and informal practices. And this guideline will not change for the remainder of the program. This can be a challenge both for participants and instructors. For participants, it is a challenge because their minds habitually may try to find ways to remove or avoid uncomfortable sensations, thoughts, or feelings (autopilots; see Sessions 5–8). Instructors, especially if they are trained in cognitive or cognitive-behavioral therapy, may find themselves wanting to work on challenging the content of thoughts and promote behavioral changes in the service of changing the experience.

In MBCT, the change in perspective and experience comes from deliberately adopting an observant stance, and seeing sensations, feelings, and thoughts as occurrences in the body that come and go. To promote this change in relating to what is happening in one's body, the instructor firmly maintains this stance of "curiosity about the experience." Ask questions such as "What exactly did you notice in your body?", "Where was this located?", "How exactly did this discomfort feel?", "When did it arise?", and "Did it stay constant for the whole time?" These questions are meant to shape the participant's ability to observe raw bodily sensations and feelings directly. The same is true for thoughts that may arise during the exercise. "When did the thought come up?" "What did the thought say?" "Did it stay the whole time?" The suggestion, whenever asked about what to do, is to "bring a curious observance to the events unfolding in the body and in the mind at that moment, no matter how boring, pleasant, or unpleasant they may be."

It is important to note, however, that accepting and observing experiences with a nonjudgmental attitude does not, of course, exclude the possibility of acting upon problems. This will also be conveyed to participants. In this program, we train the ability to stay with the experience, without engaging in our habitual tendency to immediately react. Staying with the experience and learning to accept and observe it brings us into a state where we can perceive more information about a situation because we don't turn away, and we take the time to look more carefully. On the basis of broader information about a problematic situation, we have the possibility to react more skillfully. It also gives us the possibility to engage in problem-solving behavior that might not usually be a part of our behavioral repertoire. To stop, to listen, and to observe—as opposed to acting immediately—provides us with a broader range of possibilities. While we do convey to participants that ultimately we want to be able to choose skillful behavior, the first step is to stop (do nothing), then observe/become aware. This aspect of the situation is something that we don't usually train much, which is why we focus on cultivating this ability in this program (also see the section on "reacting vs. responding" later in this session). With this in mind, after the Mood Diary check the second session begins with the Yoga–Body Scan that was introduced in Session 1.

YOGA–BODY SCAN

The purpose of the Yoga–Body Scan is to pay attention to physical sensations in the body and to begin the process of observing them. This exercise brings about many of the experiences that participants strive to become more mindful about. This includes negative, judgmental thoughts, uncomfortable feelings and sensations, and the mind's habitual or strategic efforts to minimize discomfort. These are not nuisances that detract from the exercise. To the contrary, they are the heart and soul of the material participants will learn to deal with over the next two months by working their way through the program. In these experiences we want participants to notice bodily or mental events, no matter how pleasant or unpleasant they may be. To capitalize on participants' fresh memories of the Yoga–Body Scan in class, we discuss the immediate experiences first, before broadening the discussion to the experiences participants had with the practice during the week. Themes connected with the yoga part of the Yoga–Body Scan include "Am I getting the postures right?", self-critical judgments and thoughts, uncomfortable sensations and feelings, overfocusing and blocking out uncomfortable experiences, getting mad at oneself, the exercise not being relaxing, and getting anxious. Common experiences associated with the body scan portion (after yoga or by itself) are described in Session 3.

"Am I Getting the Postures Right?"

"Doing it here in class again helped a lot," Michelle responded after the instructor had asked about participants' experiences in class. "At home, I wasn't sure whether I am getting the cat and cow part right. Seeing it here in class again will help a lot to get it right when I do it again by myself." Michelle's experience was shared by others who had looked at the drawings and listened to the recording. This still had not provided enough details about each posture to be sure that they were doing it right. This provided a welcome opportunity for the instructor to inquire about Michelle's thoughts and feelings during the yoga exercise in class. In order to get the postures and sequence of postures right, Michelle carefully watched the instructor and compared the memories from her practice of doing the yoga exercise at home with the way the postures were done by the instructor. At times she made mental notes to change her way of doing it when she noticed that she had done things differently, feeling quite pleased with herself that she had done it exactly right. When participants share these experiences, we invite them to bring awareness to these very experiences during the exercise (e.g., setting an intention, comparing memories, feeling good about doing it right, feeling disappointed when doing it wrong) and simply observe and notice them as events in their minds and body. We emphasize the point that there is no right or wrong way of doing this exercise. The purpose is to engage in movement and allow oneself to notice how moving through the postures feels in the body and whatever else may be present at the time (e.g., self-critical thoughts, questions, feelings).

Many of the questions regarding the yoga part tend to be technical. "How much should I stretch?", "Is this the right way of doing it?", "What if I can't do this part?", "Is it OK to do it this way?" Participants who have experience with other yoga exercises often inquire about the breathing. "When should I inhale and when should I exhale?," "Does breathing matter for this exercise?" All these questions offer insight about what is going through people's minds while they are doing the exercise. These experiences are explored with genuine curiosity. As part of this exploration we tend to continuously point out to the group that it is not about doing it right. Rather, the exercises serve as a vehicle so that participants can practice becoming aware of the sensations, feelings, or thoughts that are present during the exercise. This then allows participants to observe them as mental events in their minds and bodies without getting tangled up in them as they are moving through the different postures.

Self-Critical Judgments and Thoughts

"I still don't like this exercise," Jennifer said after the discussion had centered on the "technicalities" of the exercise. "The fact that I can't even do a simple exercise like this is just disheartening." It turns out that during the exercise, Jennifer (who was somewhat overweight) pictured herself and what she looked like doing it, breathing heavily, trying to work the different postures, and how "ridiculous" she would look like to the other group members "getting her fat body into the different positions." "I cannot tell you how awful that felt," she said. This kept going through her mind while she was trying hard to keep up with the sequence of postures but then channeled into rumination during the body scan. "Trying to keep up with the movements was somewhat distracting, so I kind of noticed this, but then when we had lied down for the body scan, it really took off," she described the thoughts going through her mind: "I can't even do this," "This is the program that is supposed to help you and here you go, you blow it right from the outset," and "There is really nothing that can help you." Needless to say, Jennifer was not able to concentrate on focusing her attention on the different body parts.

Jennifer's experience is common when a negative thought is triggered and the mind starts to engage in its well-grooved patterns of rumination. Often yoga then distracts from the thoughts, but as the need for focusing attention on the "how-to" of the postures and orchestrating the movements is replaced by lying still, rumination can take center stage. As with questions and thoughts about "doing it right," we ask participants, as best as they can, to just acknowledge and notice what is going on in their minds and in their bodies, and include this probe into the field of their awareness, while they are moving through the different postures. This allows them to welcome whatever experience unfolds as they are taking the different postures. If this involves negative, self-critical thoughts, we ask participants to simply acknowledge their presence but then continue with the exercise and allow themselves to focus on the physical sensations that come with moving.

Other participants may be doing the movement exercise against the backdrop of ongoing negative thoughts or rumination that may not have anything to do with the exercise, but still fold into their experience. "I know I should concentrate on the here and now and noticing how it feels doing the yoga, but I just can't seem to stop thinking about this job I have applied for." Holly explained that they did not call her back after her job interview, and as days passed after her initial interview she found herself getting increasingly occupied with not getting a call for a second interview. "Right now this is constantly on my mind, and I can't seem to think about anything else," Holly mentioned. Further inquiry revealed that not getting a second interview for Holly not only meant that her financial situation would not improve, but to not get a job for which she was well qualified was a blow to her self-esteem. As with self-critical negative thoughts triggered by the yoga exercise, we simply ask participants to allow themselves to acknowledge these thoughts and feelings and then gently continue with the exercise, noticing the sensations that are induced by the movements and without blocking out any self-critical thoughts or uncomfortable experiences.

"Unwanted Sensations and Feelings"

Moving the body in this fashion may create uncomfortable or even painful sensations, such as tightness in the muscles. The intention of the Yoga–Body Scan includes paying attention to physical sensations in the body. First, as part of the instructions, we ask participants to be gentle with themselves, and we continue to remind participants about this theme throughout the discussion. This is no competition in which the person with the strongest bend wins. Rather, the Yoga–Body Scan is an invitation to experience the sensations in the body when participants engage in the movement exercise. This way we also remind participants to respect their body's boundaries and be self-caring by not overdoing it.

Nonetheless, when strong sensations arise, the task remains the same: simply bring awareness to that region, and, as best as participants can, note carefully the sensations that arise. We ask participants to include the raw sensations into their field of awareness and not to block them out even if they are uncomfortable. Questions regarding the quality of the uncomfortable sensations (sharp, dull, steady, and fluctuating) can help participants attend to the raw quality of these sensations, rather than drifting into thinking about these sensations and what they mean. Painful sensations can trigger rumination, such as wondering what one is doing wrong or why one can't even do this simple exercise. If this happens, we ask participants to acknowledge that their thoughts have drifted into rumination and then gently refocus their attention on the physical experience of the exercise. Unwanted sensations also trigger a sense of aversion (i.e., not wanting them). This is part of the body's fight–flight reaction to avoid things that are harmful to us. The natural tendency is to move attention away from those sensations, trying not to notice them, perhaps to narrow the focus and shift it away from the sensations that attention is drawn toward. If this is the case, we ask participants, as best as they can, to include these uncomfortable sensations into their field of awareness in addition to those that are brought on by moving and stretching. This allows them to notice the raw quality of these bodily sensations.

Importantly, we also emphasize that self-care is critical when painful sensations are being encountered. Participants are encouraged to try out variations of the postures they can comfortably do. Discernment is important and should be cultivated in order to learn to differentiate between sensations that are simply uncomfortable but not harmful versus positions that are harmful and require modifications to protect the body/health.

Overfocusing

"I think I had a pretty good experience," Michael said. "I was able to fully concentrate on the moment and experience being in my body. This was great to just notice my body and be able to tune out everything else." More careful exploration yielded information that during the yoga exercise, Michael had narrowed his attentional focus on the bodily sensations that came with the movements. Whenever any thoughts or distractions arose (e.g., noticing the person next to him or wandering thoughts) he would quickly and forcefully refocus his attention on some body part or some sensations in his body to block out any further thoughts. If this happens, we invite participants to widen their attentional focus and allow all bodily experiences during the exercise to be noticed, whether that be physical sensations, feelings, or thoughts and to observe the experiences that unfold moment by moment with an open, inviting stance. As much of this deliberately narrowed focus serves to shut out unwanted distractions, one may also suggest bringing attention to that very intention and making this part of the observation.

Along the same lines, other participants describe that they tense the muscles extra hard, such that the sensations are dominant and become the sole focus of attention. Or they already felt tense before the exercise and then worked extra such that the sensations triggered by the movement exercise served as a welcomed distraction by capturing their attention. For others, releasing energy has become the primary purpose of the exercise and the focus of their attention. In all these cases, attention is moved away from something that deserves to be noticed and observed. Hence, we invite participants to widen their field of awareness and allow themselves to notice all raw bodily or mental experiences that may unfold in a given moment. Likewise, we also encourage curiosity to observe the goals or expectations that lead to the intention to move attention away from some feelings or bodily sensations.

"Getting Mad at Oneself"

Frustration and anger are other feelings that may arise as participants move through the yoga exercise. This can be triggered by negative thoughts about one's own "performance" or how one feels during the exercise (compared to how one "ought" to feel). "It happens each and every time," complained Stephen. "I really try hard, noticing everything, but I can't seem to fully be in the moment. There is always something that distracts me, pain, thoughts, mind wandering, you name it." As with the other experiences described before, we invited Stephen to allow himself to observe these experiences as part of the exercise without getting tangled up in them. What thoughts were going through his mind? How did he feel? What kind of sensations did his frustration come with, and how did the experience change as it turned into anger? What thoughts were associated with the anger and where were the sensations located?

As participants uncover their experiences, we suggest that they may also want to become more aware of their intentions and expectations that may be present as they are starting the exercise. Is there an expectation that they would like to achieve a certain state of how they feel? What is their expectation of how to do the exercise right? All of these experiences can—and in Stephen's case, did—become the object of a mindful exploration as he continued to practice yoga throughout class. Stephen discovered as his level of frustration throughout the exercise would rise, he would get into his inner monologues, "asking himself if he could not even do this exercise right, what then could he even do?" This intensified his feelings of frustration and anger. In this case, we suggested that he gently acknowledge the angry thoughts ("angry at myself that I can't reach a perfect state"), then gently allow himself to notice the sensations that come with the movement and the frustration.

"This Is Not Relaxing!"

"But I thought yoga should be relaxing," Taylor complained, seemingly disappointed about the discussion about uncomfortable sensations and self-critical thoughts getting into the way with making yoga an enjoyable experience. Taylor's expectation follows the common perception that yoga is supposed to make people relaxed. We, like other programs, emphasize that relaxation can be an admittedly desirable by-product of the exercise, but that it is not the primary purpose of doing it. The goal is to learn to observe raw physical sensations that come with engaging in the movement and to allow oneself to be with these sensations, even if they are uncomfortable. As preconceived notions about the exercise ("relaxing") may trigger thoughts and feelings that take attention away from the exercise ("Am I doing this right?", "Why am I not getting relaxed?"), a second goal is to learn to bring awareness to these mental and bodily experiences. Participants should learn to recognize when they set in, acknowledge them as mental events ("Here is my 'I should be relaxed by now' thought"), give them the space they are asking for, but then gently allow themselves to continue the exercise and notice the sensations of movement (and whatever other sensations are present at the time of the exercise).

"I'm Getting Anxious!"

Yoga induces physical sensations through movement and also increases cardiovascular activity (heartbeat, etc.). Likewise, focusing on bodily sensations induced by movement can further increase the salience of physical sensations associated with anxiety. For participants with anxiety disorders, these sensations can provoke more tension. "This exercise made me really tense." Courtney said. "Sometimes, I would notice my heart beat quite forcefully and that reminded me how it is when I get one of my panic attacks." In fact, Courtney had taken a pause during the exercise, only following through at the beginning and at the end. "I just had to slow down," she explained, "otherwise this would have been too overwhelming." Respecting one's limits is an implicit part of self-compassion that we model for participants as part of the exercises. Noticing how much one can do at a given time is an important skill we would like participants to learn during these exercises. Therefore, we ask participants to sense and respect what their limits are at any given time.

This is especially important for participants with anxiety disorders. However, with this in mind, like any other experiences, the instructor inquired about the sensations, feelings, and thoughts that Courtney experienced during the exercise. She noticed that when she was getting anxious, she would think about how she would describe the sensation and the feeling. Where was it located in her body? Did it stay the same all the time? Did it change? What kind of thoughts did she notice? As with any other unwanted experience, we encourage participants to bring a sense of curiosity to the sensations and feelings they experience, allowing themselves to notice and observe those while respecting the limits of what they feel they can do at a given time.

OBSTACLES TO PRACTICING

Inevitably, some participants will describe their difficulties getting themselves to do the Yoga–Body Scan. We use this as an opportunity to explore what unfolded at the time when the participant had planned on doing the mindfulness exercise. Common issues are (1) not being in the mood for doing the exercise (e.g., being tired, or reacting to the idea of doing the exercise as aversive) and (2) something else seemed more important at the time. When participants describe that something else was more pressing at the time, or they did not feel like doing the exercise, they are aware that they had planned on doing the exercise but then feelings and thoughts were present that led participants away from practicing. What better opportunity could there be than to use that moment to begin observing those very thoughts and feelings?

"I just can't seem to get myself to do the body scan," Justin noted, looking frustrated. "I thought that the best time would be to do it before dinner, but then either I am too hungry and feel that I would not be able to concentrate, or I get a call, or I have to take care of one more thing before we can eat." "Why don't we choose one of those situations you think you still remember well," the instructor asked, inviting Justin to process this moment. Justin picked the "got to get this one more thing done one," and he and the instructor explored the experience at that moment. "To the best that you can remember," the instructor asked, "what was going through your mind at the time?" Justin paused, then said, "Well, I know that I was supposed to do the Yoga–Body Scan, but I also needed to write this e-mail to my colleague to get him the info he needed for the meeting the next morning. I did not want to do it after dinner, because this is my time to unwind, but then I knew that I needed to cut the body scan short if I work on this e-mail first." "How did you feel at that moment?" the instructor asked. "Kind of tense, just very pressed to get this e-mail out of the way," Justin answered. "Where is this feeling of pressing located in your body?" the instructor asked. "Kind of in my stomach and in my chest. I did not wait this out for very long," Justin said. "I just got going on the e-mail because it was just more important." The instructor and Justin explored the inner landscape of his body and his mind as his conflict between e-mailing his colleague and completing the body scan unfolded (the characteristics of the pressure feeling, where exactly it would be, and what other thoughts were around). He invited Justin to make this moment of conflict a moment of mindful observation.

> *Instructor*: "As you will likely encounter conflicts like this again, perhaps you might want to take this moment and note what is unfolding in your mind and body, bringing some curiosity to the feeling and the sensations that are arising, noticing the 'I need to do this' thought, that is present at that very moment. Nothing that needs to be done about it, just allowing yourself to notice what is there at that time. In fact, by turning a moment such as this one, where a scheduled practice is difficult to complete, into one of paying attention and bringing awareness of what is going on, you are engaging in the very practice of mindfulness you are meant to practice with a formal exercise."

Note, also, that the instructor did not immediately jump into problem solving, such as finding a different time or place for the practice. Moments when the practice does not work out can be used for noticing and observing the very thoughts and feelings that are present at that time. If the exercise is aversive, then we ask participants to bring curiosity to this aversive feeling and explore the raw sensations associated with it as best as they can. Aversive feelings and thoughts may arise when participants anticipate that the exercise will be boring or may trigger anxiety with certain body postures. Paradoxically, by making the moment when they notice the aversion about the exercise a period of mindful observation, participants practice the very mindfulness they were formally scheduled to practice. One of the suggestions that often results from these discussions is to do the exercise despite "something else being more pressing." If this thought continues to be present during the exercise, we simply ask participants to acknowledge the thought as a mental event—"Here is my 'I got to get this done' thought"— and then gently redirect themselves to observe any feelings and sensations they may experience at that time. This provides participants with a welcome opportunity to practice observing and noting thoughts, feelings, and sensations as mental and bodily events while doing the exercise.

What if participants forget to do the exercise altogether? Forgetting happens not only with the Yoga–Body Scan. It happens much more frequently in the context of doing the "informal" exercise the Breathing Space, which means "coming into the present and checking into what is going on at a given time." As part of their homework, we asked participants to do this brief exercise, in which they move from one situation to the next. In fact, forgetting in this context, at least in the first few weeks, is much more common than remembering. Therefore, our first concern is to find ways for people to remind themselves to do the Breathing Space when they complete one activity but before starting the next.

One way to increase remembering is to mentally walk through participants' routines again, almost like pretending they were making a film about themselves, with the camera following each of their steps. Each time we can pause and highlight it when a behavioral chunk is coming to an end and the next one starts. For example, "Going downstairs and making coffee" is the transition from one behavioral chunk (going down stairs) to the next (making coffee). Then, while mentally walking through this scene, pause at the end of the first chunk (going downstairs) in order to set the intention to do a Breathing Space before starting the next chunk (making coffee). *Before I go downstairs, into the kitchen to make coffee, let me do a Breathing Space at the bottom of the stairs.* In fact, when leaving the day's session, we ask participants to actively "scan" their activities for transitions, and to set intentions whenever possible to increase the likelihood that they may remember to do a Breathing Space. In addition, for transitions that appear on a regular basis (e.g., going for lunch), we may schedule reminders using participants' smart phones. Likewise, random reminders can also be placed, signaling oneself to pause and to ask: "Where am I, what is going on right now? Let me do a Breathing Space."

An additional way of reminding oneself is to place colored sticky notes at places where transitions occur. Another way of increasing the likelihood of remembering is to ask participants to repeat the mental walk-through and flag the transitions from one chunk to the other at least once a day, thus repeatedly setting the intention to do the Breathing Space. This way, when encountering the actual transition in daily life, the real context (being at the bottom of the stairs) may trigger the memory of the mental walk-through and the intention to do the Breathing Space. Most of these techniques can also be used to help participants remember doing the formal exercises (e.g., reminder cues, mental walk-throughs). For example, to not get lost in their routine, participants may visualize coming home, winding down, and then setting the intention of doing yoga and visualizing how they are following through, perhaps even in the face of not being in the mood for doing yoga.

AWAKENING: THE BREATHING SPACE

How are participants' experiences with coming into the present in daily life? The themes range from "awakening," getting a "nice break," to "painful stuff coming to the forefront." "It is amazing how much one is absent," Veronica acknowledged when she returned to group the second week. "You are doing something, being immersed in it, and then, all of a sudden, you realize that you were completely gone, either focusing on your work, or wrapped up in some thoughts that had carried you away. And then you pause for a moment and listen, and then inevitably move on to the next thing before you get woken up again. But, I must say, it has definitely become easier. I just feel I am more aware of things that are going on." For Stephen, the Breathing Space had become a way of taking mini-breaks. "Pausing for a moment and noticing what is going on is like slowing things down," he noted. "Just being in the moment, noticing what is going on at that time, not focusing on anything else or doing multiple things. I really liked this." Michelle, on the other hand, was not as fortunate. For her, not feeling in sync with her husband was very difficult to tolerate. This was brought to the forefront when doing the Breathing Space. Ordinarily, she would habitually distract herself, but the Breathing Space would re-increase awareness of this feeling. "I just don't like feeling it, although it just never seems to go away."

Especially when participants become aware (or more aware) of uncomfortable experiences, we invite them to use that opportunity to stay in observant mode and bring some curious attention to what is going on in that moment. Participants should note what kind of thoughts are going through their minds at that time, and, if some sensation or feeling in the body calls out for attention, to allow themselves to go there and bring some curiosity to it (Where is it located? How does it feel: sharp, edgy, dull? And what happens with it over time as one brings some observance to it?). At the end of the discussion, the group participants do a Breathing Space guided by the instructor (for instructions, see Session 1, Box 1.4) to reorient themselves back to the present.

MINDFULNESS TO ROUTINE ACTIVITIES

To further increase participants' awareness of what is going on in the present moment, we introduce the concept of mindfulness concerning routine activities to the group (see also Segal et al., 2002, 2013).

> *Instructor*: "With our next exercise we are going to take it one step further. So far we have raised awareness to what is going on as we transition from one activity to the next. Now, we begin to pay keen and curious attention to selected activities as you are doing the activity. As you have noticed, a lot of the activities you are doing happen quasi-automatically. They are overlearned, and we don't need to pay much attention anymore. This is convenient because it saves mental energy. But this also means that often negative thoughts, rumination, and/or mood elevation have already unfolded quite a bit before we realize that it might be time to intervene. Therefore, with the next practice, we try to heighten our awareness of what is going on in the present even further."

Being in the present makes it easier to detect warning signs (worsening of mood symptoms), as well as problematic thoughts and feelings in the never-ending stream of consciousness. As group participants have experienced by now, the mind is constantly wandering, and for many of us not in the here and now. However, being more in the present will help participants to detect the worsening of mood symptoms and associated thoughts and feelings sooner.

In order to further develop this "being in the present" or "moment-to-moment" awareness, we now ask participants to choose a routine activity that they perform daily, which they can use to bring the same attention to as they have experienced in the Raisin Exercise. By "routine activities" we mean activities that normally involve little or no conscious attention (i.e., they are highly overlearned) and are often performed without having to bring much focused attention to them in order for them to be properly executed. For example, have you noticed that you usually walk up and down the stairs thinking about where you want to go or what you need to get? Likewise, eating a sandwich or a meal often does not require a lot of conscious, focused attention. For instance, even when driving their car on the highway for a longer period of time, people may find themselves drifting off with their thoughts, having a harder time paying attention to the road. We ask people to bring the quality of awareness that they applied to the raison in the first session to one routine activity they perform every day. They should observe this activity as if they were doing this activity for the first time, noting and observing it, as well as their sensations, thoughts, and feelings associated with it.

Commonly chosen activities include:

- Eating a meal/snack
- Drinking a soda/tea/coffee
- Brushing teeth
- Washing the dishes
- Loading the dishwasher
- Setting the table
- Doing laundry
- Walking around the house
- Entering the house
- Going upstairs
- Going downstairs

MOOD DIARY AND WARNING SIGNS

Next, group participants and the instructor review the Mood Diary. Inquiring about the Mood Diary can be another opportunity to explore thoughts and feelings because participants have probably encountered obstacles using it. Keeping a Mood Diary focuses participants on their mood, and participants may not like this focus because it may trigger automatic thoughts, bringing the issue of mood to the forefront. As Michelle pointed out, "I really don't like the idea of keeping a Mood Diary. It reminds me about the mood, and I really don't like thinking about this." Further inquiry yielded the admission that she was afraid that the Mood Diary could get her right back into rumination cycles. "I need to keep this diary and have not been able to control my mood. What if this gets worse?" For MBCT this creates another opportunity to relate to this thought in a different way, like observing the mood shift and the thought "What if it gets worse" as a mental event without engaging it.

For other participants it may just be an "I can do this later thought" that crosses their minds as they remember that they should fill out the Mood Diary. In those cases, this is also an opportunity to become more aware of such thought as a mental event and then to proceed to fill out the Mood Diary. Other participants simply forget to use the diary. It may have made it into their pocket or bag but never over to the nightstand, where we suggested they place it. For those participants, additional reminder cues are often helpful. For example, they could attach the *filling out of the Mood Diary* to an activity they always do before they go to bed. This could be brushing their teeth or switching off the light. A participant may decide to place a sticky note underneath the light switch ("diary") as a reminder to fill out the diary. For other participants, asking their spouse to be the reminder is also an option if both participant and spouse feel comfortable with it.

Also, note that we are not "married" to the format of the Mood Diary. Sometimes participants are very creative and develop their own system that essentially serves the same purpose, like using their smart phones or Excel spreadsheets. We tend to advise participants to keep the system simple because usually, after a short-lived phase of excitement from creating a sophisticated mood monitoring system, most of them discontinue using it. Therefore, we tend to guide people toward simplicity.

Warning Signs

In this session we broaden the concept of mood monitoring and direct participants' attention to warning signs. As discussed earlier, warning signs are mood symptoms, which, if they worsen, signal that the mood is spiraling up or down. After re-reviewing the concept (introduced in Session 1), and giving a few examples, we ask participants to pair up and discuss which warning signs for both hypomania/mania and depression they are already aware of. During the group discussion, the instructor goes around and answers questions and helps to clarify issues. After the pairwise discussion, examples of warning signs are discussed in the group. Participants will be asked to include their warning signs in Handout 8: Worksheet for Warning Signs and Action Plans.

Common warning signs for hypomania/mania include:

- Having difficulties falling asleep or waking up early
- Beginning to feel more confident, energetic, or motivated

- Wanting to engage in more pleasurable activities
- Feeling more talkative
- Becoming irritable
- Entertaining plans and ideas one would ordinarily not entertain
- Beginning to ruminate about pleasurable activities or achievements
- Finding oneself engaging in ideas on the spur of the moment; being unusually spontaneous
- Having paranoid or religious thoughts
- Things starting to have more "meaning"; feeling like one has a deeper understanding of the world and things in it
- Thoughts beginning to speed up
- Becoming more distractible
- Talking more than usual
- Doing more things (being behaviorally more active) than usual
- Engaging in dangerous activities (driving after drinking; doing drugs)

Common warning signs for depression include:

- Feeling down or depressed
- Losing interest in things
- Not enjoying things
- Feeling more irritable
- Feeling keyed up and restless
- Feeling overwhelmed
- Feeling hopeless
- Worrying about things
- Experiencing more negative thoughts
- Starting to ruminate more
- Thinking life is not worth living
- Having more difficulties concentrating
- Doing fewer things, being less outgoing

Each participant has his or her own unique set of warning signs for depression or hypomania/mania. Most participants have coped with the presence of some of these symptoms either all the time, or at least intermittently. Therefore, it is often not the simple presence or absence of these mood symptoms that makes them a warning sign. More often, we found ourselves helping participants to determine what frequency, duration, or intensity mood symptoms made them predictive for the mood spiraling up or down.

For example, Justin explained that for him a warning sign for hypomania would be that he has this feeling of "giddiness" and wanting to play pranks on people because he thought that this was funny. This typically preceded other symptoms, such as feeling more talkative or experiencing speeded thoughts. Once this pattern was identified, the instructor asked him how often this feeling would need to be present in order for it to represent a warning sign. As Justin pointed out, once was not enough. But based on his recollection of previous episodes with mania, Justin thought that the threshold should be kept rather low and opted for "feeling like playing pranks on people" for 2 days in a row as a warning sign for upcoming hypomania or mania. Elizabeth, on the other hand, identified decreased sleep as her biggest warning sign. As she described, initially, she would try to fall asleep but her body would feel too "wired." Next her need for sleep would diminish. "Once decreased need for sleep sets in, I am way too much in it." For Stephen, the "grim reaper feeling" in his back (tingling sensations he would feel, saying that he is there) would become more intense. For Michael, a warning sign was when feeling religious and relating to other people through religion increased in meaning and importance.

On the depression side, the intensification of negative automatic thoughts or a certain type of negative thought can be a warning sign. As Jennifer revealed, "I know I tend to be hard on myself. Thus, negative judgments about myself frequently come up for me and lower my mood. However, when it gets coupled with this nagging feeling that things won't get better and that I am stuck with this forever, then that usually means things are going downhill. This can be frightening," she said, "but if it starts to come back more than just once a day, then I usually know that might be in for one of my gloomy periods." For Brian, on the other hand, having more difficulties to "get going in the morning" was a warning sign. "If this happens more than just once, it is not a good sign." Once participants have identified their warning signs, they are asked to include those signs in Handout 8 (Worksheet for Warning Signs and Action Plans). Participants are asked to contact the instructor and/or their psychiatrist if any of these mood symptoms became present.

"But what if I am not sure?" In fact, not being exactly sure whether a change in mood is a sign that things are turning for the worst is a common phenomenon and can sometimes lead to anxious overfocusing on the mood. In this case, we simply ask participants to point out what they have noticed, along the lines of being "better safe than sorry." This gives both the participant and the instructor the opportunity to discuss the issue. If it remains unclear, the decision may simply be to continue to watch and be prepared if other changes signal further worsening. Next we do a brief 15-Minute Body Scan without a yoga component.

Box 2.1. Body Scan (15–20 minutes)

(Note for the instructor: [. . .] indicates a pause.)

- Please move into a comfortable position, lying on your back, either on a mat, or on a blanket on the floor. Having the legs and feet a comfortable distance apart, with the feet falling away from each other, the arms alongside the body, palms facing upward. If you feel comfortable to do so closing the eyes, but you are also welcome to keep the eyes open during this practice, if you feel that helps you to stay awake. You can also come into a sitting position, if you would like. Sitting up can help us stay awake through the practice of the body scan.

- Now bringing awareness to the body lying on the floor, and to the flow of the breath. Noticing how the breath is flowing into the body as you inhale and leaving the body as you exhale . . . sensing the rising of the abdomen with each inhalation . . . and the falling back towards the spine with each exhalation . . . not needing to change the breath in any way. Just being with its natural flow . . .

- And now moving attention from the breath down through the pelvis through the legs all the way down to the feet and bringing attention to the toes . . . being with the sensations that are possible here in the toes . . . noticing any sensations you are encountering here . . . perhaps tingling or itching, there might be sensations of warmth or coolness, or other sensations . . . simply being with whatever is present here, right now . . . if you are not noticing any sensations at all, that is fine. Simply being with what is present in the toes however they are.

- Now, letting go of this part of the body and moving awareness from the toes to the soles of the feet . . . being with whatever sensations are present in the soles of both feet right now . . . and now moving attention to the tops of the feet . . . and now the ankles . . .

- We are not trying to create any particular experience. Just being with what is naturally happening right now. Sometimes we can notice that we are having certain expectations. If you notice this, simply be aware and as best as you can let them go, coming back to the bare sensations themselves.

- At the same time, you can become aware of the breathing . . . lying here, breathing, and being aware of the sensations in any particular part of the body.

- If you notice that your focus has wandered away, allowing yourself to notice this, for a brief moment, where attention has gone and then gently bringing your attention back to the area of the body we're focusing on.

- Now letting go of the feet and moving awareness to the lower legs. Feeling the contact of the lower legs with the floor . . . the pressure where the lower legs are making contact with the floor, perhaps also noticing sensations where the legs touch clothing, . . . whatever is present here right now . . . you may also be aware that there are part of the lower legs where there is no contact with the floor . . . simply being present . . . and now letting go of this part of the body.

- If you find the attention is being carried away by intense sensations and feelings in the body, give yourself permission to bring awareness to those sensations as they are present in the body right now. Noticing where they are located, how they feel. And then, when you're ready, coming back to wherever we are now directing attention in the body scan . . .

- Now moving awareness to the knees, the back of the knees, the knee caps . . . noticing whatever is present here, right now. Becoming aware of sensations with the knees, . . . and continuing up into the sensations in the thighs . . . feeling perhaps the contact of the thighs with the floor . . . noticing how the weight is distributed here . . . there might be feelings of warmth or coolness, . . . feelings of heaviness or lightness, perhaps, . . . some itching or tingling, or anything else . . . moving close to the sensations that you are encountering in this part of the body . . . being attentive to whatever is present.

- Now letting go of this part of the body and moving up into the pelvis . . . becoming aware of sensations in the buttocks. Feeling the weight of the buttocks and the pelvis on the floor . . . . encountering these sensations without any expectations and without any judgments if that's possible. There is no right way or wrong way to feel. This practice is about feeling whatever is present in this moment . . . now moving awareness to the lower belly, the abdomen . . . maybe aware of sensations of the internal organs, encountering movement within the body . . . breathing here with awareness of sensations.

- Now letting go of this part of the body and bringing awareness to the lower back. As you bring awareness to this part of the body you may notice that it may or may not be in contact with the floor . . . noticing any sensations in this region and meeting them with an attitude of curiosity and gentleness . . .

- Now continuing up into the middle and upper back . . . noticing those parts of the middle and upper back that are in contact with the ground . . . sensations of heaviness, lightness, warmth . . . how the weight is distributed . . . moving close to the sensations in the middle and upper back . . . meeting this region of the body with an openness and curiosity as if you had never met it before . . . learning to get to know the body the way it is feeling right now . . .

- Now, letting go of this region of the body and moving to the front, bringing awareness to the chest, the rib cage . . . aware of the movement of the rib cage with breathing, . . . perhaps even noticing the sensations of the heart beating. The heart, which is pumping blood through the body, . . . perhaps here also beginning to meet the body with a sense of gratitude for the work that it is doing for you, . . . and now letting go of the chest and rib cage . . . letting this part of the body dissolve in the field of attention . . .

- And moving attention toward the shoulders and the neck. This is a region of the body where we often accumulate a lot of tension. So, becoming aware of sensations of tension in this part of the body, or whatever sensations are here, warmth, tingling, heaviness, tightness or looseness, numbness, or ease . . .

- And now letting go of this part of the body and bringing awareness to the arms. Noticing sensations in the shoulders, and the arm pits, . . . those parts of the upper body that are in contact with the floor, . . . sensations in the elbows and lower arms, perhaps contact with clothing . . . now bringing awareness to the wrists, the hands and fingers, with the same attitude of curiosity encountering sensations in the hands and fingers, the thumbs . . . perhaps feeling moisture, tingling, or pulsation in the hands . . . whatever it is, just being here with the sensations as they are. Accepting them. No need to change anything. We are just getting in touch with reality as it is in this moment in this body.

- Now, letting go of this part of the body and moving awareness up into the head. Becoming aware of the contact of the head with the floor, . . . feeling the skin on the head . . . bringing awareness to the face, noticing sensations along the forehead, the eyebrows, and eyes, aware of any sensations of tension around the eyes, . . . possibly feelings of relaxation as you are lying here on the back . . . in a mode of being rather than doing . . . present to sensations in the cheeks, the nose, aware of sensations at the nostrils related to breathing, . . . and now feeling the lips, the tongue, inside the mouth, . . . and now moving attention outside the mouth, along the jaw, toward the ears, the earlobes, and now expanding awareness to include the entire face and head . . .

- And from here, slowly further expanding the field of awareness to include the body in its entirety . . . widening the field of awareness to include the face and head, the shoulders, the upper, middle, and lower torso, both arms and hands, the legs, and the feet, feeling the body in its entirety, whole . . . and also becoming aware of the flow of breath in the body, . . . there is nothing to be done right now . . . nowhere to go . . . just being here . . . being aware of what-ever is present in this moment as we are making the time for stepping out of the constant mode of doing as we are usually in and making time for just being here, . . . cultivating an awareness of the present moment . . . everything is just the way it . . . there is nothing that needs to be changed about this moment . . .

- And as we are ending this practice, expanding awareness further outside the body, as well, noticing sounds around you, the air surrounding you, . . . and if you had your eyes closed, slowly opening them, and gently bringing movement back to the body, wiggling the fingers and the toes, bringing movement into the arms and legs, . . . perhaps stretching out the entire body . . . you may wish to congratulate yourself, for having made the time for coming out of the constant mode of doing, making time for simply being, coming closer to the way you really are . . . complete and whole, just as you are . . .

RESPONDING VERSUS REACTING

One of the issues most often confusing to participants about the idea of thoughts, feelings, or bodily sensations as passing mental events is when to observe these or when something should be acted upon. As Michelle pointed out early on in the program: "I realize that my mind often blows things out of proportion, and then I get revved up and cannot stop think-ing about it. From that perspective, it makes a lot of sense to be observant and not jump into action mode. But then, is this what we are supposed to do with everything? Sometimes, things are real. You can't just observe everything and pretend it goes away by itself! Yesterday, for example, my daughter comes home from school crying and tells me that this teacher who has been picking on her for a while has called her out again. This has happened numerous times with this teacher. I don't like her to be treated like this. Now, am I supposed to just observe this and not do anything about it? This does not make sense." Jennifer had a similar experience: "Yesterday at the club, there was this girl at the front desk again. She is rude to everyone. Normally, I avoid interacting with her completely, but yesterday I needed to find out the e-mail for the person who deals with membership issues. So I asked, and from what I can tell, she was rude again."

Both Michelle and Jennifer have a common question that most, if not all, participants in this program encounter sooner or later: "When do I observe and when do I act? When do I treat a thought or a feeling as something 'real' or as a 'mental event'?" After all, there are real problems that need to be taken care of. We cannot treat a real problem as just "some mental event," observe it, and pretend it just goes away by itself (although sometimes this happens). Conflicts do come up and it makes sense to solve them when possible. However, not all thoughts blow things out of proportion. Sometimes, we are being treated unfairly, rudely, or with lack of respect. And letting everything sit there and not address some of it may make people feel frustrated and helpless. So when do you observe and when do you act? Moments such as those described by Michelle and Jennifer are an opportunity for participants to bring mindfulness to them, by observing how the blood rushes and the knot in the stomach when one gets angry or noticing the frustration and the bodily sensations that come with it. Or perhaps even noting the reaction tendency to want to yell and scream, "No, you cannot treat me this way." And, as participants bring mindfulness to these difficult moments, they gradually gain the freedom of responding rather than reacting.

As Jennifer pointed out later in the program, "It has become a very different experience for me when I deal with upsetting situations now, compared to how it used to be. Take the front desk situation: I would tell the woman with a tense voice that this is not acceptable to me and that I would like to speak with the manager. He would then talk to me and try to smooth the situation over and I would feel that I am not being heard again. I would just get more upset and angry, and that would stick with me all day. These days, when I have a moment like this, I try to let the rush of anger cool off. It is actually kind of an interesting experience when you see this coming on and the thoughts kicking, the blood rushing, and the cramp in my stomach that I have learned is so indicative of me getting started again. Observing this interestingly creates this distance between me and the situation. Trying to resolve or address it in that moment has never yielded much other than me getting more upset and angry. This does not mean that I necessarily let it slide. But it helps me to address it in a way that is more productive for me, calmer, perhaps more solution-oriented. I actually ended up talking to the manager at some later point and asked him what was up with this girl at the front desk who seemed to be rude to almost anybody. He then ended up telling me in confidence that lots of people have already complained about her and that they were in the process of addressing it. I am sure that this is not anything he would or could say when he is being called in to mediate the acute situation when I am fuming!"

In the moment, when something is happening we ask participants to bring mindfulness to it, so that they are aware of what is happening. This puts them in a much better position to make a decision about what to do. This is what is referred to as "responding." Our usual way of dealing with things is reacting—using highly ingrained, overlearned ways of dealing with a situation that are handy. We quickly "react" either because this is what we have learned from previous situations or because of an innate tendency to react that way. Therefore, mindfulness can be a powerful tool to change from reacting to responding, no matter whether a thought is blowing things out of proportion or a conflict is real.

HOMEWORK

For homework we ask participants to continue with their Mood Diary and begin to pay attention to warning signs (Handouts 5 and 8). Increased moment-by-moment awareness as practiced by the Introduction to the Breathing Space when participants switch from one activity to the next, as well as mindfulness to routine activities are meant to support this process of raising awareness toward warning signs. Should warning signs arise, participants are directed to contact the instructor. Action plans for how to deal with warning signs will be developed in the next session. As a formal exercise, participants are asked to make daily time for the Body Scan that was practiced in session (audio track 3) and record their experiences (Handout 7). As with the Yoga–Body Scan, we work with participants to map out when and where participants would like to do the Body Scan exercise (Handout 6). The session ends with doing an Introduction to the Breathing Space.

The End of the Honeymoon

PARTICIPANT HANDOUTS FOR SESSION 3

- Handout 5: Mood Diary (in case a participant forgot to bring his or hers)
  - Handout 7: Homework Sheet
  - Handout 8: Worksheet for Warning Signs and Action Plans
  - Handout 9: Worksheet for Trigger Situations
  - Handout 15, p. 1: What Can I Do When I Start Feeling Down or Depressed?
  - Handout 20, p. 1: What Should I Do When I Notice Warning Signs for Mania?

ABOUT THIS SESSION

If you just sit and observe, you will see how restless your mind is. If you try to calm it, it only makes it worse, but over time it does calm, and when it does, there's room to hear more subtle things—that's when your intuition starts to blossom and you start to see things more clearly and be in the present more. Your mind just slows down, and you see a tremendous expanse in the moment.
—STEVE JOBS (in Isaacson, 2011, p. 253)

With the third session, participants have gotten an idea of what it means to practice mindfulness, as well as the time and effort that comes with participating in this program. With "realism" rising ("The end of the honeymoon"), we have seen the first participants miss sessions, come late, or not attend at all. Some participants have practiced a lot, while others have barely gotten around to doing any of the exercises. The third session is often a critical juncture in the program because disappointed participants are at risk of dropping out. Therefore, continued support, encouragement, and problem solving around the obstacles encountered by participants are part of today's session. In terms of group exercises, we introduce the Mindfulness of the Breath Exercise after practicing the Body Scan. Participants continue to work on raising everyday awareness (mindfulness to routine activities and Breathing Space) including detecting warning signs for mania or depression. In this session they develop action plans about what to do when warning signs arise. In addition, we go one step beyond warning signs and ask participants to begin their journey of becoming more aware of factors ("triggers") that contribute to the occurrence of warning signs. Recordings for home practice after this session include Mindfulness of the Breath (audio track 4) and the 3-Minute Breathing Space (audio track 5).

WELCOME BACK AND MOOD DIARY CHECK

As in the previous week, before the start of the group, the instructor briefly checks each participant's Mood Diary individually and inquires how things are going. This check-in will become a routine over the coming weeks as participants return to the weekly group meetings. If signs of hypomania and mania are noted, the instructor assesses the participant's ability to participate in the group. If able, he or she may briefly discuss with the participant how to be with the experience during the group meeting (see guidelines for how to be mindful with symptoms of mania, Session 6 and Handout 20). For example, after she had smoked marijuana in the week before the group meeting, Sara became manic (see Chapter 4). She was enthusiastic and wanted to share her experience about how mindfulness was "helping her through her manic phase." The instructor also suspected that the conversations in the group would provide Sara with stimulation that would increase her urge to talk. Therefore, Sara and her instructor decided to bring mindfulness to this urge (observe where it is located in the body, with curiosity but without following it). Sara and the instructor also agreed that he or she may at times redirect her to mindfulness when she might talk in group for too long.

OBSTACLES

For most of the obstacles participants encounter, instructors simply ask participants to bring awareness to the moment that may get them derailed and problem-solve with them around priorities and memory issues to ensure participants are on time and get a sufficient "dose" of practice (see Chapter 4: Individual Sessions, as well as Sessions 1 and 2). But what can we do if participants, despite their best efforts, do not seem to "get around" to the formal or informal exercises? Two common scenarios involve "doing too well" and "going through a rough time."

"Doing Too Well"

Scott had been very excited about the program at the outset. He had been diagnosed with bipolar disorder relatively recently, following a manic episode that landed him in the hospital. The year after his manic episode had been difficult, with lots of mood swings. At the time when he signed on with the program, he had been doing very well for quite a while, took his medication regularly, had few, if any, side effects, and felt that things were on a good trajectory. He had been excited about the idea of "doing something for himself such as yoga and meditation." But when it came to practicing, he barely "found the time" to do the yoga exercise, body scans, or take the time to do the Breathing Space, even when he was aware of it. "Whenever I think about it, I just don't feel like doing it, because I just feel fine," he said, when we discussed the issue in an individual session.

Indeed, if a participant's mood is really stable, and he or she has not experienced that this stability may be a temporary break before things get worse again, an important motivator for mindfulness may be missing. While the idea of mindfulness, preventing relapse, and mood stability may resonate "intellectually," at the same time it is harder to connect with it "emotionally." Also, participants who "feel well," may not want to get reminded about mood symptoms, warning signs, and triggers (i.e., it feels aversive). This is one of the things that MBCT does. What can the participant and the instructor do? For example, one could simply acknowledge the fact that it is more difficult to see the benefit when things are going well, but that this is exactly the reason why this time of well-being is the time to get mindfulness on board. More often, however, we have found ourselves "redefining the target," like deemphasizing mood and warning signs (while keeping them on the radar), and emphasizing the observance of daily thoughts, feelings, and sensations in the service of learning to relate to those differently. This redirection can also include learning how to deal differently with a work assignment one may not like or relating to the frustration about a date that did not go well. Redefining the intention of the mindfulness practice for this participant may help him or her to gain skills for how to buffer stress or to cope with daily hassles, no matter what it does for bipolar disorder. In our experience, it is most important to find the subjective tangible benefit that resonates with a participant to keep him or her engaged in the program. At times, compromising on formal exercises is what happens. Scott stayed in the program but focused on Breathing Spaces. Only when some mood symptoms returned did the value of longer sitting meditations began to resonate with him.

"Going through a Rough Time"

For Lindsay, her mood became labile shortly after she started the program. "Not sure what it is," she said "but everything seems to set me off." Lindsay started to experience mixed mood symptoms (symptoms of both depression and mania), which can be extremely difficult to tolerate. She would feel depressed and irritable at the same time, as well as keyed up, wired, and as if she had been plugged into an outlet. Her thoughts felt speeded and jumpy. "I can't deal with this anymore, this is just too much," she confessed when she met with the instructor individually after the second week. While she tried to do the Yoga and Body Scans, she would usually give up after a few minutes. "Everything just feels too overwhelming at this point," she said. In response to her distress, Lindsay's psychiatrist added medications to her mix of drugs. For Lindsay, the Breathing Space became her "lifesaver." She and the instructor practiced the Full Breathing Space in the individual session. Being able to ground herself by attaching her attention to the breath and following it with a single focus became a way of finding something to hold on to in the midst of inner turmoil. Her symptoms continued for weeks. Only slowly and gradually would things begin to calm down as she and her instructor jointly refined the Breathing Space for her. She would practice to stay "out of racing thoughts" and "let painful feelings in" as they unfolded. "Breathing Spaces 24/7 is what I did," she announced when looking back to that period. "The anchoring was most important, but then learning not trying to fight all this turmoil was the hardest. It is difficult to see at the beginning, but if you hang in there, things will calm down eventually."

BODY SCAN

At the beginning of this session, the group practices the Body Scan exercise (see Session 2, Box 2.1, for the instructions) without any lead-in yoga phase. As with the Yoga–Body Scan, we discuss participants' more immediate experiences with the Body Scan in today's session first before discussing the issues that may have come up doing the Body Scan as part of their homework. The instructor can provide general guidance as follows: When the mind wanders away, and you become aware of it, note where the mind has wandered and then gently redirect attention toward the body part that is in focus. If negative, self-critical thoughts arise, or if you find yourself getting caught up in rumination, simply notice where the thoughts have gone, label this as a thought, and then gently redirect the attention to the body part in focus. Likewise, when feelings or sensations arise that call attention in the body, bring gentle and curious attention to the raw sensation, observing this sensation for a while before gently shifting the attention back to the body part in focus. Do not try to block out or disregard that sensation if it is still there, but allow it to be there as it is while following the exercise. The following themes typically come up for the Body Scan.

Mindwandering

A common occurrence during the Body Scan is thoughts wandering away from the focus of the exercise. As this happens, we simply ask participants to determine what thoughts were present at that moment and to view them as mental events unfolding in the mind. We also ask them to pay attention to the moment when the thoughts wandered away from the body part that is "under" investigation: becoming curious about that very moment when the thoughts begin to wander. What do participants notice? Each time a participant is or becomes aware that his or her thoughts have wandered away, we invite him or her to curiously note where the mind has wandered and what the thought is saying: labeling the thought as a mental event (e.g., "thinking about dinner later"), and then gently redirecting the attention toward the body part that is the focus of the observation as part of the Body Scan. Participants may have to repeat this process of becoming aware, noting, labeling, and redirecting their attention as many times as this process occurs.

Negative Thoughts and Judgments

"This was like the beginning of yoga all over again," Michelle said, when asked about how she experienced the Body Scan. "I was not sure whether I was doing it right, and then, at times, I did not know what to do when certain sensations came up." Experiences such as those described by Michelle are a welcomed opportunity to explore and highlight thoughts as mental events. As we probed further, Michelle described that after the initial thought ("Am I doing this right?") the thoughts had gone on to putting her down, saying "that she could not even do a simple exercise bringing attention to her body parts," "this should be easy," and "I am the one making it complicated again." Note, that instructors, unlike in cognitive-behavioral therapy, will not attempt to challenge the content of thoughts. They simply praise participants for becoming "aware" that these thoughts were present during the exercise, label them as a mental event that can be observed, and invite them, at that moment, to continue to curiously observe what the mind is "saying" and where it is going like this. Labeling thoughts can be done by saying to oneself that there is a "self-critical negative thought occurring in the mind" or a "thought that tries to put one down."

We highlight that part of the reasons why we are practicing things such as yoga or the Body Scan is because they tend to provide us with some of the experiences that we want to learn to become more mindful about, such as negative thoughts, distressing feelings, and uncomfortable sensations. From this perspective, this is setting the stage for bringing observance to those mental and bodily events that occur during the exercise. After having brought observance to the negative, self-critical thought, participants can simply return to the body part that is now being observed, in order to continue with the exercise. But whenever a negative or self-critical thought occurs in the mind, and one is becoming aware of it, one should simply repeat the exercise of recognizing and labeling the self-critical thought as a mental event.

"But what if the thought is real?" Michelle asked. "Often I do feel that I can't get things right and this is really frustrating." This moment may be tempting for instructors to ask more about how she is doing the exercise to confirm that she is actually doing it "correctly." In this program, we simply ask her to treat this thought as a mental event, that may occur whether or not she is doing the exercise right. The thought is a mental event that she can learn to recognize, observe, and to disengage from regardless of whether it is right or wrong, real or not.

Rumination and Worry

"I could not concentrate on the Body Scan at all," Veronica confessed, looking frustrated and disappointed. "I just kept thinking about 'what if I can't get this proposal of an advertisement right.' The whole day, I have been going over what I should do, how to make this right for the meeting tomorrow, but I am not sure, and I don't think it is good enough. I tried to concentrate on paying attention to my legs, but I just kept wondering about tomorrow, and how the meeting will go." As in the case of negative thoughts, the instructor greeted Veronica's experience with a warm welcome and as an opportunity to observe rumination when it is present. We maintain the stance of curiosity, wanting to know more about the rumination. "What was the mind saying?" "What kinds of thoughts were there?" Veronica noticed that she was talking back and forth from trying to reassure herself that it would be OK, to her mind asking "What if it is not?" This was intermixed with thoughts such as "I can't deal with this anymore" and "This is never going to end."

In general, in these kind of moments, we encourage participants to bring curiosity to the mind and to what it is saying at that moment, and to take the opportunity to observe the mechanics of their rumination. We also ask them to bring curiosity to the negative thought that the rumination or worry is trying to resolve. For Veronica, implicitly woven into the stream of rumination and worry was the "fear" that what she would present the next day would be met with criticism, her boss would put her down, and that she would receive a bad evaluation. This, again, is a mental event, and raising awareness toward the negative (or catastrophic) thought that is embedded in the stream of rumination or worry is an important step in the process of learning to disengage. As with self-critical negative judgments, after bringing curious observance to it and acknowledging the thoughts as mental events, we then ask participants to simply bring their attention back to the body part that is being felt/observed, and to repeat the process whenever they find rumination carrying them away from the exercise.

Positive Rumination

"I could not stop thinking about the date I am having tomorrow," Sean described. "I am so excited. My mind just kept going over how fabulous this will be and felt the excitement just sizzling in my body." That week,

Sean's mood had been elevated. It did not just stop at being excited and not being able to stop thinking about the date he was having. With his mind playing the dating scenario, he felt euphoric, full of anticipation, and eager to talk. This all also became part of his Body Scan experience. As with negative rumination or worry, once participants become aware that their minds have wandered, they should begin to observe where it has gone, what the thought is saying, label it as a mental event, and then redirect the attention to the body part that is being observed at that time. We also asked Sean to bring direct observance to the "wanting to engage in the thought." For Sean, the thought about the date was highly pleasant. The fantasy about the date was desirable. When his mind began to wander, we asked him to bring curious observance to that feeling in his body, the pleasure, anticipation, and wanting. Where was that located? With what sensations did it come? How was it expressed in his body? For Sean, the Body Scan exercise this week became an exercise of allowing himself to observe the pull, the sensations associated with wanting but without engaging in it. He then also began to gently redirect himself away from pleasurable images and thoughts that his mind might send him in anticipation of his date, rather than engaging with them. "Now does this mean I can never think about pleasurable things?" he asked. Not at all. This skill of being able to observe the wanting for pleasure without getting tangled up in it and being able to disengage from the mind creating pleasurable and tempting scenarios is central when one is vulnerable to developing mood elevation. This is not meant as a skill to abandon all pleasurable activities at all times.

Painful Sensations

Just as paying attention to physical sensations is at the heart of the Body Scan, sooner or later, uncomfortable or painful sensations will arise. As Taylor pointed out, "Paying attention to the body really brings my joint pain to the forefront, and this is really hard to take." Naturally, there is the tendency of not wanting to be uncomfortable or of wanting to get away from uncomfortable sensations. In this exercise, we ask participants to take an observational stance, bringing awareness to the region that is calling attention and to pay attention to the raw sensations that are unfolding in that particular region in the body. We ask "What kind of a pain is this?", "Is it sharp, dull, or throbbing?", "How is it over time as one continues to pay attention?" Often, pain or uncomfortable sensations trigger thoughts about the pain. "It feels like I can't deal with this anymore especially on those days where it is bad." It is important to also notice when thoughts about the pain have taken the mind away from the actual task of observing the raw sensation. They should note the rumination that may unfold at that moment, but then, in the spirit of the exercise, gently and deliberately bring themselves back to the task at hand, observing the body part that is currently in focus.

Being Irritated, Anxious, or Bored

"I got really irritated with this," Jennifer complained. "I could not keep my attention on the body and it kept wandering off." When this complaint was explored further, she described this "feeling of frustration" rising when she had to bring her attention back to the body after her thoughts had wandered, with her frustration rising each time she had to do it again. The exploration went to where this was located in her body, how it felt, what type of sensations were associated with it, their time course, and so on. When sensations or feelings are dominant in the body, as they were for Jennifer, we guide our participants to bring curious attention to it. This is similar to the Raisin Exercise, where they approach the familiar raisin with a renewed sense of curiosity as if they had never experienced it before. But they also want to recognize that this may be difficult (i.e., aversive; see also the topic of attachment and aversion in Session 4). Therefore, we ask them to practice self-care, to respect their own boundaries, and to be aware of what they can do at a given time.

The same is true for feelings of anxiety or boredom if they call atten- tion to the body. Especially at the beginning, allowing oneself to observe uncomfortable and perhaps anxiety-provoking sensations in the body is easier when one gives him- or herself permission to step out of the exer- cise at any time or go back to the body as a whole. For some participants, thoughts dominate when anger, irritation, or anxiety arise. If this is the case, they should begin to observe these thoughts as mental events, noting their content, perhaps even the pattern they display (always, again) and then to gently redirect themselves to the body part that is being observed at the time.

Whenever a participant experiences frustration, anger, anxiety, or symptoms of mood elevation at the time of the group meeting, during an exercise, or during discussion, this always opens the door to practice mindfulness exploration right in that moment. It can be challenging and require skill to help the participant become aware of what is going on in that moment. For example, when Jennifer became frustrated and angry during the Body Scan, she initially remained in that mode during the dis- cussion. "Observing my toes, what is this good for? I don't get this." "I am sensing some annoyance, is this right?" the instructor asked (signaling that he understood where Jennifer was coming from). "Yes, you do," she said, with an edgy tone in her voice. "Forgive me for asking," the instructor responded, "but because we are practicing being with uncomfortable and difficult feelings and thoughts without getting tangled up in them, would you give us permission to explore what you are noticing in your body right now?" With this response, the instructor signaled to Jennifer that he understood that she was frustrated in this moment. He also briefly gave her an explanation of why he wanted to explore this frustration and anger further and also asked for Jennifer's permission to do this with her (he gave control back to her). This, in turn, helped Jennifer to step out of her anger enough to start the process of exploration.

Using this opportunity, we then started to look in detail into how her frustration and anger during the exercise had risen to the point that she "snapped" during the discussion. First, she noticed frustration and the sensations associated with it, told herself she should observe, and had thoughts occurring about "how stupid this was." Then, she redirected herself back to the body part in focus, getting more frustrated when her thoughts wandered away again. This was followed by angry thoughts, "Why she was not able to do even such simple thing such as watching her knee, and that nothing worked in her life and this class was no different." Having the opportunity in class to explore this cascade of feelings, sensations, and thoughts, and to see the anger autopilot unfold is a gift. For Jennifer, discovering this sequence was eye-opening. After the group meeting, she spoke to the instructor individually and was thankful. "This is what happens to me all the time. I get annoyed, cannot shake it off, and then I snap. I can see the value in learning to not only become more aware of it when it happens, but to also learn to step aside into observational mode and not get involved."

When Feelings Are Intense

When feelings and sensations in the body are intense and aversive, and one does not want to feel them, taking an observational stance and approaching that sensation with a sense of curiosity is a difficult task. It will get easier over time, but at the beginning it can be overwhelming. Wanting to avoid those feelings and sensations is the normal way of dealing with anything that is intense and uncomfortable. As we introduce this different way of approaching uncomfortable bodily experiences, we convey the message that there is nothing dangerous about having uncomfortable sensations or feelings in the body. At the same time, the instructions emphasize perceived control: guiding participants to respect their boundaries and to be gentle with themselves as they are engaging in this exercise—this act of self-compassion is especially important when experiences are distressing and difficult. They give themselves permission to go away from the sensation, widening the attentional window to the whole body, or, perhaps, stepping out of the exercise altogether. In our experience, this sets the stage for participants' willingness to observe and approach what they would ordinarily much rather avoid and begin the process of exploration that will continue throughout the rest of the program (see Session 5: Emotion-Focused Meditations).

Going back to an anchor in moments that feel overwhelming is another element. As part of the Body Scan (and later in this session Mindfulness of the Breath and the 3-Minute Breathing Space) the breath serves as an anchor to which participants may always return. Attaching their attention to the breath and following each inhale and each exhale until they feel ready to open the attentional window again and perhaps approach the feeling and its sensation again with a renewed sense of curiosity. If using the breath is anxiety-provoking (as it can be for participants with panic disorder), they can use sounds as another anchor, such as the ticking of the clock, or some noise that is present outside that one can closely follow.

Becoming Relaxed and Falling Asleep

When the Body Scan does come with strong sensations, feelings, or rumination, it is commonly praised for its relaxing quality and ability to help participants fall asleep. Yet, as we (and other programs) to point out, this is not the purpose of the exercise.

> *Instructor*: "As desirable as relaxation or sleep is, we are not doing the Body Scan for these reasons. To the contrary, the purpose of the exercise is to observe physical sensations and whatever else arises in the body at the time, such as thoughts or feelings. From that perspective, the purpose of observation is the observation itself. There is no other goal we are trying to achieve. Now, we may be able to observe feeling relaxed, or we may observe becoming sleepy, but at the heart of this exercise is learning to directly observe raw physical sensations that arise in our bodies at any given moment. Imagine you start doing this exercise because you often become relaxed, and there is one day when you don't. Let's say you become frustrated and tense in that moment after trying too hard. What we will ask you to do in that moment is to bring attention to the sensations that are associated with it, and ask you to observe this, without doing anything else with it. We may also ask you to become more aware of the intention you are setting when you are doing the Body Scan ('I am doing this to become relaxed'). As you can see, the heart of the exercise is observation itself, to physical sensations, or in the broader sense, whatever else arises in a given moment."

BREATHING SPACE AND MINDFULNESS
TO ROUTINE ACTIVITIES

Breathing Space

Following the discussion of the Body Scan, we explore participants' experiences with the Breathing Space when they shift from one activity to the next. Are participants finding themselves getting reminded about coming into the present and doing the Breathing Space when they switch from one activity to the next? Or are they still mainly relying on external reminders? What have they noticed when doing the exercise? During the process of exploration with the group the instructor should keep a few key ideas in mind.

1. At this point of the program, with regular Breathing Space practice, participants should find themselves becoming increasingly reminded by themselves to come into the present when they shift from one activity to the next. For some participants this occurs faster, but for others it takes more time. One way to foster this process is to attach this exercise to shifts that occur every day, thereby ensuring the regularity with which the exercise is done. Reminder cues work by association. That is, if one does an activity in a certain place at a certain time every day, then the context (place, time) will begin to serve as a reminder cue itself. Therefore, one should choose activities that happen every day and do the Breathing Space after the first activity and before starting the second activity. This way the place and time, but also the act of ending the first activity, will begin to remind the participant to do the Breathing Space and come into the present. If this process is not unfolding, then selecting designated pairs of activities (e.g., activity 1: brushing teeth, then activity 2: taking a shower) and placing reminders to cue the Breathing Space (e.g., sticky note on the mirror). If these external reminders are still needed, it also helps to change those once in a while. The sticky note on the mirror will lose its reminding quality if it has been ignored.

2. Reasons abound for not doing the Breathing Space. Even with a brief and simple exercise such as the Breathing Space, the mind may find reasons to not want to do it, such as having no time, being in a rush, or other things feeling more important than pausing in that moment. If this happens, we simply ask participants to note what is going on in that moment. For example, if they are pressed for time, what thoughts are there in that moment, how does it feel in their bodies? Pausing in that moment and checking in with themselves as they find themselves "not wanting to do the exercise" is doing the very exercise they are "not wanting to do."

3. It is not unusual for participants to modify this exercise in some ways that work better for them. For example, several participants in our groups took a deep breath when they got reminded about checking in with themselves. The breath then became the cue to switch to an observational mode. These modifications are fine. The purpose of the exercise is to come into the present and to notice what thoughts, feelings, and sensations are present right then and there. The way this is achieved, from our perspective, is not important.

4. For participants who continue to have difficulties getting around to the formal exercises (Yoga–Body Scan, Body Scan), we try to maximize the frequency of the Breathing Space Exercise. The more they do it during the day, the better it is. We also try to reduce guilt and keep motivation up; if participants feel they are failing in the program, they may drop out of group. Therefore, if it becomes clear that a participant, for whatever reason and with all the provided help, is not getting to the formal exercises, then maximizing the informal exercises is what we do. One of the central purposes of mindfulness is to learn to recognize and disengage from difficult thoughts and feelings that may worsen depression or lead into hypomania. Which vehicles that ultimately help participants to achieve this goal is not important.

Mindfulness to Routine Activities

The experiences associated with paying attention to a particular activity range from "time slowing down," "the moment being richer," and "noticing things one did not notice before" to "getting distracted" and "falling into old habits."

As Daniel described, who had chosen to be mindful when brushing his teeth, "You begin to notice all the sensations that come with the brush rubbing your teeth and your gums. The pressure, sometimes more, sometimes less. And also the taste of the toothpaste is much more vivid. And time seems to slow down, as you are only focusing on this one task." He also noted the tendency to go back to the old way of doing it. "Inadvertently, you find yourself speeding up, after you slowed down initially," Daniel said. "It just happens, and then suddenly you realize that you are back to the old way of brushing your teeth." Michael had the same experience after choosing eating his lunch. "The flavors were much more colorful compared to my usual way of eating." Usually, Michael would read the newspaper online while eating lunch to keep up to date with what was happening in the world. "Now, I sit there with my meal and nothing else, and you pay attention to every bite, you notice the texture of the food much more than before. But then, all of a sudden you find yourself getting distracted, thinking about something you need to do after lunch, and all of a sudden you are back to your old way of eating. Having sped up, not really paying attention what you are doing."

When participants describe becoming aware of getting derailed during the exercise, we simply ask them to come back into the moment and renew their effort to pay direct attention to the activity they are doing. Experiences such as those shared by Daniel, and Michael are also used to connect the exercise back to the goal of mindfulness. The goals to purposefully pay attention to the moment in order to be able to know what is going on. This way, participants will learn to detect warning signs for depression and hypomania/mania earlier and will have a chance to intervene. Likewise, as discussed later, going beyond warning signs and becoming aware of thoughts, feelings, and behaviors may prevent the mood from spiraling out of control. As part of their homework, we ask participants to choose another routine activity and be mindful with it the same way they did it in the previous weeks. For participants who had difficulties remembering, the strategies outlined in Sessions 1 and 2 should be used to increase the likelihood that they will follow through.

MOOD DIARY: WARNING SIGNS AND ACTION PLANS

Next, the group turns their attention to warning signs and action plans. In the last session participants included their own warning signs for hypomania/mania and depression in Handout 8 (Worksheet for Warning Signs and Action Plans). As in the last session, group members pair up and discuss whether (1) they became aware of any warning signs they had not noticed before (if yes, they should be included in the Mood Diary), and (2) whether participants encountered any warning signs during the week and how they handled those.

For Brian, paying attention to his warning signs paid off in the previous week. "I am often under pressure to review things quickly, because the contracts need to go out, and they are usually time-sensitive. Of course people are getting them late to me and then expect me to turn them around in just a few days. This is something that often makes me irritable. And there is a point when I start stewing. Not just being annoyed, stewing. I had noticed this before, but not spelled it out that clearly, as we did in group last week. With several days like this, I typically spiral down into depression. Hating my job, my life, and so forth. Now, given that I am doing this program, I figured I need to do something. Just calling in sick would make me feel guilty. So that is not a good solution. I ended up talking to my boss and told her that I am not feeling well and won't be able to get all those contracts done in time. We worked it out so that some of my colleagues picked some contracts up, and this way I felt OK about it."

In this session, participants begin to develop action plans for periods when warning signs for hypomania/mania or depression come up using Handout 8 and the white board. Elements of an action plan are first discussed among participants as pairs, and then discussed with the whole group. We typically write all the elements on the white board, thereby creating a master plan that can then be individualized with each participant during the individual sessions. The action plan typically specifies (1) when it should be initiated (e.g., after the second night of difficulties falling asleep and increased activity levels) and (2) concrete behavioral guidelines (i.e., "What do I do when warning signs arise?").

Action Plans for Mood Elevation

The purpose of setting the action plan in motion at the time when warning signs arise is to prevent warning signs from spiraling into full-blown hypomania or mania. Common warning signs for mania include increased energy, feeling overly confident, increased motivation to engage in pleasurable activities (i.e., increased reward sensitivity), feeling "plugged in," "wired," or irritable, speeded or jumpy thoughts, developing plans on the spur, having more ideas, the mind being quicker and more fluid, feeling more talkative, talking more than usual, "odd thinking" (e.g., more paranoid); things (people, activities, topics) starting to have special meanings (e.g., religion), having (more) difficulties falling asleep or staying asleep, or reduced need for sleep. When these symptoms set in, participants should do the following (see Handout 20):

Behavioral Strategies
- Contact group instructor and psychiatrist; investigate medication options.
- Reduce activities.
- Do something that requires little thinking and focus (e.g., watching movies, gardening, taking a walk, listening to music, reading if you can).
- Reduce stimulation—avoid doing things that require a lot of task switching.
- No multitasking. Do one task at a time.
- If needed, give up access to pleasurable web activities.
- Surrender your credit card and passwords (better safe than sorry).

- Have other people change your passwords.
- Try not to act on anger/irritability even though you may feel that your anger/irritation is justified. This does not mean that you cannot take action at a later stage, but acting on anger often increases irritability for the day.
- Do Breathing Spaces.

Implementing these behavioral changes can be challenging because they may make participants feel uncomfortable. Not going out, even though one really wants to, can come with feeling bored or sad ("Why can't I?"). Likewise, a participant may notice that he or she wants to "spend" energy but "can't," now being stuck with the feeling of excess energy. Likewise, if "odd thinking" comes up (feeling paranoid or that things have special meaning), it is often difficult for participants to see these as "mental events" ("But it does feel real!"). If warning signs arise, participants will work with their coaches to bring mindfulness to these experiences in addition to implementing the behavioral aspects of the action plans (e.g., Breathing Space; strategies for being mindful with difficult feelings and thoughts—see guidelines about how to be mindful with signs of mood elevation (Session 6).

Action Plans for Depression

Warning signs for depression commonly include an increased lack of motivation, lack of energy, feeling tired or sluggish, decreased interest in activities, decreased interest in food/eating, self-critical thinking, feeling guilty or worthless, caring less, ruminating about how bad things are, more difficulties concentrating, talking less to people, withdrawing from people and activities, thoughts that life is not worth living, hopelessness, suicidal thoughts (starting up or increasing in frequency), increased sleep difficulties (falling or staying asleep), or feeling tense or irritable. When these symptoms set in (or worsen), participants should do the following (see Handout 15):

Behavioral Strategies

- If possible, increase your activities—choose simple things, nothing complicated. Do something that used to be fun, might be fun, or gets you involved in some activity. This is not the time to shoot for major accomplishments! Getting small things accomplished is key! Do things that are soothing to you.
- If it is hard to focus, do something that requires little thinking and

focus (e.g., watching movies, gardening, taking a walk, listening to music, reading).

- Irritability can be part depression. As with manic symptoms, if you feel irritable, coach yourself not to express anger/irritability to others even though you may feel that your anger/irritation is justified. This does not mean that you cannot take action at a later stage, but acting on anger often increases irritability for the day.
- If your mind tends to ruminate (going over things repeatedly), choose simple activities that get you involved in something (gentle, mindful redirection coupled with engaging in tasks tends to work best for rumination).
- Remember, doing something that you may not feel like doing is difficult! Give yourself credit for trying!!

Although positive activities and mindfulness with positive activities is systematically practiced starting in Session 8, participants who are depressed at this point in the program start activity scheduling as part of their individual sessions from the beginning (see Chapter 4). Participants who notice increases in depressive symptoms will be directed to increase their activities, as behavioral activation is one of the most effective treatment strategies for depression. Even though participants may have only practiced mindfulness for a few weeks (or possibly not at all), if depression symptoms arise, we work with participants to bring mindfulness to them (for guidelines, see Session 5 and Handout 5).

When Action Plans Aren't Set in Motion

Most of the participants who have encountered multiple episodes of depression and/or hypomania/mania have an implicit plan about what to do when their symptoms get worse. Often, however, these plans do not materialize or are set in motion way too late. This is particularly true for episodes of hypomania or mania. Why? For one, increasing mood-stabilizing medications often comes with feeling drowsy and sedated. Some of them (especially second-generation antipsychotic medications) carry the risk for weight gain. Both effects are typically not welcomed. Participants also may fear losing a good stretch (if hypomania is pleasurable, not irritable). They may feel overconfident that they will be able to handle it or think that mood elevation will calm down by itself. Some have difficulties discriminating feeling good from feeling too good. When considering whether to set action plans in motion, one or more of these issues can prevent someone from getting in touch with his or her psychiatrist. Increased feelings of depression, on the other hand, may prompt requests to boost (or start) "antidepressants" quickly, although the efficacy of "antidepressant" medication for bipolar disorder is largely undetermined.

When action plans are discussed as part of the group discussion, we ask participants what kind of emergency plans they implicitly (or explicitly) had in the past (if any) and what has kept them from exercising them. As part of the discussion we highlight the following thought patterns as mental events and potential obstacles to successfully implementing action plans.

- Fear of side effects
- Fear of losing a good stretch
- Feeling overconfident that one can handle it
- Thinking it goes away by itself
- Difficulties recognizing elevated mood (feels "normal")

We alert participants to the pattern of these thoughts: (1) minimizing (I can handle it—mood elevation) or magnifying the consequences ("I won't be able to handle it"—depression), and (2) subjectively minimizing or magnifying the likelihood of the consequences ("It will go away by itself"; "I will go downhill from here for sure"). Note, however, rather than challenging these patterns (as would be done in cognitive-behavioral therapy), we simply ask participants to direct their awareness to these thought patterns and their potential consequences as they try to weigh their options whether to contact their psychiatrist and/or group instructor.

MINDFULNESS OF THE BREATH

Next the group begins the first formal sitting meditation, which is Mindfulness of the Breath. Participants may sit either on a chair or a meditation cushion, crossing their legs. Most important, however, is that participants find an erect, yet comfortable position. For participants with back pain, sitting with the back against a wall may provide additional support. This exercise will be brief at the beginning (10–15 minutes). In class we briefly discuss the experiences participants have with this exercise (see beginning of Session 4 for common discussion points). Especially for participants with bipolar disorder who have concentration issues (sustaining focus for a longer period of time), it can be aversive to do this sitting meditation for a longer period of time. While aversion is something that can be observed (see Session 4), if the exercise is too aversive at the beginning, participants may avoid it altogether. Therefore, for homework we ask participants to start with a duration that feels doable. For homework, participants are asked to start this sitting meditation once per day. Gradually they can stretch the practice time a little longer each time they practice (i.e., ignore the end of the recorded instructions and continue with observing the breath). Alternatively, participants have also done two or three briefer practice times at the beginning of learning the practice before doing longer sitting meditations.

Box 3.1. Mindfulness of the Breath (10 Minutes)

(Note for the instructor: [. . .] indicates a pause.)

- Taking a comfortable sitting position. Sitting on the floor on a cushion or on a blanket that you can fold up a couple of times. Sitting comfortably upright, with the spine straight but not rigid. Allowing the knees to sink down toward the ground, with the legs comfortably folded. Or you might choose to sit on a chair, if that feels better to you.

- And now bringing awareness to the legs and feet, becoming aware of the contact points of the legs and feet with the ground or chair, . . . feeling them sink into the ground. Allowing their weight to sink into gravity.

- Bringing awareness now to the hips. You may wish to slightly tilt the pelvis forward, so that the back can rise out of the stable position of the pelvis. Allowing the spine to lengthen and the shoulders to soften . . . Having the head in a dignified and balanced position, with the chin slightly lowered toward the collarbone, so that the neck and upper back are in an upright position and the chest can open up to the front.

- You can have the hands either resting on the knees or folded in your lap. Letting the weight of the arms and the hands sink into the legs . . . And now bringing awareness to the face, allowing the face to soften, allowing the mouth, the tongue and lips to relax, and relaxing the eyes, having the eyelids closed if that's comfortable for you. Allowing the forehead to relax and soften.

- And now bringing awareness to breathing. Feeling the way the breath naturally flows into the body, and the way the breath leaves the body. Loosening the belly, so the breath can naturally flow into the belly without any hindrance . . . Just becoming aware of the natural flow of the breath, without changing or modifying it in any way . . . letting it flow and being aware of the way it flows . . . Coming into direct contact with each inhalation, and each exhalation.

- You might feel the breath most distinctly in the nostrils, the nose area, or maybe you experience it most vividly in the chest or belly region . . . putting your attention wherever you feel it most distinctly without needing to change it in any way. The breath is happening by itself, and you are just being with it it . . .

- You can also know how you are breathing at the moment, aware of the quality of the breath, the pace, the duration of a single breath . . . long or short, deep or shallow, however it is feeling right now . . .

- Sooner or later you will notice that the mind has wandered off, that it is no longer with the breath, but has been drawn to some other events, like thoughts or feelings, or other kinds of sensations, or sounds around you . . . whenever you notice this, just bring attention, bring awareness back to breathing. Do this with patience, and, and as best as you can, without judging yourself. Rather, congratulating yourself for having noticed that the mind has wandered off . . . and gently and firmly returning attention to the breath that's happening right now, whether an inbreath or an outbreath.

- Redirecting attention back to the breath whenever you become aware that the focus has shifted, perhaps to a thought, a memory, a fantasy, planning, or comparing . . . no need to give yourself a hard time. Simply return to this breath . . . becoming aware of the process of breathing. As if you were riding the waves of the breath . . .

- See if you can encounter the breath with an attitude of curiosity. It might be a very new experience to move so close to the breath. Becoming so intimate with your breathing . . .

- There is nothing else to do right now, just paying attention to breathing, being aware of breathing.

- And noticing: where is the mind right now? And if you notice that it has wandered off, bringing it back gently and firmly to being with the breath.

- And as we are ending this practice, expanding awareness outside of the body, becoming aware of sounds around you, of the air and temperature around you, of the space and the room around you . . . slowly opening your eyes, and gently bringing movement back into the body.

TRIGGERS: BEYOND WARNING SIGNS

Being aware of warning signs is an important first step—but we do not want to stop there. Mood symptoms (warning signs) often do not occur (or worsen) out of the blue. By being aware, participants are often able to identify situations, thoughts, feelings, and behaviors that lead to the occurrence of warning signs. This is what we refer to as "triggers." Specifically, the continued or recurring presence of a trigger makes the occurrence of warning signs more likely. Therefore, the next step is raising awareness for triggers relating to warning signs. Much of this detective work will continue throughout the rest of the program, as participants gradually develop a better awareness of which situational, behavioral, and thought–feeling patterns trigger (worsen) mood symptoms. To get the ball rolling, we open the topic up for group discussion and collect examples of triggers participants already recognize.

"When my wife gets obstructive, this is a huge trigger for me," Stephen noted, instantly connecting with the theme. "Every once in a while when we have a discussion, I just don't seem to get through and I hit this stonewall with my wife and my daughter. When that happens, it is incredibly frustrating. Usually there is no resolution. I get the silent treatment for at least a few days and my head is spinning, wondering what I said or did." Further exploration yielded that this would typically result in disrupted sleep, which would make Stephen feel "wired, and energized." "It is not a good scenario," he said. "At this point, my psychiatrist and I knock me out with sleeping pills to avoid mood elevation. But then I feel hung over all day." At the end of this exploration, Stephen had his homework laid out for him. As he could not quite describe what would lead him to interpret his wife's and daughter's behaviors as "obstructive" and what he thought and how he felt in that moment, the instructor asked him to use the next "obstructive situation" to pay attention to his thoughts, feelings, and behaviors as the discussion with his wife and daughter would unfold.

For Michelle, a similar trigger (having a conflict with her boyfriend) triggered feelings of sadness, hopelessness, and even thoughts about suicide if things "would not get resolved." Like Stephen, she could not quite put her finger on what it meant that "it would not resolve." She was asked to begin to bring attention to her feelings, sensations, and thoughts in situations when conflict with her boyfriend would arise.

For Elizabeth, positive performance feedback from her supervisor could trigger an escalating cycle of hypomania. "After positive feedback from my boss, I typically feel more energetic and happy. Then I get more projects going. When I have more going I tend to switch back and forth between multiple tasks a lot. On those days, I am pretty energized at the end of the day. This makes it harder to calm down at bedtime and I get less sleep. With a few days like this, my need for sleep goes down, which is one of my warning signs."

Like we did with Stephen, Michelle, and Elizabeth, we ask participants to start paying attention to moments when they notice their mood shifting, like feeling distressed, frustrated, angry or anxious, or moments where they notice rumination setting in. For those situations, we ask them to come into the present and begin to notice the situation, their thoughts, feelings, and bodily sensations, and behaviors. Because remembering those is difficult, we ask them to complete a worksheet which allows participants to record the situation, feelings, thoughts, and behaviors they notice so that they can refresh their memories in group as well as individual sessions (Handout 9: Worksheet for Trigger Situations). Going forward, the focus will be threefold: (1) becoming more aware of situations, feelings, thoughts, and behaviors that are in some way associated with warning signs/worsening of mood symptoms; (2) omitting/phasing out situations and triggers that participants can avoid (stimulus control); and (3) bringing mindfulness to those situations that cannot be avoided. That means bringing in mindfulness early when participants notice negative (or hyperpositive-manic) thoughts arise, or when they find themselves slipping into depressive, manic, angry, or anxious rumination. Both in group and in individual sessions, instructors and participants work together through the process of mindful problem solving (see Chapter 4) in order to achieve this balance. Common trigger situations include, but are not limited to:

- Conflict at work, with spouses or partners
- Situations where the participant feels expectations are too high
- Changes in routines
- Changes in time zones
- Seasonal changes
- Achievements
- Disappointments
- Situations with uncertain outcomes

THE 3-MINUTE BREATHING SPACE

The group ends with an expanded version of the Breathing Space (adapted from Segal et al., 2002, 2013) that includes two new elements. After coming into the present and noticing what is going on at a given time, participants are then asked to anchor themselves around the breath by following the inbreath and the outbreath for a moment, before widening their attention again to be present and open to whatever is unfolding at that time. For homework we ask participants to practice this more comprehensive Breathing Space at least three times per day (audio track 5). This will be the Breathing Space that participants will utilize starting in the next session when trigger situations arise.

Box 3.2. The 3-Minute Breathing Space

(Note for the instructor: [. . .] indicates a pause.)

- The first part of the Breathing Space is becoming aware of what is going on with you right now. Becoming aware of what is going through the mind. As best as you can noticing thoughts as mental events. Also becoming aware of any feelings that are around at this moment . . . allowing any discomfort or unpleasant feelings to be with you, rather than pushing them away or shutting them out. Just acknowledging them. And also noticing the sensations in the body . . . Are there sensations of tension? . . . Again, just allowing yourself to be aware of them . . . Simply noting them. Whatever it is you are noticing right now, thoughts, feelings, or sensations, simply allowing yourself to just notice whatever is going on right here.

- The second step, now that you have stepped out of automatic pilot, is to collect your awareness by focusing on a single object: the movements of the breath. Focusing attention in the movement of the abdomen, the rise and fall of the breath . . . spending a minute or so focusing on the movement of the abdomen, moment by moment, breath by breath, as best you can. So that you know when the breath is moving in, and you know when the breath is moving out. Just anchoring awareness to the movement of the breath at the abdomen . . . gathering yourself: using the anchor of the breath to really be present.
- And now as a third step, having gathered yourself to some extent, allowing awareness to expand. As well as being aware of the breath, also including a sense of the body as a whole. So there is more spacious awareness . . . A sense of the body as a whole, including any tightness or sensations related to holding in the shoulders, neck, back or face . . . following the breath as if your whole body is breathing. Holding it all in this slightly, softer, more spacious awareness.

Adapted from Segal et al. (2002, 2013). Copyright 2002, 2013 by The Guilford Press. Adapted by permission.

HOMEWORK

For homework we ask participants to continue with their Mood Diary and continue to pay attention to warning signs (Handouts 5 and 8), do Breathing Spaces when participants switch from one activity to the next, and be mindful with the chosen routine activity daily. In addition we ask participants to do the full 3-Minute Breathing Space at least three times per day (audio track 5). Should warning signs arise, participants are instructed to enact their action plan and if needed contact the instructor (Handout 8). As a formal exercise, participants are asked to practice Mindfulness of the Breath daily (audio track 4) and to record their experiences (Handout 7). Trigger situations encountered during the week are recorded on the Worksheet for Trigger Situations (Handout 9).

Aversion and Attachment

- Handout 5: Mood Diary (in case a participant forgot to bring his or hers)
- Handout 7: Homework Sheet
- Handout 8: Worksheet for Warning Signs and Action Plans
- Handout 9: Worksheet for Trigger Situations

ABOUT THIS SESSION

This session is about attachment and aversions: the mind's judgments of liking or not liking and how they relate to warning signs and participants becoming manic or depressed. This will become part of participant's observation as he or she continues to practice mindfulness. Throughout the previous week participants have begun to observe triggers that may lead to warning signs. We now begin the process of working with those moments more mindfully. Participants will use Breathing Spaces when they encounter trigger situations and work on responding to those situations more skillfully. This journey will continue for most of the program. We also review action plans for depression and mania and the difficult choices that participants often need to make to set those in motion. As part of the formal exercises, we broaden the focus of attention from the breath to the breath and body. For home practice the Mindfulness of the Breath and Body Exercise is included as a recording (audio track 6). Obstacles to practicing receive continued attention; this involves discussing the balance of formal and informal exercises and, for some participants, whether continuing with the program is in their best interest if they have rarely come to the group sessions and barely practiced.

WELCOME BACK AND MOOD DIARY CHECK

As the fourth session is beginning to unfold, participants have settled into a familiar routine of the brief check-in when they arrive for group. Warning signs and mood symptoms are noted as well as any other change that is noticeable compared to the previous week. As needed, participants and the instructor may decide to meet after class or during the week to discuss any concerning developments. At any time, as participants become aware of warning signs that they had not recognized previously, they are included in the Worksheet for Warning Signs and Action Plans (Handout 8) and will be monitored by the participant going forward.

AVERSION AND ATTACHMENT

Part of this session's practice and discussion will be the topic of attachment and aversion: liking and not liking. Our mind judges our experiences as positive or negative. At the heart of rumination is the brain believing that things ought to be different. These judgments of good or bad, positive or negative, set the stage for rumination. Anything can become the object of judgment: thoughts, feelings, sensations, or behaviors. Judging an experience as bad, negative, uncomfortable, or dangerous creates a feeling of aversion (undesirable, not wanting, wanting to avoid, wanting it to be different, wanting it to be over). Judging experiences as positive, pleasant, or good creates a feeling of attachment (wanting, wanting more, not wanting it to be over, desire). Many mental and behavioral activities seek to reduce what is disliked, undesirable, or perceived to be dangerous, or to maintain or increase what feels pleasant or desirable. These mental activities may include rumination, avoiding thoughts or feelings, distraction, and attempts to suppress thoughts and feelings, as well as all other behaviors that functionally seek to decrease (or eliminate) unwanted experiences. Such behaviors also include positive rumination, fantasizing, and engaging in pleasurable activities that induce, maintain or increase positive feelings. As these mental and behavioral activities are utilized and practiced more frequently, they become overlearned. Finally, they take the form of the well-oiled mental/behavioral grooves ("autopilots") participants are familiar with and find difficult to stop. Therefore, as participants continue to practice reflecting upon wanted and unwanted experiences, we now highlight the importance of objectively becoming aware of and observing these feelings of aversion and attachment as they unfold. Therefore, going forward the sitting meditation will include the instructions that participants should not only notice the thoughts, feelings, and sensations they are experiencing, but also observe whether these thoughts, feelings, and sensations carry aversion or attachment.

WIDENING THE SPACE

In the first Sitting Meditation (Mindfulness of the Breath), participants practiced to focus their attention on a single object, the breath. When thoughts disrupted their focus (either through mindwandering or rumination), participants practiced observing where the mind had wondered to, acknowledging the thought and its content, then, gently shifting their attention back to the breath as the sole object of observation. When bodily sensations or feelings took attention away from the breath, participants were encouraged to approach those sensations and feelings with curiosity as they came up, and to observe and notice them, as much as they felt comfortable doing so, and then also gently shift their attention back to the breath as an anchor. Over the next sessions, we will bring additional elements into this sitting meditation. They will include widening the attentional focus to include the sensations of the body as a whole, in addition to following the sensations of breathing (Mindfulness of the Breath and Body).

Then the focus will be further expanded to include observance of sounds and thoughts (Mindful Sitting of Sounds and Thoughts; Session 5) in order to create a wider space from which experiences can be viewed and observed within the body. As feelings and thoughts continue to catch attention, trigger rumination, and foster suppression or distraction, the meditations designed to widen the space will be complemented by a series of Emotion-Focused Meditations (starting in Session 5). During these meditations, participants will continue to practice observing and accepting feelings and thoughts without getting tangled up in them (Sessions 5–8). All of these exercises are geared toward building participants' abilities to find space within themselves from where they can understand uncomfortable, challenging, or distressing experiences as elements that are a part of a wider space within themselves. Today we start this part of the journey with Mindfulness of the Breath and Body.

MINDFULNESS OF
THE BREATH AND BODY

This sitting meditation should last for approximately 10 to 15 minutes. This is shorter than in Segal et al. (2002, 2013) and accommodates individuals with concentration difficulties. Participants for whom this is too long should have permission to step out of the exercise whenever they feel they need to. Typically, this option helps participants to stay with the practice longer because it is clear that it is their own decision when to step out or take a break. Participants who can do a longer sitting meditation are encouraged to do so as part of their homework. Those who find longer sitting meditations aversive should begin meditating for homework for a shorter length of time than when practicing in class, and gradually lengthening the sitting meditation exercise.

Box 4.1. Mindfulness of the Breath and Body (10 Minutes)

(Note for the instructor: [. . .] indicates a pause.)

- Taking an upright and comfortable sitting position, either in a chair or on a cushion on the floor. Sitting with a straight back, and allowing the shoulders to relax and soften. Now bringing awareness to the points of contact of the legs, the feet, and the buttocks with the floor or the chair; feeling into that contact and allowing the weight to rest on the contacts; aware of the position of the pelvis on the cushion, or on the chair, and the spine rising out of the pelvis, into the upright sitting position, opening the chest to the front so that the breath can fully flow into the body; and allowing the face muscles to relax.

- And now bringing awareness to the flow of the breath. Feeling the sensations that arise with breathing. You can be with these sensations either in the abdomen, the chest, or the nostrils, wherever you feel them most vividly. Simply becoming aware of the constant rising and falling of the breath. The breath rising with each inhalation, and falling back with each exhalation . . .

- Whenever you notice that the mind has wandered off, very gently and kindly escorting it back to the sensations of breathing in the current moment. Guiding your attention, as if you were taking a little child by her hand and very gently guiding her back to the place where she should be. This is an opportunity to meet yourself with a kind, friendly, and loving quality . . .

- Becoming aware of this very breath that is happening right now, in this present moment. Breath by breath . . . Paying attention to breathing is a way to anchor awareness in the present moment . . . the breath is always happening right here, right now . . .

- And now, for the next period of this meditation, we're going to expand the field of awareness, including physical sensations throughout the entire body. While being aware, in the background, of the movements of the breath, you can change your primary focus, becoming aware of a sense of the body as a whole and the sensations in the entire body . . .

- Becoming aware of sensations in any parts of the body, buttocks and legs, as they are making contact with the floor, maybe the hands and arms, as they are resting on the knees or in your lap . . . sensations in the torso, the chest, head and face . . . or establishing an awareness of the body as a whole, sitting here, in this very moment, breathing . . .

- Whenever you notice that awareness has wandered off from sensations in the body, you might want to congratulate yourself for having "woken up" to the present moment. Taking a moment to notice how that feels to come back to the awareness in the present moment, as opposed to having gotten lost in thoughts or fantasies. The mind has the tendency to get drawn into stories, plans for the future, or memories of the past. This is a very natural tendency of the mind. In meditation, we practice the willingness to let go of the stories, for the sake of coming back to the reality of this moment, as it actually is . . .

- Very gently and lightly, resting awareness on the sensations in the body, and on the flow of the breath.
- It is possible that some sensations can be intense, or even painful, such as discomfort in the back, knees, or shoulders, or other parts of the body. You may find that the attention gets drawn to these sensations, and away from the intended focus on the breath or body as a whole. If that is the case, you can experiment with intentionally bringing the focus of awareness into the region of intensity and gently exploring the quality of the sensations here: What do these sensations feel like? . . . Where exactly are they located? You might notice that they change over time in their intensity, or they might even change in their entire quality. They might feel different from moment to moment. Allowing yourself to fully feel it. Is it sharp, hot, prickly? Does it throb, is it diffuse? Our typical reaction when we experience pain is to turn away from it, to feel that we don't want it. See if you can approach the sensations with openness, with curiosity, and maybe even acceptance . . . Turning toward them, rather than turning away . . . Even if that feels unknown, see if you can find a different way of being with painful or unpleasant sensations . . . always being gentle and compassionate with yourself. Only exposing yourself to as much of the experience as feels right at any moment. If the sensations become too intense, feel free to slowly move the body, very gently, with intentionality and awareness . . . or, to come to the breath and stabilize there . . . returning to explore the strong sensations as you feel ready. And now, after a while of having explored these sensations, coming back to the awareness of the breath, and the awareness of the body in its entirety . . .
- Resting in this gentle contact of the attention with the sensations in the present moment. Right here, right now.
- And now, as we bring this meditation to an end, slowly opening the eyes, and at your own pace bringing movement back into the body.

Adapted from Segal et al. (2002, 2013). Copyright 2002, 2013 by The Guilford Press. Adapted by permission.

Discussing participants' experiences with this sitting meditation will bring up some familiar topics, some of which have already been discussed as part of the Yoga and Body Scans. These include "mindwandering" and the idea of "not having thoughts during meditating." Likewise, meditating is a way of "calming the mind," and a way to "relax." These topics are discussed with the group.

Mindwandering and Having No Thoughts

Mindwandering is normal. It is how the mind works, and this should be explained to participants over and over again. Our minds work by association. One thought triggers another, which in turn triggers another thought, which may come with a feeling, which triggers another thought or feeling, and so forth. This way we each experience an ongoing stream of consciousness, ebbing and flowing, which never ends. When we direct attention to the breath and sensations in the body ("holding them in awareness"), our attention will be captured by thoughts and wander away. This is an entirely normal process. It is also not the purpose (or even possible) not to have any thoughts (or feelings) at a given time. Minds and bodies, by nature, have thoughts and feelings. How many thoughts, and the intensity of feelings and sensations, may depend on the time of practice and what is going on at that time. This could be compared to a highway with a fast flow of cars, or a small neighborhood street, where a car drives by only once in a while. But there are still cars. In fact, what we practice during the sitting meditation exercise is not to become devoid of thoughts or to block thoughts out. We practice in order to become aware of when our attention wanders, to recognize where it goes, and then gently and kindly to bring ourselves back to the breath or the body as a whole. Therefore—no matter how many times one needs to do this—if the mind wanders, and one becomes aware of this, then one should note where the mind has wandered, acknowledge what it says, perhaps labeling this as a thought, and then gently and kindly returning one's focus to the breath and the body.

Meditation as a Way to Relax

Most people associate meditation with relaxation. However, relaxation is a by-product of meditation that may occur at times, but often it will not—especially when times are tense and one conducts the sitting meditation on a day that was stressful, or perhaps was filled with distressing things. In this case, the mind may be filled with thoughts and the body full of tense sensations. It is unlikely that just because one is engaged in sitting meditation, the mind will instantly calm and the body will relax. Rather, the sitting meditation will give the practitioner a different way to relate to the stream of thoughts and the sensations and feelings in the body. Meditation will provide the opportunity to be a kind, attentive observer rather than an active participant in whatever is going on. Thus, as a by-product, meditation may calm things. But consider the opposite: actively trying to calm the body and the mind. Trying not to have thoughts. Trying to relax the feelings and sensations one is experiencing. Paradoxically, this often yields effects opposite to relaxation, making one more tense and distressed.

Self-Critical Thoughts and Uncomfortable Sensations and Feelings

As with the Yoga–Body Scan and Body Scan, during sitting meditations, participants will find themselves facing negative, self-critical thoughts and uncomfortable sensations and feelings. Self-critical thoughts may either be triggered by the exercise itself (e.g., "I cannot even do this simple task"), or the exercise may be conducted against the backdrop of a day rife with negative thoughts and rumination. If this is the case, the exercise is a welcome opportunity to practice. As for negative thoughts, we ask participants to clearly notice them for what they are: a negative, perhaps self-critical thought that has occurred in their minds: a mental event. It does not matter whether this thought is right or wrong, or whether it is believable or not. It is a mental event, and as part of the exercise it is labeled and treated as such. Then, after congratulating oneself that one has become aware of this negative thought, the exercise calls for gently redirecting the attention to the breath and the body. By the time the negative, self-critical thought has been identified, it may already have triggered rumination. Participants may suddenly find themselves in the midst of rumination when they "wake up" and recognize where their mind has taken them. As one participant, Taylor, described, "We are dealing with my son's school about the IAP plan and things are not going well. It does not look like he is getting the support he will need and I can't stop thinking about what else we can do." At this point, as best as one can, recognize the negative or catastrophic thought ("My son is not going to get the help he needs"), acknowledge it as a thought, perhaps remaining with the thought for a moment, examine it, and then gently redirect the attention back to the breath and the sensations of the body. Negative thoughts may also carry uncomfortable feelings and bodily sensations. If feelings and sensations in the body demand attention, then, as directed by the exercise, bring a kind, gentle, and curious attention to that region and then, as best as possible, allow oneself to observe the sensations in that region of the body.

In today's session, we introduced the concept of aversion and attachment. Therefore, we not only ask participants to notice the sensations, but also whether they have aversion attached to them. Aversion includes sentiments of wanting this feeling, this sensation and/or this thought to go away. This aversion, the not wanting to have this thought, feeling or sensation, often triggers rumination. Therefore, becoming aware of this aversion, where it is in the body, and how it feels, from now on will be an integral part of the sitting meditation exercise.

Mood Elevation

Likewise, the sitting meditation may be practiced against a backdrop of mood elevation. The mind may be creating new plans and ideas, and one may feel more confident and energetic, wanting to engage in the ideas that the mind is floating. As Luis, another participant, pointed out, "Finally I feel I got my energy back. It's been way too long, and I got to get going on things. . . ." Feeling that the energy is "back," heightened confidence, having plans and ideas, all come with attachment. One may wish to engage in and pursue new goals. If these sentiments are present during the sitting meditation, the exercise itself introduces a barrier. We ask participants to sit and observe, and not to move or engage. This can turn wanting into aversion. If one wants to begin something and cannot, this may become uncomfortable. Therefore, if a participant experiences this during the sitting meditation, we ask them to bring a gentle and kind attention to the tension in their body (where it is, how it feels, etc.). In doing so, participants may become aware of the attachment and the aversion as it unfolds in the body. The Mood Diary may have already given a hint of what that participant's experience may be during the sitting meditation in this particular session, and the instructor can help the participant become more aware of what is going on in this moment.

It is important to notice those attachments and aversions, and allow oneself to observe, but not to engage in any feeling or sensation of energy. Deliberately choosing not to engage and remaining in this observant mode allows one to just note the sensation and any attachment or aversion that comes with paying attention in this way. Why is it important to become aware of the attachments and aversions associated with mood elevation? As we will see later, when discussing trigger situations (like the aversion to negative self-critical thoughts), the attachment to positive thoughts and feelings (wanting, wanting more) may increase in activities that increase mood elevation (e.g., being more active, engaging in more pleasurable activities). Anger and irritability often come with a mix of aversions and attachments. Aversion may be associated with frustration. Attachment may be associated with the wish to express that one has been treated disrespectfully or unfairly. This desire may already be playing out in rumination: thoughts and fantasies about how one will "get back at others" or "set them straight." Again, the task here is to notice and become aware of these thoughts, feelings and sensations as well as the aversion and attachment: acknowledging frustrated or angry thoughts as mental events and then bringing oneself back to the breath and body, paying attention to the raw sensations that are associated with frustration and anger, while becoming aware of the sensations of aversion associated with the pull to express oneself.

When thoughts are more fluid or perhaps already feel speeded, we ask participants to notice that the thoughts are wandering, but not to "catch" each individual thought or try to follow where the thoughts are going. Rather, for speeded thoughts, our advice is to adopt a certain "lightness" when one has noticed that the thoughts have wandered away again. This will happen frequently when thoughts are speeded. Therefore, one must gently acknowledge "mindwandering" and "speeded thoughts" but then gently redirect attention to the body as a whole or the breath as an anchor.

Anxiety

Feeling anxious is another common experience that may be present during the sitting meditation exercise. This may be triggered by the sitting meditation practice, being in a group of people (social phobia), or preexisting worries about something, for example, that a panic attack may come up. Participants with anxiety disorders may choose to pay attention to sounds as their anchor if the breath is anxiety-provoking. When participants find themselves carried away by worry, we ask them to notice what the worry thought is, and, as for all other thoughts, label it as a mental event, an occurrence in the mind. Attention may also be drawn to feelings and sensations in the body: the uncertainty that is an integrative part of worry, perhaps some physical sensations. This is aversive and may have already triggered the mind to look for solutions, which in turn may lead to going in circles, revisiting options, ultimately never arriving at a point that seems to be acceptable. Noticing the aversion that comes with one's fears is part of the exercise. Likewise, aversion may lead to the mind trying to "distract" itself from the catastrophic or worry thought.

Therefore, we direct participants, as best as possible and as much as they can, to notice the catastrophic or worry thought, and label it as a mental event, but then when acknowledged to redirect their attention back to the sensations associated with the anger in their body. Bringing a gentle, curious observation to the aversion that is present in the body allows participants to observe it. However, if at any point, sensations, feelings, or thoughts become overwhelming, participants should know that they may give themselves permission to step out of the exercise

CONTINUED OBSTACLES TO PRACTICE

Within the first month of mindfulness, patterns of participation in the group will begin to unfold. Some participants, despite good intentions, may barely have attended group or individual sessions. Other participants that may have begun with enthusiasm may now see how much work is involved and slowly begin to fall off. Others may have "good" weeks and "bad" weeks in terms of how much they practice. Some may have experienced intermittent crises that were addressed as part of the individual sessions and may be "trailing behind in practice." Still others may continue to attend but barely practice outside of the group. How do instructors work with these different patterns?

For participants whose attendance is spotty, and who neither engage in formal nor informal practices, it makes sense to ask whether this is the right time for them to participate in this program. When considering this question, as instructors, we carefully weigh the interests of all group members. As the program proceeds, group cohesion develops. Group members begin to trust one another, disclose personal material, and mutually support each other while working through obstacles and dealing with setbacks. For participants with irregular attendance, it is difficult to become part of this core. Therefore, while they might still benefit from occasionally attending the group, their participation may not be in the best interest of the group. For members who have dealt with intermittent crises, whose attendance may have suffered because of this, we will use the individual sessions to catch them up so that they may stay connected with the group and the content of the program. For other participants, who, despite their best efforts and intentions, do not complete the formal exercises (sitting meditations), we focus on maximizing Breathing Spaces throughout the day.

That said, exploring the reasons why formal practice does not materialize and problem-solving around those obstacles remains a central strategy. However, if despite these efforts, a participant continues to struggle in this area but seems to be able to utilize the Breathing Space in daily life, this is where we place the emphasis (see Breathing Space practice below). Continuing to emphasize formal exercises is effective only up to a certain point, so long as the message increases the likelihood of engaging in the formal exercises. If despite this consistent reinforcement, a participant does not do it, he or she may conclude that he or she cannot do the work and this may lower his or her motivation to continue with the program, and may ultimately lead to dropout. Therefore, we attempt to send a "dual message." While strongly "advertising" the benefits from the formal exercises, we also convey consistently that the "daily life, informal (Breathing Space)" portion of the program was specifically developed to promote a way of getting a "dose" of mindfulness that can be easily built into day-to-day activities. While participants who do not engage much in the formal exercises at home may not benefit as much from the program as those who do, they will likely still benefit from engaging in the Breathing Space throughout the day. Another pattern that will have started to unfold at this point will briefly be discussed with the whole group: getting on and falling off.

Getting On and Falling Off

How are new habits, or ways of being, acquired? First, as all active participants will have seen, it involves declaring an intention of doing something new or different. Then, one must remind oneself of this intention (or be reminded of it) and begin the practice, gradually learning one's way, with things getting easier over time. But often, all of a sudden, when a behavior seems established, people fall off. We are not sure why this happens. One likely reason is that old ways of doing are not simply erased (or extinguished). Rather, people learn new behaviors in a given context (e.g., to brush your teeth mindfully in the morning). The context (time of the day, place, etc.) becomes a reminder for the behavior (brushing teeth mindfully). Now there are two ways of brushing teeth at this particular time and place. There is the old way of tooth brushing (quickly, not paying attention), and the new way (slowly, mindfully). These two habits compete with each other. Often, compared to the new way of doing things (i.e., more mindfully), older behaviors are more overlearned (i.e., more ingrained). Therefore, they have a tendency to reoccur.

We review this problem with group members so they may become aware of this tendency of old ways "creeping back in" and supplanting new habits. First, if this has already happened (and it happens a lot), we want participants to know that this is absolutely normal and understand the reasons why it happens. Second, we ask participants to become aware of this phenomenon, so that when they notice it, they will renew their efforts to engage in the new behavior.

BREATHING SPACE AND MINDFULNESS OF ROUTINE ACTIVITIES: STAYING PRESENT

Breathing Space

In this section, we will review participants' experiences with the first part of the Breathing Space (audio track 2) when they shift from one activity to the next. Ideally, participants will find themselves increasingly reminded about coming into the present when they switch activities. For participants for whom this is not the case, we will use the strategies for raising awareness outlined in Sessions 1–3 as part of their individual sessions. In this group session, we will begin to tie in "coming into the present" with the thoughts and feelings participants encounter in their mindfulness practices. Specifically, part of the reason to be in the present is to detect mood symptoms (warning signs) and/or self-critical negative or overly positive thoughts early, in order to bring "mindfulness" to them.

> *Instructor*: "As you are coming into the present, you may notice thoughts, sensations, and feelings in this moment. Allow yourself to become aware of whatever is going on in this particular moment and congratulate yourself that you have just woken up. Allow yourself to notice thoughts as mental events crossing through your mind, perhaps,

as you have by now done many, many times, labeling them as mental events. 'Thinking.' Likewise, allowing yourself to become aware of any sensations or feelings in your body that may catch your attention. Observing what is present without getting tangled up in it. With all of this present, also now, going forward becoming more aware of aversions and attachments in your body. Being aware of wanting to feel or think about something, or not wanting to feel something. As you know, this is often the entry into the autopilot of endless rumination and the mood spiraling up or down."

We would like to know whether group members have started to catch themselves when difficult thoughts or feelings or rumination are setting in. Therefore, we ask group members to share their experiences. As one participant, Brian, described, "Since I have started practicing this, I have become aware of the slight shifts in my mood. As you know, I review contracts and I have noticed how at times my mood goes slightly up or down during the day, and have started to adjust for this." When asked what that actually meant, he explained, "The late morning, around 10 A.M., is our busy period, when a lot of e-mails are coming in and requests to get things reviewed on time. This can get overwhelming quickly. Since I have noticed this, I pause, and let it all sink in. But then I also have started to change my behaviors. I collect the requests, and I now tell some people that they have to wait until after lunch. Why after lunch? Because this is when I feel most sluggish, and that reminds me quite a bit of being depressed. It is hard to get going. At this point it actually helps to have a few contracts on the schedule, because it activates me again. Although it is sometimes not that easy to get back in the swing, but when I am in, it feels pretty good." Becoming more aware of his thoughts and feelings ("overwhelmed") as well as his subtle mood shifts during the day ("sluggish") allowed Brian to shift his behavior in a way that he began to have more productive days. This in turn made him feel more empowered and optimistic.

Another participant, Michelle, had begun to notice when negative thoughts would enter her mind. "Last night my daughter called and my live-in boyfriend talked to her. I overheard the conversation and found myself thinking 'What a great relationship the two have,'" but also that 'she does not talk to me like this.'" You can guess what the next thought was: 'She does not like me as much as my boyfriend,' because we don't talk like this. Of course, I also noticed a pain in the pit of my stomach. So I did the Breathing Space, just walked away, let the thought sit there and did what I had planned on doing anyways. The thought stuck for a while, but I let it sit there, invited it in, but left it there, although I noted the pull to review the conversation, to ask my boyfriend why she had called him, and so forth, but then I got distracted. Usually, this would have been a huge cascade with me crying in the end, feeling awful and my boyfriend being completely unnerved again."

For group participants such as Brian and Michelle, using the Breathing Space as they transition activities and practicing to be deliberately present during routine activities gradually improved their ability to detect shifts in moods as well as automatic thoughts. We believe that this awareness is critical for bringing mindfulness to triggers that shift the mood to prevent the mind from going down the overlearned path of depressive or manic rumination. As we will see during the discussion of trigger situations, going forward, participants will be asked to bring the full 3-Minute Breathing Space to those moments when they notice they are being triggered.

TRIGGERS: GOING BEYOND WARNING SIGNS

Next, the group participants will continue their detective work on triggers (situations, thoughts, feelings, and behaviors) that may lead to the occurrence or worsening of mood symptoms (warning signs). We ask participants to use the Worksheet for Trigger Situations (Handout 9) to remind themselves about trigger situations and the associated thoughts, feelings, and behaviors. The phone conversation that Michelle overheard between her boyfriend and her daughter is an example of a trigger situation. For Michelle, interpersonal situations, in the broadest sense, were a trigger. Any interaction with her boyfriend that led her to feel like they were not in sync could send her into a tailspin. Often, interacting with others, such as her boss and coworkers, yielded the same result. For Michelle, these situations triggered negative thoughts ("I will get a divorce," or, with respect to her coworkers, "We won't get along anymore and I will feel awful all the time"). The negative thoughts would then start her rumination autopilot: wondering whether she did something wrong, whether she said something wrong, and endlessly reviewing the situation trying to find some solution. It is in the initial moment, when Michelle notices a shift in her feeling of "being at odds or not being in sync with others," when we would like her to become more aware of the negative thoughts going through her mind. Recognizing the mental event is a necessary step to bringing mindfulness (the Breathing Space) into the moment.

For other group participants, such as Elizabeth, her own behavior (i.e., multitasking) could trigger the "appetite" for more tasks, as well as feeling energetic and driven. This, in turn, would trigger positive rumination, increased ideas, and plans. Therefore, Elizabeth learned to recognize (and avoid) too much multitasking as a trigger situation, and began to bring mindfulness to moments when she noticed that particular shift in the way she felt. Other triggers may be external, such as seasonal changes. Participants may be more likely to develop symptoms of mood elevation in the spring and the summer, as opposed to the fall or winter. For Elizabeth, multitasking during the winter could make her feel overwhelmed, whereas the same tasks could trigger mood elevation in the summertime. Therefore, for both instructors and participants, identifying and working with triggers often involves some detective work. As participants progress through the program, the increased awareness toward shifts in thinking and feeling will come in handy as they begin to systematically address trigger situations.

We ask participants to pair up in dyads, compare their notes, and discuss what types of trigger situations they may have noticed for themselves, before opening the discussion to the whole group. Both Stephen and Michelle updated the group about their trigger situations. "I ran into the issues being unresolved with my boyfriend again," Michelle stated. "What's interesting about it is that it does not even have to be a conflict. It can be anything that signals to me that we are not in sync." She had also noticed thoughts and feelings triggered by this "feeling out of sync." "First, I wonder what is going on. Often, I am actually not sure whether I am picking up on something that is real or not. I usually then try to interact with him, looking for signs that everything is OK: a smile, a touch, just something that tells me we are good. When I don't get this then I start worrying." Michelle also noticed negative thoughts beginning at that time. "I wonder whether I said something wrong, or what I may have done and then start going over all the things we had talked about that day which could have made him feel upset. At the end of this, I feel exhausted, tired, like I can't take it anymore, just wanting to end it. My boyfriend usually does not even notice what is going on, until I break out in tears. Of course, 90% of the time, it's just something else that has nothing to do with me." As the instructor probed further, Michelle also described how anxious she was, thinking that she had done something wrong. She described feeling tense and a pulsating knot in her stomach. "I cannot stand this!" she exclaimed, noting that this tied into her feelings of aversion that had been part of the session. The instructor invited her to observe this feeling of anxiety and aversion in her body further, and to explore and observe whether there could be any other thoughts in her mind that might explain why "doing something wrong" might trigger such strong feelings of anxiety and aversion.

Another group member, Stephen, also had experienced a situation in which his wife and daughter were being "obstructive." "It was interesting being so aware of it, because I think I caught it sooner this time," he noted. "My daughter wanted to go out with her friends on a Saturday night. I did not have an issue with this, but for a 15-year-old, I thought coming home at midnight was too late. As you can imagine, my daughter disagreed, but my wife supported her, arguing that it is a Saturday." The instructor inquired about the thoughts and feelings Stephen experienced in this situation. "It was actually interesting, because I just got the thought 'They are being obstructive again,' and got immediately very frustrated. Something like 'Here we go again' was in my mind. I know these situations so well at this point. So I try to explain my point, trying to be very calm, but it seems there is no reasoning with them at this point." As the instructor inquired about what he actually felt in his body at that moment, Stephen explained that the frustration felt like sinking. He described a sensation of bodily heaviness with a sharp angry tension in his abdomen, and blood rushing to his face. "I actually allowed myself to observe this, as I was going through it, and I noticed the frustration and anger kicking in, and that I was hitting the moment we had talked about in group last week." Further exploration yielded that thoughts and labels such as "obstructive" were relevant particularly when his wife and daughter were in agreement from the beginning of a discussion, and Stephen would have a "strong opinion" in opposition. "I just don't think it's right for a 15-year-old to stay out that late, even if it is a Saturday night." As Stephen reflected upon the situation, he realized that he worried that "something might happen to her if she is out that late."

"It really sounds like there are multiple things going on, if I hear you right," the instructor summarized. "Thoughts that something could happen to her if she stays out that late, thoughts saying 'my concerns are not being heard,' and 'this is a pattern,' all of which are associated with feeling frustrated, anxious, and getting angry." The instructor invited Stephen to continue with his mindful observation and allow himself to note what would unfold when his wife and daughter would be on the same page. He also invited Stephen to direct his attention to his behavioral reactions when situations like this unfolded.

"Multitasking seems to be one of my issues setting me up for mania," Elizabeth noted, "at least in the summer." Elizabeth worked as a laboratory manager for a research group at a large teaching hospital. "It seems, as more and more things are making it on my to-do list, I am getting more and more wired. Then when I come home, it is difficult to wind down and I often have trouble falling asleep because all these work issues keep going through my head. If I have more than a couple of days like this, I need to drug myself with Benadryl, otherwise I can't fall asleep and get manic." As the instructor inquired about the situations when tasks were being added to her to-do list, it became clear that Elizabeth was organized in her work activities. Elizabeth would plan the day ahead of time and seemed to be able to realistically estimate how much she could accomplish in a given day, "But then, Postdoc X wants me to do this, and Postdoc Y wants me to do this, and of course, the earlier the better." Due to these last-minute requests, Elizabeth would frequently experience getting derailed and trying to fit too many tasks into a given day, and try to do multiple things all at once. When the instructor asked Elizabeth to reflect upon her thoughts and feelings at the moments when she is asked to do yet another task, Elizabeth responded, "Well, it needs to get done. Not doing it is just not an option, and I don't want to be the one holding things up. And I can do it obviously." Her record of the situation listed thoughts like "I don't want to do it," but "it needs to get done," "feeling frustrated," and "overwhelmed," yet she continued to accept these tasks without limiting them or pushing them back to another time. Therefore, the instructor asked Elizabeth to specifically direct her attention to the thoughts and feelings that were present when she did accept task assignments even though she felt it was "overwhelming." This also provided a bridge into the discussion of how to cope with trigger situations going forward.

How do you handle trigger situations? We employ two strategies:

1. If possible, a participant may simply choose to avoid the trigger. This is a form of stimulus control and may work well if the trigger is external (e.g., an avoidable situation). For example, for Stephen, having discussions with his wife and daughter at night would interfere with his sleep if he felt frustrated and angry. Therefore, he and his wife opted to move their discussions earlier into the afternoon. Unfortunately, however, often things are not that simple. Avoiding a trigger may come with adverse consequences. For example, canceling "ineffective meetings with one's supervisor" may avoid the trigger, but result in adverse long-term consequences (possible bad job evaluations and job loss). Avoidance may also trigger additional negative thoughts and feelings. For Elizabeth, the idea of not accepting additional assignments on a day when she already felt overwhelmed and stressed did not seem to be possible. "I can do it, I really can. It's just a matter of how to work it in."

2. For situations in which participants notice they are feeling stressed, sad, frustrated, depressed, angry, irritated, energized, euphoric, or anxious, we ask them to initiate the 3-Minute Breathing Space. This exercise provides a means of coming into the present, connecting with the feelings and bodily sensations that are present at that very moment (including those that are aversive), anchoring themselves, and then choose how to move forward mindfully. As stated by Segal et al. (2002, 2013), the end of the Breathing Space is presented as a period of deliberate and mindful choice. "What should I do next in this situation? How can I best take care of myself right now? What do I need for myself right now?" (Segal et al., 2002, p. 279;

Segal et al., 2013, p. 350). The answer to these questions depends on the situation, as well as the thoughts and feelings that are present at that very moment.

For Elizabeth, this meant two things. At first, we asked her to direct her attention to the thoughts associated with potentially not accepting assignments at work. This way, she realized that her thoughts followed a pattern saying that "she was not doing a good job if she did not get all her tasks done" and "that she would lose her job if that happened more than once." She also began to experiment with the situation by pushing back assignments and asking for more time. "This was challenging, but it also opened my eyes—most things aren't that urgent. Nonetheless, I still get these thoughts, but I have become much better at seeing them for what they are, products of my mind, rather than reality." As mindful, self-compassionate next steps are different in every situation, we help participants develop their own, personalized approaches using mindful problem solving (see Chapter 4 and Sessions 5–8). In each of the following four sessions, participants will learn more about the patterns associated with the autopilots (thought–feeling patterns) associated with depression, mania, anger/irritability, and anxiety. Concurrently, participants will continue to practice sitting meditations and Breathing Spaces to increase their ability to observe, but not get tangled up in, automatic thoughts or feelings that could start autopilots that lead into depression, mania, anger/irritability, and anxiety.

WARNING SIGNS AND ACTION PLANS REVISITED

Next, the group will turn their attention back to warning signs and action plans. By now, participants should have a basic understanding of their warning signs and have a basic action plan for what to do when warning signs occur. At this point, we pair participants up and ask them to take turns describing their warning signs and action plans, both for mania and depression. Instructors will join the discussions among the pairs. Two topics to highlight are: (1) Are warning signs always the same? (2) Should action plans be flexible?

Are One Person's Warning Signs for Depression and Mania Always the Same?

Unfortunately not. Let us consider Elizabeth. For her, anxiety was a warning sign of both depression and mania. "When I get anxious, it can go both ways. Either I spiral up and start feeling kind of wired and speeded. That is when I need to be extra careful, because it impacts my sleep and when that is impacted, I am really at risk for becoming manic. However, it can also go the other way. I may start feeling anxious and then start feeling overwhelmed. That has the potential to turn into depression rather quickly." If a warning sign can signal impending mood elevation or depression, it is difficult to know what to do, as the action plans for mania and depression in many ways call for opposite behaviors (e.g., decreasing behaviors vs. increasing behaviors). What can participants and instructors do? Often, the context, including other warning signs, can be helpful to discern whether one's mood is heading toward mania or depression. For example, for Elizabeth, the season made a difference. In the spring and summer, feelings of anxiety would typically lead to feeling more keyed up and energized, whereas during the fall and winter the same feelings would trigger feeling overwhelmed and ruminating that things are not going her way. Also, we have learned that carefully listening to the content of the anxious (or catastrophic) thoughts is helpful in terms of predicting where things are heading. Anxiety about having too much work and not enough time is likely to be associated with feeling overwhelmed and getting depressed. Feeling anxious about "wanting to get her experiments done and not get distracted by other work" carried the risk for working long hours, disrupted sleep, and mania.

Should Action Plans Be Flexible?

Action plans must always be made in a way so that they can be adapted to what is needed. For example, if warning signs are detected early, the intervention may be less dramatic compared to what will need to happen if signs are overlooked for too long. One participant, Trevor, contacted the instructor after he had missed a group because he had visited his mother, who was battling cancer. Not only was this an emotionally difficult time for Trevor, he also had to travel to a different time zone. After a few days, he noticed that he had difficulties falling asleep, was waking up early, resulting in only a few hours of sleep each night, but otherwise, he was still holding up well. After a discussion with his psychiatrist, a benzodiazepine that Trevor had taken in the past and tolerated well was added at night to help him fall asleep. In the morning, instead of rising immediately upon waking, he would do the Body Scan and continued to rest until his usual time to get up.

For the next few days, Trevor seemed to be doing fine. In his first week back, however, with family conflicts unfolding, he found himself getting keyed up, feeling tense, having speeded-up thoughts, and speech that was louder and more pressured than usual. This time the intervention was more comprehensive. Trevor's psychiatrist increased his mood stabilizer, and his family agreed to postpone discussions of topics that were likely to lead to conflict. Trevor also reduced stimulation. While he went back to work, he made sure that despite his time off, his workload was reduced for the next 2 weeks. No frequent task shifting. No multitasking, as this tends to increase speeded thoughts and distractibility. Breathing Spaces, Body Scans, and Sitting Meditations were part of his daily routine. Over the next 2 weeks, Trevor's mood returned to normal. Could a more intensive intervention earlier on have prevented Trevor from experiencing mild mood elevation 2 weeks later? Perhaps if this was a consistent pattern, but it wasn't for Trevor. Therefore, the initial intervention of a benzodiazepine and Body Scans appeared to be appropriate to the level of warning signs he experienced. However, if over time, it becomes apparent that an early, stronger intervention (e.g., medication boost, higher dose of mindfulness) is the best course of action to prevent mood dysregulation, then this is what participants need to consider.

DIFFICULT CHOICES

As Trevor's example illustrates, enacting action plans to prevent mania (or depression) can come with difficult choices. It is often due to these choices that an action plan is not set in motion. Trevor found asking for a reduced workload after taking a week off, when his coworkers were waiting for him to come back to address bottlenecks, was extraordinarily difficult. "I owe this to my colleagues," he protested when we discussed what needed to be done in order to engineer a soft landing. Like medication ("Take sedation now in order to prevent worse symptoms later"), participants often face the choice between two nonpreferred options such as (1) not reducing the workload and face the possibility of becoming manic, or (2) reducing the workload and feeling guilty because one is not fulfilling one's duties. We make participants aware of this problem as they develop their action plans. Of course, not all eventualities about action plans can be mapped out in advance. Therefore, we also ask participants to become mindful of those moments when they are contemplating setting an action plan in motion, but are hesitating. What thoughts and feelings are holding them back? Becoming aware of thoughts and feelings that might interfere with an action plan's initiation increases the likelihood that a participant will follow through despite the obstacles. As Michelle pointed out, "It feels good to be engaged in this book exchange. It is exciting and I like it. But when I get overly excited and too many books in the mail, I still don't want it to end. It just is a good feeling that I would like to keep. Having become explicitly aware of this particular draw that keeps me from doing what I need at that time has been helpful to slow things down at those times."

MINDFULNESS OF THE BREATH AND BODY II

Before reviewing the homework for the coming week, the class will do another Sitting Meditation, "Mindfulness of the Breath and Body" (for instructions, see Box 4.1) followed by a brief discussion of the experience. This exercise can be slightly longer than the Sitting Meditation conducted at the beginning of the class.

HOMEWORK

For homework we ask participants to continue with their Mood Diary and continue to pay attention to warning signs (Handouts 5 and 8), do Breathing Spaces when participants switch from one activity to the next, and be mindful with the chosen routine activity daily. In addition we ask participants to do the Full 3-Minute Breathing Space at least three times per day and when they encounter trigger situations. Should warning signs arise, participants are instructed to enact their action plan and if needed contact the instructor (Handout 8). As a formal exercise, participants are asked to practice Mindfulness of the Breath and Body daily (audio track 6) and record their experiences (Handout 7). Trigger situations encountered during the week are recorded on the Worksheet for Trigger Situations (Handout 9). The session ends with doing a Breathing Space.

Depression and Acceptance

OVERVIEW

- About This Session
- Welcome Back and Mood Diary Check
- Mindfulness Sitting with Sounds and Thoughts
- Acceptance
- Triggers: Going Beyond Warning Signs
- Breathing Space
- The Depression Autopilot
- Breathing Space
- Choice Points: How to Move Forward When Feeling Down or Depressed
- What If Problems and Thoughts Are Real?
- Emotion-Focused Meditation: Difficult Feelings
- Homework
  - Mood Diary and attention to warning signs
  - Alternate: Mindful Sitting with Sounds and Thoughts (audio track 7) and Emotion-Focused Meditation: Depression (audio track 9)
  - Continue to become more aware of trigger situations
  - Use the 3-Minute Breathing Space with Acceptance (audio track 8) for coping with trigger situations
  - List of troubling thoughts and feelings

INSTRUCTOR MATERIAL FOR SESSION 5

- Script for Mindful Sitting with Sounds and Thoughts (Box 5.1)
- Script for the 3-Minute Breathing Space (Box 3.2)

- Script for the 3-Minute Breathing Space with Acceptance (Box 5.2)
- Script for Emotion-Focused Meditation (Box 5.3)

PARTICIPANT HANDOUTS FOR SESSION 5

- Handout 5: Mood Diary (in case a participant forgot to bring his or hers)
- Handout 9: Worksheet for Trigger Situations
- Handout 10: The Depression Autopilot
- Handout 11: Exercise 1 for Session 5
- Handout 12: Automatic Negative Thoughts
- Handout 13: Cognitive Biases in Depression
- Handout 14: Exercise 2 for Session 5
- Handout 15: What Can I Do When I Start Feeling Down or Depressed?
- Handout 16: List of Troubling Thoughts and Feelings

ABOUT THIS SESSION

Acceptance of unpleasant thoughts, feelings, and sensations is the central theme of this session. Paradoxically, bringing acceptance to aversive experiences may change that very experience people would much rather avoid. We discuss how automatic negative thoughts and feelings create a vicious cycle that may lead back into depression. Mindfulness may halt this process. Participants continue to work with trigger situations. Emotion-Focused Meditations are introduced as a meditation practice that may get participants to a place where they can remain centered when strong, unpleasant, and aversive feelings and thoughts arise. For home practice the exercises Mindful Sitting with Sounds and Thoughts (audio track 7) and Emotion-Focused Meditation (audio track 9) and the 3-Minute Breathing Space with Acceptance (audio track 8) are included as recordings.

WELCOME BACK AND MOOD DIARY CHECK

As in the previous sessions, before we start the sitting meditation, we will conduct a brief check-in when participants arrive for group. Warning signs and mood symptoms are noted, as well as any other noticeable changes since the previous week's session. As needed, the instructor and participants may decide to meet after class or during the week to discuss any concerning developments. At any time, if participants become aware of warning signs they had not recognized before, they can begin to monitor them on an ongoing basis. As in the previous weeks, the group starts with a mindfulness exercise.

MINDFUL SITTING WITH SOUNDS AND THOUGHTS

After checking the mood diary, the group starts with a sitting meditation in which the focus of attention is broadened to the experience of sounds and thoughts.

Box 5.1. Mindful Sitting with Sounds and Thoughts (10 Minutes)

(Note for the instructor: [. . .] indicates a pause.)

- Once again, coming into a sitting position that is upright and stable. Taking a posture that supports the state of mind of being fully alert and relaxed. Begin by bringing awareness to the posture of the body, the contact of the legs, the feet, and the buttocks with the ground or the chair; feeling into that contact and allowing the weight of the body to rest . . .

- Now, focusing attention on breathing. Bringing awareness to the sensations of the breath. Following the constant rising and falling of the breath. Rising with every inhalation, and falling back with every exhalation . . . (*Longer pause to let participants settle the attention on the breath*)

- And now, if you wish, changing the focus of attention and shifting to hearing. Allowing awareness to open and expand, so there is an awareness of sounds as they arise . . . no need to classify or identify the sounds that come to the ears. Simply remaining with the bare sensation of hearing. What does it feel like to be hearing? . . . You might notice that the mind automatically judges the sounds, perhaps classifies them as pleasant or unpleasant, interesting or uninteresting. Whenever you notice such tendencies of the mind, see if you can simply come back to hearing itself . . .

- No need to search for any particular sounds. Just being aware of any sounds that are present at this moment . . . obvious sounds, or perhaps more subtle sounds . . . and also becoming aware of the spaces between sounds, or aware of silence.

- When you find that you are thinking *about* the sounds, simply reconnecting with the direct awareness of their sensory qualities. This might be patterns of pitch, timbre, loudness or softness . . . coming to bare sound itself . . . simply hearing.

- And while you are being with sounds, see if you can also be aware that you are doing so. Hearing and knowing that you are hearing. Right here, in this present moment . . .

- Whenever you notice that awareness is no longer focused on sounds, gently acknowledge where the mind has moved to, and bringing awareness back to sounds as they arise and pass from one moment to the next . . . (*Longer pause*)

- For the next period of practice, once again we will be changing the focus of attention. Letting the sensations of breathing, and the awareness of sounds move into the background, and bringing awareness to the process of thinking. While we often consider thinking a disruption of focus during meditation, we are now going to bring the process of thinking itself into the focus of attention.

- Not following the content of the thoughts, but rather establishing an awareness of thinking. Becoming aware of the constant moving of the mind, a thought entering into the field of awareness, lingering for a brief moment, and passing on, making space for the next thought to come.

- Just as you have done with sounds, now, as best you can, bringing awareness to thoughts that arise in the mind—noticing them as they are arising, passing through the space of the mind, and eventually disappearing . . . no need to make thoughts come or go. Just letting them arise naturally, in the same way that you related to sounds arising and passing away.

- If you would like, bringing awareness to thoughts in the mind in the same way that they might if the thoughts were projected on the screen at the movie theater. You sit watching the screen, seeing a a thought or image arise. Paying attention to it so long as it is there "on the screen," and letting it go as it is passing away.

- And as you are sitting here, watching the process of thinking, perhaps you notice a sense that you are not the thoughts. Thoughts are coming and going, but you are not identified with them, . . . you remain in the awareness of thoughts as events in the mind . . . (*Longer pause*)

- And as this meditation comes to an end, taking a moment to expand awareness to the entire body. Being aware of the body in its entirety, sitting here. And being aware of the flow of the breath. And now, whenever you are ready, slowly opening your eyes, and bringing movement back into the body.

ACCEPTANCE

A new key element that will be explicitly emphasized from now on is acceptance. "Acceptance" means actively responding to thoughts, feelings, and sensations by allowing them or letting them be before rushing in and trying to fix or change them (Segal et al., 2002, p. 221). This involves thoughts, feelings, and sensations that are uncomfortable (i.e., may elicit aversion) and those that are pleasurable (i.e., come with attachment). Why should participants want to learn to actively bring acceptance to difficult thoughts, feelings, or sensations? Bringing acceptance into the well-established, over-learned link between aversive negative thoughts, feelings, and sensations and mental activities geared toward ending these aversive experiences will ultimately interrupt those autopilots that worsen mood (see "Depression Autopilot" in this session). The same is true for hyperpositive thoughts, feelings, and sensations that are desirable (i.e., come with attachment) and trigger positive rumination (e.g., thinking about how good it feels, what one could do), thereby fostering mood elevation and increasing the risk for mania (see Session 6). Unconditional acceptance, on the other hand, supports the biological processes that lead to a decreased intensity of undesirable (or desirable) feelings.

Consider the following example: You are in your car and there is a song on the radio that you really dislike. It triggers a strong aversive reaction, and you do not want to listen to this song. Ordinarily, you might change the station, in order to find something that is more pleasant, but this time you deliberately decide to bring acceptance to the uncomfortable experience of listening to this song. Now imagine we replay this particular song to you over and over again, and each time you take this as an exercise in bringing acceptance to uncomfortable feelings. Interestingly, you will find that after listening to the song many times, this feeling of aversion will get weaker and easier to tolerate. Decreasing the intensity of emotion with repeated exposure is called "habituation." It also works with pleasurable experiences. Remember a song you instantly loved and got excited about? Perhaps you bought the CD (or downloaded it) and listened to it over and over again? You might still like the song, but the instant rush and intense liking is gone.

Unconditional acceptance has other benefits besides promoting the process of habituation. Our mind tends to be associative in nature, meaning that any given thought will trigger another thought, sensation, or feeling, which will trigger yet another, and so on. This creates a constant ebbing and flowing, or occurrence and disappearance, of the thoughts and feelings in our minds and bodies at any given time. One way to keep a thought or feeling present in the mind and body is to focus one's attention on it, think about it, or work with it in some way. If we don't pay attention, then it will dissolve in the many other thoughts that we have and then we will likely forget that we ever had that thought. Do you remember what you thought about on your way to work today?

When thoughts and feelings are particularly uncomfortable or desirable, they capture our attention. If a thought is undesirable, we may argue with it ("I did the best I could"), reinterpret it ("This was an unsolvable task, and I did not have enough guidance"), dispute its content ("I should not think this way"), or try to move attention away from it ("Let's not think about this"). If a thought is desirable and pleasurable (i.e., certain thoughts and feelings that may lead one back into mania), we may be tempted to keep it alive by reflecting on how good it feels, how capable and confident one may be, and contemplating future projects and success. Paradoxically, for both types of thoughts and feelings, all of these mental activities will likely make the thought and feelings "stick" and counteract their natural tendency to dissipate (or move on to the next thought or feeling). However, thoughts and feelings will dissipate if we only bring acceptance to their presence in a given moment.

Bringing acceptance to thoughts and feelings has another beneficial effect. Thoughts may predict the future (e.g., "I will go crazy if my anxiety gets worse," "I am going to fail," "This uncomfortable energy rush will never stop"). By treating these thoughts as mental events and, as best as one can, bringing acceptance to them, one may discover that many of them do not come true, even if one does nothing (besides accepting the thought). Of course, accepting unpleasant experiences is difficult. Therefore, in this session and over the next three sessions we will practice accepting unpleasant experiences in Emotion-Focused Meditations.

How do you accept aversive and pleasurable experiences? In this program, we use the process outlined in Segal et al. (2013, p. 275). In daily life, using the Breathing Space, or during Emotion-Focused Meditation exercises, we ask participants to bring acceptance to difficult feelings using a two-step process:

- *Step 1* is to become aware of whatever is predominant in one's moment-by-moment experience. If the mind is repeatedly drawn to a particular place, thoughts, feelings, or bodily sensations, then the task is to intentionally bring awareness to that place in that moment.

- *Step 2* is to become aware of how one is relating to whatever arises in that place and to stop trying to change things. That is one deliberately focuses one's awareness on the place in the body where the raw sensations that are related to the emotions are the strongest. One may use the breath as a vehicle to do this. Breathing into that part of the body on the inbreath. Opening and softening on the outbreath before then beginning to let go of any aversion or attachment. Say to oneself, "It's OK, whatever it is, it's OK, let me feel it." And then stay with the awareness of these bodily sensations, breathe with them, accept them and let them be, staying in this mode as long as needed.

TRIGGERS: GOING BEYOND WARNING SIGNS

Participants will continue with their detective work on triggers (situations, thoughts, feelings, and behaviors) associated with warning signs, which they started in the previous session. We ask participants to pair up in dyads, compare their notes, and discuss what types of trigger situations they have noticed in their own lives and how they handled those moments. After the one-on-one discussions, we will open the topic up for discussion as a group. Michelle provided a follow-up on her boyfriend. "I did my Breathing Space and then sat with this awkward feeling a little longer and allowed myself to observe the feeling and the thoughts going through my mind. Thinking that something is wrong between us triggers a whole cascade of catastrophic thoughts: he is going to leave me. I am going to be alone, with no support, all by myself. We will need to sell the house. Quite a movie my mind plays at times like this. And the aversion to these thoughts is so strong that it feels almost impossible not to find ways in my mind to refute that something is wrong." Michelle also recognized the mismatch between the movie "playing" in her mind and reality. "Ninety-five percent of the time, it has nothing to do with me. Nonetheless, the movie keeps playing." In today's session, the instructor invited her to bring acceptance to the sensations associated with that awkward feeling in her body, aversion, and continue to practice watching her thoughts, without trying to fix them or push them away.

Like Michelle, Stephen noticed something interesting when he used the Breathing Space and observed his thoughts and feelings during discussions with his wife and daughter. "The moment I sense this 'obstructiveness,' my mind goes into overdrive. I have thoughts like, 'I am not going to let you push me around. This needs to be fair game. All parties need to be heard. This is unfair.' With this comes this frustrated–angry feeling and the 'I won't let you do this to me' thought. So, I am really in fighting mode by that point, and I think this is something where I should let myself step back, and allow myself to listen first, before trying to push my agenda through."

Taylor, who had a tendency to be late for group, shared her experience of being late as a trigger situation. "Being late is a problem for me. Not only that it happens all the time, but it usually kicks off rumination, and on bad days it gets the depression going. So, this is from about an hour ago when I was on my way to group, and I thought I was good with time. Then I hit this traffic jam on the highway. Now that I have started to watch this, I have become much more aware of the thoughts that are kicking in at that time: 'I am going to be late for group.' 'Here we go again, this is supposed to help me and I cannot even be on time for this.' 'I am going to miss important things in group.' 'I just seem to boycott everything that might be able to help me.' 'How can I fix this? I need to get a grip on this.' 'I am such a loser.' But then I realized that this is a situation where you want me to do the Breathing Space, step back, and observe. And that was actually quite helpful. So I was sitting in the middle of a traffic jam, mad at myself like hell, and I am breathing. In an eerie way, just allowing myself to let unfold what would unfold was a relief. It occurred to me that whatever would happen would happen, as there was nothing I could do. Ordinarily, I would have tried to get off at the next exit, tried to find my way through town, just trying to make up the time I lost, but today I was just sitting there, breathing, thinking 'whatever would come of this.' This also calmed the storm in my mind, as there was nothing I could or needed to do to fix this."

We invited Taylor to bring the Breathing Space to other situations when she was late and ruminating about it. Additionally, we asked her to direct her attention to the precursors of being late, to the thoughts, feelings, and behaviors that contributed to her tardiness. We also used Taylor's experience to bridge the discussion to our next topic: learning more about the mechanisms of autopilots. What is happening in people's minds when they ruminate, or become euphoric, irritable, or anxious? As several participants described, trigger situations like Taylor's tend to start the highly overlearned, ingrained, ruminative grooves that we call the "autopilot." The autopilot describes habitual, overlearned patterns of the mind that are activated when people encounter events that trigger negative, positive, anger-related, or catastrophic automatic thoughts. Depressive ruminating; euphoric fantasizing; angry, irritable stewing; or anxious worrying that goes around and around all may be part of this overlearned behavior. If triggered often enough, it can lead to worsening of mood and ultimately depression or mania. Participants' experiences with autopilots associated with depression, mania, anger, and anxiety are addressed in this and the upcoming three sessions (Sessions 6–8). Because ongoing, chronic depressive symptoms (or autopilots) are the most pervasive problem for most participants with bipolar disorder, we address depression first.

BREATHING SPACE

Before the depression autopilot is discussed, the participants will practice a 3-Minute Breathing Space guided by the instructor (for instructions, see Box 3.2). This serves to reorient participants back to the present, check in with themselves, and ground themselves. Then the class is ready to move forward in the discussion with renewed, open, and accepting awareness.

THE DEPRESSION AUTOPILOT

Most, if not all, participants have experienced trigger situations eliciting negative thoughts, which may increase in frequency and lead to depression. Going forward, negative thinking will be explicitly highlighted as a thinking pattern characteristic of depression. In this session, we address how self-critical thoughts and feeling down can spiral into depression. The instructor guides this discussion by using Handout 10, "The Depression Autopilot." We give this handout to participants as a summary of the discussion at the end of the session. If a whiteboard is available, we draw the depression autopilot on the whiteboard. We typically begin the discussion with automatic negative thoughts.

Automatic Negative Thoughts

To illustrate the nature of automatic negative thoughts, we give participants Handout 11 with the following scenario (see also Segal et al., 2013, p. 312):

> *Instructor:* "You work at a company and just handed in a report to your boss. You feel you have done a really good job with this report, and look forward to discussing it with your boss. A few minutes after you handed it in, his door opens. He does not have the usual smile on his face and asks whether you have a minute to meet. What do you think?"

Common responses from participants include "What did I do?", "He is angry at me," "I must have done something really wrong," and "I screwed up the report." Then, group participants will learn the reason that the boss is not smiling: he just learned that his mother was seriously ill. He wanted to discuss with you whether you could take on some of his responsibilities for the next few days while he visits her. A characteristic feature of depression is the occurrence of automatic, negative thoughts. They are *automatic* in that they habitually occur without any effort. These thoughts are *negative* in the sense that they are unfavorable interpretations or predictions (e.g., "I can't get anything done," "No one likes me," "This will not work out,"). For people who experience ongoing or an intermittent depressive mood, their minds are biased to generate automatic, negative thoughts. This bias is present when they are depressed and also present when individuals with a history of depression are not currently depressed.

An example of this occurs during the mindfulness exercises. Most, if not all, of the participants have experienced self-critical thoughts during the Yoga–Body Scan, the Body Scan, or the various sitting meditations.

Participants also report experiencing negative, automatic thoughts during trigger situations. As part of this discussion, we ask participants to share the negative thoughts they may have encountered as part of the program thus far. Examples of negative thoughts can be listed on the whiteboard. As in Segal et al. (2013), negative thoughts listed in the Automatic Negative Thoughts questionnaire (Handout 12) are then handed out and can then be used to illustrate that these thoughts are part of depression, and reflect the continued risk of relapsing into depression.

Next, we work with participants to establish how these thoughts bias their thinking. Specifically, we ask participants whether they recognize certain patterns in these thoughts. Common patterns, among others, include *black-and-white thinking, misfortune telling,* or *"should" statements.* After discussing examples recognized by the group, Handout 13 can be used to review cognitive biases commonly encountered by people with depression and relate it to participants' experiences. Each participant will have his or her own "favorite" negative thought patterns. As part of the discussion we ask participants to identify which ones they have encountered before. We ask participants to be aware of self-critical negative thoughts as they arise in daily life or during mindfulness exercises, and label them accordingly: "Ah, here is my misfortune teller thought again."

Most participants will be able to easily recognize the connection between negative thoughts and how they feel. As Diane said, "Well, if you ask me how I feel when I think about my life right now, then I'd say 'it sucks.' I guess that's the connection to the feeling you are talking about." The take-home message is that group participants are vulnerable to experiencing depression-related negative thoughts, regardless of whether they are currently depressed, and that these thoughts make them feel bad. The more these thoughts occur, the more often participants will feel down, depressed, or unmotivated. At a certain point, a threshold is crossed into what is called a major depressive episode. However, the connection from thoughts to feelings is not unilateral. Feelings influence thoughts as well.

Mood-Congruent Information Processing

To illustrate the connection from feelings to thoughts, we use Isabel Hargreaves's moods and thoughts exercise (see also Segal et al., 2013, p. 312). Each participant receives a piece of paper describing a short scenario, and we then ask participants to write down their thoughts about the situation (Handout 14):

> *Scenario 1:* "You are feeling happy because you and a work colleague have just been praised for good work. Shortly afterward, you see

another colleague in the office and he or she rushes off quickly, saying he or she couldn't stop. What do you think?"

Common responses include that he or she might be in a rush, does not have time to talk, or has something important to do. Next, we ask participants to turn the page and read a second scenario:

Scenario 2: "You are feeling down because you have just had a quarrel with a colleague at work. Shortly afterward, you see another colleague in the office and he or she rushes off quickly, saying he or she couldn't stop. What do you think?"

In the discussion that follows, the tone of the interpretations commonly shifts. Explanations include "He must have heard about the argument," "He does not want to be seen talking to me," "He is on the other colleague's side," "I am being singled out," "I am an outcast," "Now I am going to get pushed to the side," and "He thinks I am an idiot for getting into this argument." This exercise illustrates that interpretations of the situation changed with the person's mood. When the reader was feeling happy, the interpretation was positive. When the reader was feeling down, the interpretation (or automatic thought) was negative.

This is a phenomenon called "mood-congruent information processing." It refers to the fact that when one is in a good mood, one will experience more positive thoughts, whereas if one feels down, one's thoughts will be more negative. This closes the loop from thoughts to feelings back to thoughts and can create a vicious cycle in which people can get stuck. As Taylor pointed out during the discussion, "When you are in this, it is really difficult to experience happy thoughts. They just don't come naturally." We then connect the vicious cycle of mood-congruent information processing with the feeling of aversion and how this sets the stage for rumination:

Instructor: "When you hear your colleague say that he or she does not have time to talk, and you find yourself thinking that he is thinking negatively of you, it's hard to imagine that you like this. Who wants to be singled out or looked at unfavorably? This is when your mind goes into automatic fixing mode. 'Could I be wrong thinking this? Am I imagining it? Could I be wrong about this? Perhaps he is just in a rush? But, no, this is just too close to the discussion I had with the other person to be a coincidence. But why is he taking it out on me? He should be angry at her.' This mental fixing rarely yields the desired solution of finding out why your colleague cannot talk and that this does not have anything to do with you. Additionally, it maintains and likely intensifies this mood-congruent information-processing vicious cycle, because it keeps the negative thoughts present in your mind, which is, after all, what you are trying to fix."

Thoughts Are Not Facts

There is another important piece of the scenarios that we discuss with the group. *Thoughts are not facts.* We ask the group what we actually know about the colleague's behavior and compare it with the interpretations of the situation. This can be done on a whiteboard, dividing it into two halves: noting the known facts about the colleague's behavior on the left side and the content of the negative thoughts on the right side. Fact is, we know that the colleague rushed off quickly and said that he or she could not talk. Fact is also that the colleague's behavior was exactly the same in both scenarios. The interpretation often goes beyond the factual information, speculating that the colleague is upset with you and wondering why. In order to connect this with participants' experiences, we will then discuss examples from situations that trigger negative, automatic thoughts and elicit further examples about negative thoughts group participants may have encountered.

Taylor realized that her negative thoughts regarding being late for group that day contained quite a bit of interpretation. "The fact is that I would miss part of the group but my thoughts made it sound like I would be failing the whole group and not get anything out of it, and that things will never ever get better." Likewise, Michelle realized, "I am rarely wrong when I notice something going on with my boyfriend, but the thoughts are taking this too far. Splitting up and separation." We use these examples to illustrate that automatic, negative thoughts are products of the mind, mental events, but not facts. We ask participants to deliberately take this stand from now on.

> *Instructor*: "As you can see, automatic, negative thoughts are not only part and parcel of depression but they can also easily lead back into depression. The first step of dealing with them differently is recognizing automatic, negative thoughts for what they are—thoughts, mental events, something that the mind produces. As you have seen from the examples we have discussed, everyone has his or her own set of automatic, negative thoughts. Often they feel believable. They seem real. There always seems to be some truth to them. Nonetheless, recognizing them for what they are before they can set the autopilot in full swing is key. As negative thoughts arise, they can feel quite painful and aversive, call for fixing, and lead into rumination and more pain. Therefore, from now on, as you become aware of negative thoughts,

as you notice yourself feeling down or depressed or perhaps already ruminating about something, we would like you to do a Breathing Space right then and there. Coming into the present, checking in with yourself, noting what is going on in terms of thoughts, feelings, and sensations. Then, as you have done before for trigger situations, anchor yourself on the breath and ground yourself, before expanding your attention to include the body as a whole and bringing acceptance especially to those feelings, sensations that are particularly difficult at that moment. The Breathing Space is a means of stepping out of the autopilot and bringing yourself back into the present and connecting with the present moment. Let's practice the Breathing Space again."

In this session, and going forward, the instructor uses the 3-Minute Breathing Space instructions, which include directions for acceptance (Box 5.2; see also Segal et al., 2013, p. 288). The ending of the Breathing Space will be a point for participants to decide how to move forward when they have concluded the Breathing Space.

> *Instructor*: "The end of the Breathing Space represents a decision point for everyone. The questions you want to ask yourself at that point is, 'How can I go forward in a way that I take good care of myself right now?" and "What do I need right now?" The answer to this question may depend on the thoughts, feelings, and sensations you are experiencing at the time, so I would like to go over a few useful guidelines that may help you with this."

The instructor and group will go over the information outlined in Handout 15 (see also below). Let's consider two examples of how participants moved forward after the Breathing Space.

For Justin, who was attending an evening master's program in landscaping, homework was a constant source of negative thoughts and depression. "I don't know where to start. For one class, in particular, it is not clear to me what the instructor wants. I keep looking at the assignments and trying to wrap my head around them, but there are so many different ways that these assignments could be done. I find myself thinking that I could do it this way, or that way, or perhaps another way, but then I get lost, think that what I am going to do will be wrong, that I will get bad grades, and then fail the course. And I need this course because it's a prerequisite for next year. It's agonizing. Often I end up not doing anything and procrastinating until the last minute and then doing something just to be able to hand it in."

Over the course of the previous sessions, Justin had recognized that his autopilot thinking was circling around the different ways of approaching projects, and trying to find the right approach, the right solution, was mixed in with increasingly catastrophic thoughts about his grades and future. He had been able to bring the Breathing Space to these moments, but was not sure of what to do next. For him, moving forward mindfully meant picking a starting activity. He would start some aspect of his homework that he knew how to do. This got him going and gave him the confidence of accomplishing something. Research has shown that getting involved in a task is a strategy that tends to protect against the "ruminative autopilot." Justin also realized that he lost a great deal of time trying to find the right way to approach homework and began to settle on an acceptable approach, while bringing acceptance to the feeling that it may not be the best way of doing it.

Holly, on the other hand, had no difficulty completing tasks and assignments, but found that her most difficult situations centered on dating. She had not been in a relationship for several years and had recently started online dating. These dating situations often made her feel depressed. "This guy, after we had talked on the phone, did not want to go for a coffee. This really hurt. I am worth going out for a coffee. How can he be so rude to already call it off after one phone conversation? I think I am a really nice person, and I think we had a decent conversation and I don't understand why just after one phone conversation he can call it off." She had been ruminating about the topic at great length. "I am trying to find reasons why and have been going over this again and again, but can't seem to understand it. I really liked him." Her strategy in dealing with the situation had been very proactive. She discussed it with her friends at length, often for hours, rallying support for herself. "My friends are all saying the same thing. He is wrong in just calling it off after just one conversation."

For Holly, mindfully moving forward did not require her to be more active. Her challenge was to acknowledge and bring acceptance to the painful thoughts and feelings that this situation had caused. Her mental and behavioral activities had centered on proving that her love interest had been wrong in declining to go out for a date and trying to fix what her mind was already saying. "I guess he is not interested in me," she said sadly, as the instructor asked her to allow herself, as best as she could, to feel the pain in her body, rather than running away or closing her inner eye. Justin and Holly's experiences illustrate that mindfully moving forward at the end of the Breathing Space may involve different things for different people.

BREATHING SPACE

Before discussing how to mindfully move forward after the end of the Breathing Space, the group practices a 3-Minute Breathing Space with Acceptance guided by the instructor.

Box 5.2. The 3-Minute Breathing Space with Acceptance

(Note to the instructor: [. . .] indicates a pause.)

- The first part of the Breathing Space is becoming aware of what is going on with you right now. Becoming aware of what is going through the mind. As best as you can noticing thoughts as mental events. Also, becoming aware of any feelings that are around at this moment . . . allowing any discomfort or unpleasant feelings to be with you, rather than pushing them away or shutting them out. Just acknowledging them. Noticing sensations in the body . . . Are there sensations of tension? . . . Again, just allowing yourself to be aware of them . . . Simply noting them. Whatever it is you are noticing right now, thoughts, feelings, or sensations, simply allowing yourself to just notice whatever is going on right here.

- The second step, now that you have stepped out of automatic pilot, is to collect your awareness by focusing on a single object: the movements of the breath. Focusing attention on the movements of the abdomen, the rise and fall of the breath . . . spending a minute or so to focus on the movement of the abdomen . . . moment by moment, breath by breath, as best you can. So that you know when the breath is moving in, and you know when the breath is moving out. Just anchoring awareness to the movement of the breath . . . gathering yourself: using the anchor of the breath to really be present.

- And now as a third step, having gathered yourself to some extent, allowing awareness to expand. As well as being aware of the breath, also including a sense of the body as a whole. So that you get this more spacious awareness . . . A sense of the body as a whole, including any discomfort, tension, or resistance . . . If sensations are there, bringing awareness there by "breathing into them" on the inbreath. Now breathing out from those sensations, softening, and opening with the outbreath. Saying to yourself on the outbreath, "It's OK. Whatever it is, it's OK. Let me feel it." . . . And now, as best as you can, bringing this expanded accepting awareness to the next moments of your day . . .

Adapted from Segal et al. (2002, 2013). Copyright 2002, 2013 by The Guilford Press. Adapted by permission.

Next, we discuss the choices participants have concerning how to move forward after the Breathing Space when participants are feeling down or depressed (see also Segal et al., 2002, 2013).

CHOICE POINTS: HOW TO MOVE FORWARD
WHEN FEELING DOWN OR DEPRESSED

Activities

When people start to feel down or depressed, they are often not motivated to do things. However, rather than waiting until motivation returns, it often is beneficial to try to do things nonetheless. Two types of activities are typically recommended: (1) pleasurable activities, and (2) mastery-based activities. This rationale follows the following logic: If you do things that are fun, meaningful, and provide you with a sense of accomplishment, then you will feel less down or depressed. But you can't wait until you feel like doing these things. Rather, it means doing them even though you are not in the mood. In other words, behavior needs to take the leading role. For this, we ask participants to think about behaviors and activities that typically make them feel good, are self-soothing, provide meaning, or generate a sense of accomplishment. As Justin's example shows, these activities or behaviors do not necessarily need to be big tasks. Sometimes an ice-breaker activity such as getting started with something you know does the trick. On the other hand, we advise participants to avoid activities that keep the autopilot going. For example, Holly had talked to many of her friends in order to rally support for herself. The thought that this individual did not want to meet her was painful, and rallying support for her worthiness was geared toward reducing the pain. However, this kept the automatic thought alive in her mind, and no matter how much Holly tried, she could not garner enough support to put it to rest. For her, learning to be with thoughts as thoughts and uncomfortable feelings was critical (see below). Her experience also illustrates that one needs to carefully consider what activities to choose, as sometimes activities can serve as an avoidance (or fixing) behavior that keeps the autopilots alive rather than helping one to step out of it.

Being with Thoughts

When thoughts dominate, it may be necessary to spend some time on them, in order to move forward after the Breathing Space. The instruction is explicit: Thoughts are mental events, not facts. Therefore, it can be helpful to observe thoughts entering and leaving the mind with a gentle interest, curiosity, and welcoming stance, without making any effort to hold on to them. This is analogous to inviting a person to stay or leave as he or she pleases. If one or more negative thoughts are dominant in the field of awareness, it may be helpful to write them down on to a sheet of paper, one by one, and look at them as an object. Or one can imagine writing them in the sky, attaching the thoughts to a cloud, and watching them from the ground. As negative thoughts tend to carry things to the extreme, it can also be helpful to ask the following questions (see also Segal et al., 2002, p. 266).

> "Are the thoughts I am experiencing . . .
>   confusing thoughts with facts?
>   jumping to conclusions?
>   painting things in black-and-white terms?
>   totally condemning myself because of one thing?
>   concentrating on my weaknesses and forgetting my strengths?
>   blaming myself for something that isn't my fault?
>   judging myself?
>   setting unrealistically high standards for myself so that I will fail?
>   mindreading/crystal ball gazing?
>   expecting perfection?
>   overestimating disaster?"

Some of these questions could lead participants to review evidence for and against some of these statements. Often, this gets them back into rumination very quickly. When this happens, we advise participants to simply acknowledge the possibility that the thought might be overly negative or catastrophic.

Being with Feelings

If feelings and bodily sensations are dominant (e.g., aversion), we encourage participants to approach these feelings and sensations with gentle curiosity. Note where the feeling is expressed in the body, note the raw sensations for what they are and bring a gentle, accepting curiosity to those feelings and sensations while maintaining a sense of the body as a whole. Perhaps breathe into those sensations, and tell yourself that it is OK to feel whatever you are feeling. By the same token, respect your abilities and give yourself permission to move attention away from the sensations and feelings if it becomes too overwhelming or difficult. You may reanchor yourself on the breath, or any other anchor that you may choose. Give yourself permission to approach and withdraw from the sensations and feelings at any time. This is especially important when feelings and sensations are particularly strong. We simply ask participants to respect what they can do at a given time. In the next session, we will begin a sitting meditation practice during which participants will practice the above approach, focusing on how to be mindful when strong feelings and sensations are present in the body.

When participants have difficulties motivating themselves and have low energy, often they try to modulate this feeling on the inside, trying to get themselves "motivated" or "energized" just to have the right level of motivation to do things. Often, however, they don't reach the "right" feeling, or the "right" energy level that would allow them to do what they wanted to do, such as getting up from the couch, out of bed, or going to the store or to work. In MBCT, we ask participants to bring awareness to this feeling of not being motivated, noting where it is in the body, and with what sensations it comes. It may be a feeling of heaviness of the limbs or perhaps feeling "mentally tired." Bringing acceptance to this feeling and to the way it is expressed in the body is the first step. Then, we ask participants to make themselves move, get up, and start what they needed to do. With awareness of the present feelings and without trying to change them, let behavior take the leading role.

We also remind participants that as they may find themselves getting derailed when the autopilot comes back, they can simply repeat the Breathing Space as often as they feel it is needed, and then go from there. The signs of depression are different for every participant. For some, the most defining features may be negative thoughts and rumination. Perhaps they may not being able to snap out of it in their usual way. Others may feel less motivated than usual and have diminished interest in things they used to enjoy, or have a hard time keeping up with tasks and activities. Others (see Session 7) may start to feel more irritable. The above template of how to move forward after the Breathing Space will be individualized with each participant so that each participant develops his or her own personalized way in how to bring mindfulness to these experiences (see also Chapter 4).

WHAT IF PROBLEMS AND THOUGHTS ARE REAL?

One participant, Michael, remained skeptical. "But what if the thoughts are right? What if a situation is really bad and thoughts are not just making this up? Last week, I had an interview, and I knew right away that I wouldn't get the job. The interview did not go well, I did not seem to connect with the interviewer, I couldn't answer some of her questions, and I knew instantly that I would not get the job, given how horribly I was doing. I actually found out this week that I did not get the job. So, the thought was right about it." Michael makes a common point. Often, negative thoughts are not completely off-base, and carry some element of truth. This is why they are believable and we take what they say for granted. Michael's observations that he did not seem to connect well with his interviewer and that he was unable to answer some of her questions were likely correct. But there was more to the thought than just that—it immediately judged his performance as "horrible" and concluded that "Michael would not get the job." This is a mix of black–and-white thinking ("horrible") and misfortune-telling ("I am not going to get this job"). And then something else happened to Michael after the job interview. "I found myself going over what I had said in the interview, over and over and over again. Trying to find out what I could have said or done differently, how I could have answered some of the questions that I could not answer, and just trying to improve my performance for the next interview that might come my way. I tried to somehow convince myself that my performance was OK, and that I still have a chance."

For the next week, Michael felt anxious and keyed up as he kept reviewing the interview situation in his mind and trying to fix it. Going forward, Michael's task became twofold. Whenever he found himself returning to the interview situation, Michael began to use the Breathing Space, becoming aware of his thoughts and feelings in that moment, acknowledging catastrophic thoughts such as "If you don't fix this, all other interviews will go badly, too." Michael practiced bringing acceptance to these images, thoughts, and the feeling of aversion as he experienced them. In doing so, Michael also realized that he could have been better prepared for some of the interview questions. Going forward, Michael decided to start a log with questions he was asked in job interviews in order to improve his interview performance. In this situation, mindfulness meant actively bringing acceptance to whatever an experience is in that moment, at the time, but does not necessarily mean that things should stay unchanged. Mindfulness requires acceptance, but also calls for mindful consideration for how we can best address existing problems.

Justin, the landscaping student, also found himself in a situation that required problem solving. Justin was not the only student in his landscaping class having problems with homework; the other students shared his frustration with the ambiguous assignments. So what could they do? We brainstormed with Justin during his individual session and created a list of several options: Muddle through? Ask the teacher to make assignments clearer and more focused? Work on the assignments with other students? In the end, Justin and his peers opted to talk to the teacher together, which yielded something interesting. The teacher deliberately made homework assignments ambiguous because he was interested in the different approaches and solutions that students would come up with.

EMOTION-FOCUSED MEDITATION:
DIFFICULT FEELINGS

In this session participants will also begin to practice Emotion-Focused Meditations. In these meditations, participants will purposefully bring awareness to difficult themes and topics that are present in their lives. The purpose is for participants to practice being more mindful of difficult feelings, sensations, and thoughts (i.e., notice them, observe them, accept them without getting tangled up in them or slipping into attempts to fix them or make them go away). This involves any feelings and thoughts related to feeling down or depressed; mood elevation; feeling angry, irritable, or anxious.

Why Emotion-Focused Meditations? Turning toward difficult thoughts and feelings and being with the experience in an observant, accepting way, without trying to modify or change it, leads to habituation. That is, the perceived intensity of the feelings associated with difficult thoughts and sensations will lessen with time. This is one of the hypothesized mechanisms by which mindfulness helps people to deal better with difficult thoughts and feelings.

The instructions for this Emotion-Focused Meditation exercise are generic in order to encompass the various experiences that participants have (see below). The material provided in Sessions 5–8 (Handouts 15, 20, 25, 27) will help instructors and participants personalize the exercise to participants who experience thoughts and feelings related to depression (see above), mood elevation (see Session 6), anger/irritability (Session 7), and anxiety (Session 8). Based on their experience with mindfulness thus far, as well as their knowledge of trigger situations, we ask participants to note topics that are difficult for them. For Michelle, this was "feeling out of sync with her boyfriend." Jennifer mentioned being treated disrespectfully by other people, "especially the employee at the front desk in the gym." These are examples of topics and negative thoughts, which we ask participants to voluntarily bring to mind during the focused meditation. During this meditation, participants bring an accepting observation to the feelings and sensations associated with that particular topic. Participants should choose a topic they feel comfortable working with, not necessarily from today's topics of depression and automatic thoughts. For Elizabeth, this meant calling to mind the feeling of wanting to do more experiments at work, which could lead her into hypomania, and bring an accepting observance to the feelings, sensations, and thoughts that were evoked. For other participants, this meant deliberately bringing on sensations, feelings, and catastrophic thoughts associated with panic or worry. Of course, if negative, self-critical, catastrophic, or angry thoughts are already present during the Emotion-Focused Meditation, then this is what we encourage participants to work with.

Box 5.3. Emotion-Focused Meditation (10 Minutes)

(Note for the instructor: [. . .] indicates a pause.)

- For this meditation, make sure that you are sitting in a comfortable and relaxed position. Being aware of how it feels to be sitting here, in this moment. Becoming aware of sensations in the body, sensations in the legs and feet, the buttocks . . . the back and torso, . . . the arms, hands, the neck, head, and the face. And becoming aware of the breath. Inhaling and exhaling as it is happening right now . . . (*Longer pause*)

- Throughout the entire meditation session, it is always possible to return to the breath at any point, whenever you feel that this is what you need.

- And when you are ready, bringing awareness to feelings, the emotions that are present in this moment.

- Bringing awareness to whatever kind of feeling is present right now. This can be any feeling. There might be sadness or anxiety, maybe impatience, anticipation, or perhaps boredom, peacefulness, or happiness, contentment, or anger. There is no right or wrong way to be feeling right now. Just notice whatever is present. Whatever it is, bringing full awareness to what you are feeling in this moment.

- Familiarizing yourself with this emotion . . . It is of course possible that there is no particular feeling present in this moment. Oftentimes, we don't experience any particular kind of feeling.

- If this is the case, and no other feelings are dominant, you may choose to bring to mind a difficult thought, sensation, or feeling that you have been struggling with. Perhaps this is a thought, feeling, or sensation that you would much rather avoid because it is aversive, or one that is pleasant and comes with wanting.

- With whatever feeling is present in the body, whether it was already here, or perhaps brought on voluntarily, now, bringing awareness to the sensations in the body that are present right now wherever they are . . . being with whatever is present . . . opening up to it . . . turning toward it, . . . maybe asking yourself where in the body this feeling is most predominant? Where is it most vividly noticeable? What kind of sensations in the body are related to it? . . .

- Now, also remaining aware of the thoughts that come with the feeling, thoughts that are related to the feeling, or thoughts about the feeling. There is no need to change them in any way. Just noticing them as mental events in the mind without getting tangled up in them, no matter what they say and how long they stick around, . . . and now gently allowing yourself to be with the feeling, the emotion, and the bodily sensations again . . .

- And at any time, if you feel it is too much, if it is too intense, always feel free to back off a bit . . . returning to the breath or returning to the sensation of sitting on the cushion, even opening the eyes if it feels too much, . . . finding out what feels appropriate right now and following that . . . taking care of yourself . . . and if it feels right to you in this moment, coming back to opening toward the feeling, toward the emotion.

- Becoming aware of the tendency of the mind to label the experience as either pleasant or unpleasant.

- And also becoming aware of the tendency of the mind to want more of the experience if it was labeled as pleasant and to want the experience to go away if it is unpleasant. Not reacting to it. Just being with it. As best as you can, bringing a kind, gentle acceptance to whatever feeling and sensations are unfolding in the body in each moment.

- You might notice that the feelings or the sensations you are experiencing are changing from moment to moment as you are being with them. They might change in intensity, or even in their quality . . . they might become a different feeling, or they might disappear overall . . . just noticing that things are different moment to moment . . . and bringing this present acceptance to each and every experience in every moment, right here, right now . . . and also aware of the flow of the breath at the same time . . . the breath coming along with the feeling, underlying the emotional quality . . . (*Longer pause*)

- And as you are sitting here, observing the feelings here in this moment, perhaps becoming aware of the fact that you are not the feelings, . . . the feelings come and go, just like clouds passing by in the sky, but you are not the feelings, not the emotions themselves. The feeling is coming and going, lingering for a while and then passing through . . . (*Longer pause*)

- And now as this meditation ends, you have the option to stay with this practice, or if you want to complete this sitting, bringing awareness back to the sitting posture, awareness to the flow of the breath, and when you are ready, opening your eyes and bringing movement back into the body.

The group and instructor then discuss the experience with Emotion-Focused Meditation. These experiences are described in Session 6. For homework every participant will choose one troublesome thought or feeling for the Emotion-Focused Meditation. In general, participants should choose a topic about which they are reasonably confident that they can work with (i.e., one that is not too overwhelming). Otherwise, there is a risk of avoiding homework because it feels too aversive. We also will ask participants to start a list of troublesome thoughts and feelings that are related to depression, mania, anger/irritability, and anxiety, so that they can begin to practice with these thoughts and feelings over the next four sessions and going forward (Handout 16). Participants may consult their Worksheet for Trigger Situations and Mood Diaries as they generate their lists of topics. We also emphasize that if troublesome thoughts or feelings are already present at the time when a participant is gearing up to practice

the Emotion-Focused Meditation, then one should practice with these difficult thoughts, feelings, and sensations instead of deliberately bringing the
chosen topic (and associated thoughts and feelings to mind). However, if
nothing in particular is dominant at that time, we invite participants to
work with their chosen difficult topic.

HOMEWORK

For homework we ask participants to continue with their Mood Diary and
continue to pay attention to warning signs (Handout 5). We ask participants to do the 3-Minute Breathing Space with Acceptance (audio track
8) when they encounter trigger situations or start feeling down or elevated
(i.e., Breathing Space for Coping). Should warning signs arise, participants
are instructed to enact their action plan and, if needed, contact the instructor (see Handouts 8, 15, and 20). Trigger situations encountered during the
week are recorded on the Worksheet for Trigger Situations (Handout 9).
Participants are asked to alternate between the Mindful Sitting with Sounds
and Thoughts meditation (audio track 7) and the Emotion-Focused Meditation (audio track 9): one meditation per day. For the Emotion-Focused
Meditation participants either work with a chosen topic or with any difficult thoughts or feelings that are present at that time of the Emotion-
Focused Meditation. Difficult thoughts and feelings for the Emotion-
Focused Meditation should be listed using Handout 16.

Mania

OVERVIEW

- About This Session
- Welcome Back and Mood Diary Check
- Emotion-Focused Meditation: Depression
- Triggers
- Breathing Space
- Why Be Mindful with Mania?
- The Mania Autopilot
- Breathing Space
- Choice Points: How to Be Mindful with Symptoms of Mania
- Emotion-Focused Meditation: Mania
- Homework
  - Mood Diary and attention to warning signs
  - Emotion-Focused Meditation: Mania (audio track 9)
  - Continue to work with trigger situations
  - Use 3-Minute Breathing Space with Acceptance for coping with trigger situations (audio track 8)

INSTRUCTOR MATERIAL FOR SESSION 6

- Script for the 3-Minute Breathing Space with Acceptance (Box 5.2)
- Script for Emotion-Focused Meditation (Box 5.3)

PARTICIPANT HANDOUTS FOR SESSION 6

- Handout 5: Mood Diary (in case a participant forgot to bring his or hers)
- Handout 9: Worksheet for Trigger Situations

- Handout 10: The Mania Autopilot
- Handout 16: List of Troubling Thoughts and Feelings
- Handout 17: Why Prevent Mania with Mindfulness?
- Handout 18: Thoughts, Feelings, and Behaviors associated with Hypomania/Mania
- Handout 19: Cognitive Biases in Hypomania/Mania
- Handout 20: What Should I Do When I Notice Warning Signs of Mania?

ABOUT THIS SESSION

Today's topic is mania: the autopilot of thoughts, feelings, and behaviors that can trigger, maintain, and intensify manic symptoms. We discuss how participants can learn to be mindful about its triggers, its warning signs, and how to be mindful if it escalates into hypomania or perhaps even mania. Unlike depression, mania often feels good, unless one is irritable. Who would not want to be confident, motivated, energetic, fluent with one's thoughts, bright, and witty? This is especially true if one feels depressed a fair amount of the time, as is the case for many individuals with bipolar disorder. Unlike in depression, many of the symptoms of mania feel desirable, come with attachment (wanting more), and promote behaviors that drive them further into mania. One reason to bring mindfulness to mania is to break this cycle in its beginning stages. Bringing mindfulness to mania's triggers, warning signs, and symptoms may not be inherently motivating, so we will review some of the reasons why participants may want to do so. But before discussing mania, we will follow up on the topic of depression covered in the previous session. This involves conducting an Emotion-Focused Meditation and reviewing participants' experiences (thoughts, feelings, and sensations associated with depression). Likewise, we discuss how participants have been mindful with triggers and mood symptoms in daily life (e.g., depression symptoms; see Session 5). For home practice, participants continue to work with the Emotion-Focused Meditation recording (audio track 9).

WELCOME BACK AND MOOD DIARY CHECK

"Finally, I am starting to feel normal again." Taylor had a smile on her face as she handed in her Mood Diary. "This was the best week I've had in months. This program really seems to be working." Her Mood Diary's checkmarks, which tended to err on the side of lower normal and would dip into the depressed range at least a couple of times per week, had been holding steady for the last week. "I also started to work on some of the projects that I had in mind for a long time. Finally I have the energy." This sounded great. Yet, something did not seem to be right. In group, Taylor repeatedly brought up how great it felt not to feel "blah" anymore, having her motivation back. Now she could do the things she had been contemplating for quite a while, but had lacked the energy to start. She also had some new ideas. The instructors became concerned. Taylor wasn't talking fast or hard to interrupt. Her sleep was not disrupted. She seemed to be able to concentrate and was not shifting topics or hard to follow. But the reflections on her change in mood were a bit too long, and she was unusually interactive and chipper in group. When we raised our concerns with her after group, she was skeptical.

"My first normal week and you think I am becoming manic?" Clearly, she was not pleased with this idea. "If this discussion is about increasing my medication, then forget about it." Taylor's experience is common. Finally, one seems to be starting to feel normal, with more energy and without struggling to motivate oneself. Yet, this shift may come with some subtle warning signs, such as reflecting on how good one is feeling, new ideas, talking too long, and wanting to work on things. Taylor agreed to be careful and pace herself. Midway through the week, she experienced difficulties falling asleep one night, and she was ready to acknowledge that she was getting elevated and was ready to put the safeguards, including mindfulness, in place. The following strategies can be employed when a participant fails to recognize warning signs of mania:

- Ask the participant whether he or she has experienced a similar situation in the past.
- Conceptualize the situation with the participant as one in which we are not certain of what is happening, and should be extra careful.
- Ask the participant to carefully monitor other signs of hypomania and mania that have been present in the past. If other warning signs occur, contact the instructor and start implementing the emergency plan.
- Alert the participant that minimizing warning signs could be a warning sign in itself.
- Call the participant during the week to check in.

EMOTION-FOCUSED MEDITATION: DEPRESSION

In this sitting meditation (for instructions, see Session 5, Box 5.2), participants continue to practice being mindful with difficult thoughts, feelings, and sensations. This mindfulness may involve thoughts, feelings, or sensations related to depression or mania, but also those associated with anger, irritability, or anxiety. Thoughts, feelings, and sensations will be different for each participant. During the sitting meditation, we ask each participant to deliberately bring a topic to mind, and accept the feelings and sensations associated with this topic, no matter where they unfold in the body. We recommend that participants practice with the same topic for several days, possibly even weeks, before moving on to a different topic. We do this because with repeated practice, it will be easier to be with the feelings and sensations that the topic brings on without getting tangled up in it, trying to make it go away, or arguing with it. Participants should choose a topic that is a troublesome thought, feeling, or sensation, but it should not be overwhelming. Sometimes, participants find it helpful to rank-order their difficult topics (see below). If we sense that a participant may be over-ambitious, we recommend that he or she start with an easier topic. If a participant is avoidant, we may encourage him or her to move beyond his or her comfort zone. If troublesome thoughts or feelings are already present on the day of the session, then the participant should practice with these thoughts, feelings, and sensations. If nothing in particular is going on the day of the session, we invite participants to continue working with their chosen difficult topic. In this session, we review participants' experiences with topics that tend to be associated with depression. Examples with manic symptoms and elevated mood can be found in the next session. In general, the discussion following the Emotion-Focused Meditation tends to include the following topics: (1) difficulty in tolerating the exercise, (2) rumination triggered by the meditation, (3) decrease in intensity of some feelings over time, and (4) avoidance. As described before, most of the topics discussed with the whole group below focus on issues concerning depression.

Difficulty in Tolerating the Exercise

Experiencing uncomfortable thoughts and feelings may trigger feelings of aversion that can be difficult to tolerate. Ordinarily, uncomfortable thoughts and feelings might trigger rumination, or attempts to distract oneself or shift attention away from the difficult thought or feeling. "This was hard," Holly stated, looking drained. When the instructor asked her to share her experiences, she elaborated. "I chose to work with the 'he does not like me' topic. I have noticed that it is a recurring pattern. When I go on dates, and I do not get an SMS, e-mail, or call shortly thereafter, I feel the guy did not like me. This not being liked is really painful for me, so this is what I chose to work with for this exercise." The instructor then asked Holly what she experienced when she reflected upon this topic. "I used the date from last week, who still has not called me. For me, the pain is in my chest. Heavy pressure, as if bricks were lying on it. I also feel panicky, thinking that it will never work out. So, I started to breathe into it, telling myself that it was OK to feel this, but everything in me wants to run away from this feeling." As Holly described her experiences, the instructor guided her to bring attention to aversion, the "wanting to run away from this feeling," and to allow herself to bring acceptance to this experience: "Give yourself permission to feel what you are already feeling, stopping the running, and allowing yourself to rest in whatever is." He also reminded Holly to be compassionate with herself as she was taking on this exercise: "At any time, if you feel that this is too overwhelming, respect what you and your body can do at this time, and allow yourself to return to the breath or whichever focus you may have chosen as your personal anchor."

"This was also quite overwhelming for me," Michelle said, as she described her experience with the exercise. She had chosen to work with her feeling of "being out of sync" with her boyfriend, as this feeling frequently preceded her becoming depressed and suicidal. "We had talked some things out over the weekend, and everything seemed to be fine, but I still had a feeling that there was something not quite OK. So I focused on that. At first, it seemed to be OK, but then I don't know what happened, all these other thoughts started to come in: 'What about my daughter? Things have been a bit strained with her, too. And what if my boyfriend is just getting fed up and playing along because he can't take it anymore? And my job, and the coworker I don't seem to click with?' This felt really overwhelming; I just wanted to run away from it all."

Knowing that moments like this can be overwhelming for participants, the instructor praised Michelle for being so courageous and allowing herself to approach this difficult topic. He also offered a path to grounding herself when she might feel overwhelmed during the exercise. "With everything we are doing it is important to respect the boundaries of what we are able to do at a given time. It is important self-care to allow yourself to return to the breath and anchor yourself around the breath when you feel that this is getting to be too much." He also invited Michelle, once she felt ready, to widen her attention again, including her whole body in the field of awareness, and allowing herself to notice and be with whatever was present at that particular moment, whether this included thoughts, feelings, or sensations, noticing and being with whatever is from the spaciousness of her body. For Michelle, the feelings and sensations of not being "in sync" appeared to dominate at the time (e.g., tingling in her fingers, a knot in her stomach), and the instructor then invited her once more, whenever she felt ready, to approach the raw sensations again with curiosity and acceptance, "noticing whatever is, accepting whatever is in this very moment." Over the next few weeks, Michelle would begin to explore this feeling of being out of sync with her boyfriend, bring acceptance to those sensations, and have her breath be the anchor she could always turn to when things became overwhelming.

Rumination

Approaching difficult thoughts and feelings, not surprisingly, can trigger rumination, or efforts to mentally fix painful feelings. Holly noticed this right away when she approached the feeling of not being liked. "It kicks in right away, but I am likeable. I am a worthy person . . . When this happened, I used the strategy that we practiced before and returned back to the breath, before approaching this feeling again. Was this right?" she asked. Reanchoring oneself on the breath when one has been carried away, or things feel overwhelming, is always an option at any time during the exercise. Holly also began to label the distressing thought as the "he does not like me" thought, and invited it into her mind while continuing to approach, as best as she could, the raw sensations in her body with curiosity and acceptance. "It is amazing how much my mind wants to go away from this," she admitted, "Just trying for some way to make it less painful, by reasoning against it."

Feelings Losing Power

Even within a single session, participants may notice that the intensity of sensations or feelings they allow to unfold decreases over time. As Holly described, "It fluctuated over the course of the exercise, always there but coming and going, like small waves, and gradually it became a little easier to be with it." Holly's observation refers to the phenomenon of "habituation." Continued and/or repeated exposure to a given stimulus that tends to elicit a particular feeling (e.g., anxiety, discomfort), over time, usually leads to less intense feelings. As Holly continued working with the "he does not like me" thought throughout the week, she found that the feeling became more bearable, less painful, and that it was easier to allow herself to let the thought arise and bring acceptance to the feelings and sensations that came with it.

Avoidance

"I find myself avoiding it. I just could not get myself to do it," Veronica said, disappointed. "Whenever I thought about doing it, I noticed myself feeling very unmotivated. Each time, I found excuses not to do it." Veronica's experience is common. Who would want to bring uncomfortable thoughts to mind and be with them? When this issue comes up, we have two recommendations for participants. First, they may have chosen a topic that may be too difficult at the beginning, leading them to feel too tense or too distressed. Therefore, it may be wise to begin with a relatively easier topic. We suggest asking participants how uncomfortable their chosen topic makes them feel on a scale of 0–10 (where 0 is not uncomfortable at all and 10 is the highest possible level of discomfort). Topics that participants rate close to 10 may not be a good starting point and a less uncomfortable topic may be chosen. Second, participants may avoid the exercise even if their topics are not overwhelming. In this case, we suggest seizing the moment. When participants are aware that the exercise is scheduled and they find themselves engaging in an inner dialogue geared to find reasons why it cannot be done, we ask them to become mindful about the moment when the dialogue is beginning. Bringing awareness to this moment where they are beginning to mentally avoid the topic means that they already have the topic in mind, and they can do the exercise right then and there if they have time.

After participants discuss their experiences as a group, we instruct them to briefly pair up and discuss their list of "hot topics" (Handout 16). Hot topics include those, that consistently come up that either trigger troublesome feelings (e.g., depression, anxiety, anger, or irritability), or may be desirable but dangerous because they may lead to mania. Going forward we will return to these topics, and the discussions about mania (this session), anger and irritability (Session 7), and anxiety (Session 8) may bring additional topics to mind of which participants may not yet be explicitly aware. As Emotion-Focused Meditations continue over the next few weeks, instructors should ensure that participants address all of their most relevant topics if possible. For example, if both mania and depression are an issue, then participants should not focus on one at the other's expense. With their chosen topic, participants will continue to practice Emotion-Focused Meditation on a daily basis for the next several weeks. In this practice, they always have two options: First, we would like them to work with topics that they have identified as troublesome. This way, they work on several difficult topics over the remainder of the program. Their second option is to work with their current feelings and thoughts if they are having a difficult time on the day of the session.

TRIGGERS

As in the previous group session, participants will continue to work with triggers (situations, thoughts, feelings, and behaviors) associated with (1) warning signs and (2) the onset of depressed feelings. In this session, before switching to the topic of mania, we review some moments when participants start to feel down or depressed. In those moments, participants' homework was to initiate the Breathing Space and begin to develop plans for how to mindfully move forward. As in the previous sessions, we ask participants to pair up in couples, compare their notes, and discuss what types of trigger situations they have experienced and how they have handled them. Following one-on-one discussions, we open the topic up for group discussion.

For Michael, the mornings were especially difficult. "I manage until the kids are out of the house, but then I have a hard time getting going. It feels like there are a ton of bricks on my body. I just can't seem to get going." Despite Michael's intentions, he would often find himself unable to go grocery shopping, which would lead to fights and arguments with his wife. "I just can't get myself motivated enough, no matter what I do. The Breathing Space has helped me to be aware of how this actually feels, and where this is in my body." Additionally, adding some movement exercises after the Breathing Space made a significant difference. Michael had liked the movement exercises, and they became a vehicle of getting him going. "I just move, and allow myself to notice movement as I am doing it. And then afterward, I continue to move, and do whatever I have to do, noting movement, and the sensations of movement as I am doing it."

By paying more attention to situations that worsened her mood, Veronica came to realize how much her supervisor at work was a source of frustration for her. "Just thinking of him drags me down. It took me a while to understand what it is about his disorganized behavior that gets to me, because I work with other disorganized people and don't seem to mind. He never specifies enough how an advertisement should look. Then, when we go over it, he makes it sound like I hadn't really listened to him. As if I could read his mind about what he wants. At this point, I would find myself going over all the different options I could try for an advertisement a million times, just to find the one he has in mind. Of course, it is never right, and then I wonder how much longer I can keep my job if I cannot do anything right." This vicious cycle had started to interfere with Veronica's ability to concentrate at work. "After last week's session, I started to plug in the Breathing Space whenever I would find myself starting to ruminate. I started telling myself, 'OK, if this is what happens, then it will happen anyways, whether I ruminate about it or not.' At the beginning, sitting with this feeling was hard, but strangely, it got easier over time." Veronica had also started some problem solving; rather than trying to guess, she started asking her supervisor more direct questions about which designs he had in mind, and found her questions to be well received.

Elizabeth had an update on her mania. "I notice that I get overwhelmed if people throw too much stuff at me, but when it is a project I like, and I am interested in, then I can easily get carried away. Now that we are moving into late spring and summer, this is definitely happening more and more." (Many participants with bipolar disorder have a higher risk for mania during the summer compared to the winter.) "Last week, when they asked me to take on this new project, I was quite excited. I started making plans, began to send e-mails to get things organized, and to set things in motion. It's this 'I am excited' feeling in my body that I need to be careful about. This 'I like this, I can do this' feeling. It feels like ping-pong, jumping up and down in my body that wants out, and like a pleasant tension in my chest and abdomen coming and going. I feel impatient, not wanting to wait. Interestingly, this week, I was aware of it when it happened and brought the Breathing Space to it, observing this rush of excitement, and allowing myself to notice and observe it without turning it into action." Elizabeth's experience provided a bridge to discussing the reasons for bringing mindfulness to triggers, warning signs, and symptoms of mania as they arise, as well as the autopilot that is associated with mania.

BREATHING SPACE

Before turning the attention to mania, the group does a 3-Minute Breathing Space with Acceptance (see Box 5.2) without the guidance of the instructor (i.e., each participant does it by him- or herself). This way, participants reorient themselves to the present and ground themselves so that they can move forward in the session with renewed, open, and accepting awareness.

WHY BE MINDFUL WITH MANIA?

Participants may not be as motivated to prevent the symptoms of hypomania and mania as those of depression. Before discussing the mania autopilot and how to bring mindfulness to thoughts, feelings, and sensations that could otherwise spiral into mania, we include a motivational booster: What should motivate participants to prevent mania? We discuss this topic as a group using Handout 17. We acknowledge that becoming hypomanic and feeling more confident, energetic, motivated, and so on, often feels good. As these symptoms arise, it is understandable that participants want to engage in mental and behavioral activities that maintain and intensify this desired state. Bringing mindfulness in at this point will likely not maintain, but rather decrease, the intensity of some of these experiences. As we shall see later, if symptoms have progressed, bringing in mindfulness can cause discomfort (e.g., not talking when you have an urge to talk). So, why would participants still want to utilize mindfulness techniques?

The key for this discussion is to not try to convince participants that they should bring mindfulness to thoughts, feelings, and sensations that trigger mania. Rather, in this discussion we will try to identify each participant's personal reasons for making this investment. We will list the reasons brought up by participants on a whiteboard. Common reasons include:

- Hypomania feels good, but it does not stay that way. That is, there is an initial period where participants feel great, productive, and high functioning. Then, people get increasingly erratic, they can't keep their thoughts straight, and it can even become painful to not be able to sleep anymore.
- Even hypomania can be dangerous if one ends up engaging in risky activities, such as spending too much money, drinking to excess, doing drugs, or engaging in other dangerous activities.
- Following hypomania/mania, participants may crash into a period of depression.
- Following hypomania/mania, even if participants do not crash into depression, they will likely be emotionally labile for weeks. That is, minor things will trigger strong emotional reactions. People get easily overwhelmed, anxious, angry, or irritable.
- Following hypomania/mania, participants may find that it is very hard to get motivated to do anything. This may last for months.
- Hypomania/mania is often followed by impaired functioning. After a single manic episode, half of the people with bipolar disorder do not return to the level of functioning that they had prior to that episode.

We ask participants to record their personal reasons for preventing mania with mindfulness using Handout 17. Next the discussion will turn to the mechanisms of how thoughts, feelings, and behaviors can spiral into mania.

THE MANIA AUTOPILOT

How can, thoughts, feelings, and behaviors trigger, maintain, and intensify manic symptoms? As in the previous session we draw the autopilot (see Handout 10) on the whiteboard. We typically begin the discussion about the autopilot involved in the development of mania by presenting the warning signs and symptoms of hypomania/mania. This is presented as a puzzle. We divide up the group into one to three smaller groups and give each group Handout 10. The figure depicts how thoughts, feelings, and behaviors constitute the mania autopilot. Warning signs and symptoms of mania are printed on small cards handed to the groups (Handout 18). Each group assigns the cards to the *Thoughts, Feelings,* and *Behavior* boxes in Handout 18.

Once the sorting process is completed, we broaden the discussion to the whole group and we invite participants to categorize each of the warning signs and mania symptoms (the instructor writes those on the whiteboard next to the corresponding box). This discussion is geared to renew and deepen the group's understanding that warning signs typically trigger a vicious cycle of thoughts, feelings, and behaviors, which lead to hypomania/mania. Therefore, we start asking for warning signs first (e.g., feeling more confident) and then add mania symptoms (e.g., being grandiose) to the schema drawn on the whiteboard. To keep things consistent, we then tend to continue the discussion with automatic positive thoughts (see below), but one may also start with feelings. Note that irritability can be a sign of either mania or depression. Session 7 is devoted to irritability and anger autopilots.

Automatic Hyperpositive Thoughts

Participants who develop hypomania or mania typically experience hyperpositive thoughts that occur without effort, hence the term *automatic* hyperpositive thoughts. These ideas are hyper*positive* in that they come with favorable or perhaps overly optimistic interpretations or predictions about one's abilities or outcomes (e.g., "It'll work out." "I can get away with this"). Automatic hyperpositive thoughts may appear to be insights into how things are coming together. Participants may perceive an increased understanding of the meaning of things. We ask participants to share with us what kind of hyperpositive thoughts they have encountered as part of the program so far, either during practice or trigger situations that were discussed in this session and the previous session. Note that feeling more confident or being more hopeful are often assigned to the "Feeling" category, but they are also mental representations of one's abilities or predicted outcomes for one's tasks and activities. For many participants, increased confidence and hyperpositive outcome expectations are the entry into the mania autopilot. Participants may also experience paranoid thoughts as part of the mania autopilot. This often happens in the context of others noticing their behavioral changes and trying to prevent the participant from making mistakes, or acting in a way that comes with negative consequences (e.g., doing drugs, spending too much money). Others' efforts can be interpreted as "They are trying to stop me," "They don't want me to advance," "They are trying to get in the way of my life," and so on. Like automatic negative thoughts, hyperpositive thoughts follow certain patterns that we highlight next using Handout 19. These include positive fortune telling, overestimation of one's capabilities, or underestimation of risk of danger.

Thoughts Are Not Facts

We will point out that similarly to automatic negative thoughts, hyperpositive thoughts are not facts either. Although one might feel more confident, one's capabilities have likely not increased. The greater sense of connectedness one has gained probably does not correspond to a change in the real world. And why would others suddenly start interfering or attempting to cause harm? We can use participants' previous experiences of what happened to their feelings of being extraordinarily confident and competent when hypomania/mania was treated or subsided. Using these examples, the instructor highlights that the idea of changing feelings represent a cognitive shift, rather than a corresponding change in the real world. Therefore, we ask participants to take the same approaches that they have adopted for dealing with automatic negative thoughts: (1) thoughts are not facts and (2) recognize the patterns that come with the automatic hyperpositive thoughts (see section "Choice Points: How to Be Mindful with Symptoms of Mania," below).

Mood-Congruent Information Processing

Automatic hyperpositive thoughts are associated with feelings of increased motivation or energy, and perhaps anxiety or irritability in the context of paranoid automatic thoughts. These feelings bias the brain to automatically generate or retrieve further automatic positive thoughts. Participants are already familiar with the phenomenon of mood-congruent information processing from the discussion about negative automatic thoughts in the last session. One's feelings shape one's thoughts and interpretations. If an individual is feeling down, their interpretation of a situation will likely be much more negative than when they are feeling happy. We can illustrate this reality by asking participants to recall experiences of euphoric mania. Often, participants will describe these experiences as addictive. This is how good it feels. We then ask participants to recall how they felt about their abilities at that time: how capable they felt, their skills, and so on. Daniel described his experience: "You think nothing can stop you. This was the time when I started my restaurant. I had no idea about the restaurant business. I had never owned one before. I am not a chef. That still did not stop me." Mood-congruent information processing closes this initial loop from thoughts to feelings back to thoughts and can create a vicious cycle of mania. Positive rumination and increased mood-congruent goal-directed activities both appear to intensify the cycle.

Positive Rumination

"I cannot stop thinking about her," Sean confessed. "She is the one. I keep getting fantasies about how great it would be to go out for coffee and dinner with her and talk to her. I find myself creating scenarios about how I could ask her out." Positive thoughts carry feelings of motivation, anticipation, and pleasure. How great it would be to take on certain tasks and activities and this feeling of attachment (wanting), similar to feelings of aversion in depression. Unlike aversion, attachment is about wanting more, and as a result, individuals find themselves fantasizing about what they want, intensifying the positive automatic thoughts and the feeling of wanting. As Elizabeth pointed out, "When an experiment catches my eye, it is hard to get my mind off of it. I can get this experiment done really efficiently and really fast. And the results are going to be great! In those situations, my mind is caught and I find myself having this constant push wanting to get it going and thinking about how great this feels. My mind almost goes on autopilot: set this up, do this, do that. And it feels great to be in the swing of things again." Engaging in these types of thoughts increases participants' feelings of being energized and motivated. Rumination can be focused on the feeling (emotion-focused positive rumination) or on the self (self-focused positive rumination) (Feldman, Joormann, & Johnson, 2008). Examples of both forms of rumination are below and are shared with the group. These types of rumination can also be a warning sign for mania and we ask participants to become aware of when they set in.

Examples of Emotion-Focused Positive Rumination
- Noticing how one feels full of energy.
- Savoring the moment.
- Thinking about how one feels up for doing everything.
- Thinking about how happy one feels.
- Thinking about how strong one feels.

Examples of Self-Focused Positive Rumination
- Thinking "I am getting everything done."
- Thinking "I am living up to my potential."
- Thinking "I am achieving everything."
- Thinking about how proud one is of oneself.

The review of the connection between positive automatic thoughts and attachment sets the stage for positive rumination that participants have experienced. The instructor describes this connection as a critical element to recognize:

> *Instructor*: "As you find yourself *thinking* that you can do things, that you are going to get great results in a short amount of time (positive automatic thought) you noticed how your body was creating this feeling of wanting: the push to get it going. This is the attachment, the wanting, the being drawn toward it we have been talking about. Now your mind goes into positive rumination mode. This is what I could do, that is what I should do to get it going. Images, sentences, that increase and intensify the feeling of wanting."

Mood-Congruent Goal-Directed Activities

When participants feel more motivated and energized, engage in positive rumination, have new ideas or plans and become attached to them, their mood-congruent behaviors often increase. Elizabeth explained her experience: "Once I feel it is worth it, I almost start on the experiments instantly, get the prepping going, set everything up. This tends to go well into the night and I get back home late. It is just a great feeling when this happens, and I feel buzzed with excitement." Sean, on the other hand, had started to take a class on dating and how to talk to women, as he felt that he was not sufficiently equipped to talk to the girl he admired. These increases in goal-directed behaviors (steps toward getting the experiment going or gaining skills in talking to women) not only keep the vicious cycle alive, but can also intensify it quite dramatically. This also accounts for some of the associated symptoms that tend to develop as participants become hypomanic or manic. For example, Elizabeth would tend to run multiple experiments at the same time, switching her attention back and forth between different tasks. Within just a few days, her thoughts would feel speeded, she would constantly switch between tasks, making her feel more and more frazzled with her thoughts, increasingly jumpy, have difficulties keeping them straight, and become more and more distractible. Because she would go home late, still thinking about what to do the next day, she would have difficulties falling asleep, further fueling the vicious cycle. Sean started to stay up late to go out on dates, and would also not get enough sleep. This led to his becoming increasingly overconfident in his abilities of asking women out and rendering him unable to tell when women were not interested in talking to him, ultimately resulting in an arrest. What should participants do when they notice warning signs?

Instructor: "As you can see, automatic, positive thoughts, feeling more motivated, energized, and wanting to do things, can easily lead back into hypomania/mania if we are not careful. The first step in dealing with warning signs differently is recognizing the automatic, positive thoughts, the increase in wanting to do things, the ideas and plans entering your mind, and positive rumination for what they are: thoughts, feelings, mental and bodily events, something that the mind and body produce. As you have seen from the examples we have discussed, everyone has his or her own personal warning signs. Often feeling this way is desirable. It feels good. There is the attachment. The wanting. Recognizing this early on before the autopilot gets into full swing is key. From now on, as you notice signs of mood elevation, we would like you to do a 3-Minute Breathing Space right then and there. Come into the present, check in with yourself, noting what is going on in terms of thoughts, feelings, and sensations. Then, as you have done before in trigger situations, anchor yourself on the breath, ground yourself, before expanding your attention to include the body as a whole, and bringing acceptance especially to those feelings and sensations that are particularly dominant at that moment. The Breathing Space is a means of stepping out of the autopilot and bringing yourself back into the present and connecting with the present moment. Let's practice the Breathing Space again, each person by him- or herself, without me giving any guidance or instructions."

BREATHING SPACE

Before turning the attention to how to be mindful with warning signs for and symptoms of mania, the group does a 3-Minute Breathing Space with Acceptance (see Box 5.2) without guidance from the instructor (i.e., each participant does it by him- or herself).

CHOICE POINTS: HOW TO BE MINDFUL WITH SYMPTOMS OF MANIA

The ending of the Breathing Space will be a point for participants to decide how to move forward.

Instructor: "The end of the Breathing Space represents a choice point for everyone. The questions you want to ask yourself at that point are, 'How can I go forward in a way so that I take good care of myself right

now? What do I need right now?' Let's go over a few guidelines that
may help you with this."

At this point, we pull out the template of the Mania Action Plan again
(Handout 20). In Session 3, participants developed behavioral strategies for
when they experience warning signs. As some participants may have experienced, implementing some or all of these strategies introduces a barrier to
participants' sense of increased motivation and energy, new ideas or plans,
and the desire to pursue them. The behavioral guidelines ask participants
not to turn their increased motivation into behavior. As a result, participants may experience aversion to not talking, aversion to not pursuing their
plans and ideas, aversion to slowing down, and aversion to only doing one
task at a time. We will now address these feelings and thoughts with mindfulness (see amended strategies in Handout 20).

Mindfulness with Manic Thoughts

Mindfulness is brought toward the *content* of thoughts (e.g., hyperpositiv-
ity, increased "connectedness," or paranoia) as well as to the *format* of
thoughts (e.g., thoughts being experienced as speeded, bouncy, jumping
from topic to topic).

Thought Content

Hyperpositive Thoughts. Participants are asked to consider thoughts
of increased confidence or downplaying risk as mental events that are
present in their minds. Bringing acceptance to their presence, without
engaging them or arguing with them. Just allowing them to be there for
the time being without turning them into behavior. Perhaps label them
as hypomanic thoughts. Reanchoring themselves around the breath, or
another anchor they choose if they find themselves getting carried away
by positive rumination and elaborating on those thoughts.

Thoughts of Increased Connectedness and Meaningfulness. We
ask participants to recognize these thoughts as what they are, products
of the mind. Again, labeling them as mental events, giving them permission to be in the mind, without mentally pursuing them, approaching
them, turning them into rumination, elaborating on them. Just allowing
them to be around. Reanchoring themselves around the breath as needed,
reopening themselves to the body as a whole and wide spaciousness afterward.

Exciting Ideas and Plans. Participants are guided to notice them as mental events entering participants minds. Giving them permission to be there without engaging them or taking countermeasures. Accepting them for what they are, occurrences in their minds. Do not pursue them. Just acknowledge them, without turning them into action/behavior.

Sexual Thoughts. We ask participants to note their presence and label them as sexual thoughts as they may enter their minds, but without pursuing them or turning them into fantasies or scenarios. Bringing acceptance to the feelings and sensations that come with these thoughts. Noticing the impulse and the attachment that comes with these thoughts and where they are in the body. Noticing the raw sensations, the draw, and the aversion that may arise with not pursuing these thoughts.

Grandiose, Religious, or Paranoid Thoughts. Often, initially, participants have the ability to recognize these thoughts as warning signs. The key is to stay away from engaging them further. Similarly to the other thoughts, they should be acknowledged as mental events. One may notice their presence, but disengage from any further processing such as rumination, planning, or elaborating. As needed, participants may redirect their attention to the breath to disengage from these thoughts, or label them as inappropriately "grandiose," "religious," or "paranoid." Participants with bipolar I disorder, for whom these thoughts are warning signs, should be advised to contact their psychiatrist immediately as the start or increase of antipsychotic medication may be indicated.

As with negative thoughts for depression, participants may want to ask themselves some questions. For example, for any overconfident, grandiose, religious, or paranoid thoughts, participants may ask themselves:

"Are these hypomanic thoughts?"
"Am I getting too confident?"
"Are these ideas that want me to do things on the spur of the moment?"
"Am I not taking consequences into account?"
"Am I overestimating the probability of a positive outcome?"
"Am I taking an unnecessary risk?"
"Is this a dangerous idea?"
"Does this get me to do too much?"
"Could this thought get me back to being manic?"
"Do my insights reflect a change in the real world?"
"Could this feeling of being connected be the first sign of mania?"
"Could this sense of meaning and insight be the start of hypomania?"

Thought Format

Flight of Ideas. If thoughts are jumping from topic to topic, we ask participants to allow themselves to notice and observe the ebb and flow of thoughts and ideas, without trying to follow or control the flow of thoughts. There is no need to catch all of the content. Rather, they may want to label the thoughts as "bouncy," and bring acceptance to their experience of thoughts coming and going,

Speeded Thoughts. Participants may want to notice the increased pace of thoughts as they enter their minds. Not trying to catch every thought, or notice all of the content; rather, labeling the flow as speedy, allowing the flow of thoughts to unfold, without trying to jump in or focus, hold onto thoughts, or slow them down. Accepting the flow for now, like watching cars on a highway, the constant flow and movement.

Feelings

How to be with "feeling" manic? In general, with mood elevation, atten-tion is usually drawn toward the feeling of wanting and the impulse of doing. We ask participants to allow themselves to go toward the feeling of increased energy or motivation, the impulse to do things, the urge to talk, and the desire to act (attachment). They are directed to note where these feelings are located in the body, bringing a curious yet accepting attention to the raw sensations that come with these bodily experiences, but not pur-suing them mentally or turning them into action. Likewise, we ask them to note the attachment that comes with it. If one has the urge to talk, we suggest not to talk, but allow oneself to notice and observe the impulse to talk, in an observant, accepting way. If a participant wants to go out, stay at home. If one wants to do multiple things, do one thing at a time, mind-fully. Not following the impulse to do things introduces a barrier and often is aversive. Therefore, participants are asked to bring mindfulness (accep-tance, observance) to the raw sensations that are associated with aversions that are present in their bodies at the time, in the same way that we asked them to do for feelings associated with depression and feeling down, when they are behaviorally restraining themselves from following impulses.

The same instruction applies toward the impulse or wanting to fanta-size about sexual thoughts and feelings that may have started to increase. We ask participants to gently disengage when they notice that they have been drawn into a sexual or manic fantasy that is fueling the impulse to engage in pleasurable or risky behavior. This does not mean that partici-pants should be passive and do nothing with this experience. Rather, we ask them to mindfully engage in other behavioral activities that do not increase energy, or the impulse, or thoughts, and shield them from too much stimulation.

For every participant, the initial signs of mood elevation are different. Some may feel increased motivation and energy. Others' thoughts may begin to disconnect, and they may not seem to be able to concentrate as well. Still others might notice a feeling of meaning that was not there before, foreshadowing mania. Using this template (Handout 20) about how to deal with the various experiences that come with warning signs and mania symptoms, each participant can begin to work out his or her own way of how to be mindful with these experiences. This is part of the homework, and should also be part of the individual sessions.

EMOTION-FOCUSED MEDITATION: MANIA

After discussing how to be with symptoms of mania, the group does a second Emotion-Focused Meditation. Participants will either continue with their chosen topic or practice with whatever troublesome thoughts, feelings, or sensations are present at the time. If possible, we will ask subjects to choose one of their troublesome thoughts or feelings associated with mania for practice.

HOMEWORK

For homework we ask participants to continue with their Mood Diary and continue to pay attention to warning signs (Handout 5). We ask participants to do the 3-Minute Breathing Space with Acceptance (audio track 8) when they encounter trigger situations or start feeling down or elevated (i.e., Breathing Space for Coping). Should warning signs arise, participants are instructed to enact their action plan and, if needed, to contact the instructor (see Handouts 8, 15, and 20). Trigger situations encountered during the week are recorded on the Worksheet for Trigger Situations (Handout 9). Participants are asked to do one Emotion-Focused Meditation per day (audio track 9) either with a chosen topic or with any difficult thoughts or feelings that are present at that time of the Emotion-Focused Meditation.

SESSION 7

Anger

PARTICIPANT HANDOUTS FOR SESSION 7

- Handout 5: Mood Diary (in case a participant forgot to bring his or hers)
- Handout 9: Worksheet for Trigger Situations
- Handout 10: The Anger Autopilot
- Handout 21: Automatic Anger Thoughts
- Handout 22: Anger-Related Cognitive Biases
- Handout 23: Exercise for Session 7
- Handout 24: Anger Discussion Questions
- Handout 25: What Can I Do When I Feel Frustrated, Angry, or Irritable?

ABOUT THIS SESSION

Why devote a whole session to anger? Anger and irritability can be part of both depression and mania. They can also be "stand-alone" issues. For example, profound irritability and anger have been documented in patients with unipolar major depression (e.g., depression with anger attacks). For these individuals, depression may come with dysphoric, uncomfortable frustration and irritability, which can quickly trigger intense anger. Hypomania or mania can be characterized by feeling irritable rather than (or in addition to) expansive or euphoric. Anger and irritability are also experienced by approximately one-third of patients with bipolar disorder even when they are not depressed or manic (Deckersbach et al., 2000). These people may be highly prone to react with anger in frustrating situations. For individuals who are feeling irritable, even minor frustration can trigger feelings of anger, angry outbursts, or angry rumination. This can create a cycle of automatic irritability- or anger-related thoughts and feelings: the anger autopilot. For home practice, formal anger-focused meditation can be practiced using the Emotion-Focused Meditation exercise (audio track 9).

WELCOME BACK
AND MOOD DIARY CHECK

As in the previous sessions, at the beginning, we check participants' Mood Diaries when they arrive for group. Changes in their mood will be noted and briefly discussed individually as needed, either before or after group. Warning signs that have been newly recognized by participants will become the subject of their ongoing monitoring going forward.

EMOTION-FOCUSED MEDITATION: MANIA

We start the group with an Emotion-Focused Meditation (for instructions, see Session 5, Box 5.3) on troublesome thoughts, feelings, and sensations related to mania. Whichever topic is most relevant for a given participant at the time of the exercise should be practiced then. For participants, the purpose of working with the thoughts, sensations, and feelings that lead to mood elevation, or those associated with mood elevation itself, over the past week, is to increase their ability to disengage from or not engage at all in these feelings. When participants encounter these feelings in real life, we hope that they will be better equipped to disengage from these feelings so that they do not lead to full-blown hypomania or mania. For example, for Elizabeth, opportunities to lead projects and experiments at work posed a particular challenge. The ability to carry a project was exciting for her, and would make her feel confident, appreciated, and create the drive to get started and succeed. This would also lead to working longer hours and coming home late, still feeling excited, which made it difficult to fall asleep. Then she would experience speeded-up thoughts and feelings as if she were "plugged in." Elizabeth's challenge during the Emotion-Focused Meditation was to observe and bring acceptance to those moments and situations, paying attention to the feelings of wanting and anticipation but not engaging them.

Participants may deliberately bring aspects of mood elevation to mind, in order to practice with them. This activity may involve bringing to mind past feelings of confidence, past thoughts of feeling connected and understanding the meaning of things, observing these thoughts as thoughts, without engaging them, bringing acceptance to their presence as mental events. Reflecting upon the thoughts and feelings associated with mood elevation provides participants with the opportunity to bring mindfulness to those experiences. Even though bringing these experiences to mind will not be as intense as the experience of mood elevation, practicing will help them to disengage from these thoughts and feelings when it is most needed. These thoughts and feelings come with being drawn toward them, attachment to them, and wanting to experience them. It feels good to feel confident and capable, which is why participants may want to engage in positive rumination and increase their goal-directed activities that lead into hypomania/mania. It is important to practice bringing experiences that create this wanting to mind, in order to become more mindful of not following that wanting. Finally, for participants who are currently experiencing mood elevation, the practice will provide hands-on experience for developing a more observant, accepting, and decentered stance in the midst of being drawn toward and into those experiences. Working with thoughts and feelings associated with mood elevation during the Emotion-Focused Meditation has its unique challenges.

"I Get Drawn into It."

One challenge may be getting carried away in positive rumination when bringing moments to mind when one felt good, excited, or hyper. For example, Elizabeth described how bringing the thought of conducting new experiments to mind would make her feel excited and create a feeling of wanting. This wanting would quickly turn into reflecting upon how capable she is and fantasizing about the things she could do (positive rumination). For her, the challenge was to observe the wanting, bring an accepting curious attention to where it was located in her body, and start to notice it as a bodily event. As part of the meditation she began to practice accepting its presence, breathing into the drive and the wanting that she was feeling, and allowing these feelings to be present without turning them into action.

"Not Following the Impulse Makes Me Uncomfortable."

Not following one's wanting and impulses to talk, even though the body is saying "Please do so," can create discomfort and aversion. Likewise, not following the ideas or plans one's mind is generating creates an uncomfortable disconnect between the mind and the body. We have all experienced moments like this, when we wanted to do or say something, but needed to wait our turn. For example, we may have wanted to make an important or urgent point but needed to wait until someone else finished speaking. Bringing attention to wanting often means observing and bringing acceptance to not wanting. Not wanting to wait and not wanting to not engage are common examples. Where is this aversion located in the body, and what raw sensations come with it? Ultimately, participants are practicing to bring an accepting observance to this mix of attachment and aversion, with whatever raw qualities it brings.

"I Have a Hard Time Catching the Thoughts."

When participants experience speeded thoughts, often trying to be observe them ends up in a race with thoughts speeding by and participants trying to catch up with them. Rather than trying to catch thoughts and discern their content, we advise participants to allow themselves to notice the speeding by, and label their thoughts as racing without trying to catch each and every one. Participants may label them as racing thoughts and perhaps see their mind as a highway where thoughts are rushing by. The same tenet holds true if participants experience their thoughts bouncing from topic to topic, perhaps in an unrelated fashion, which is called "flight of ideas." We advise participants to just allow themselves to notice and observe without trying to hold on to their ideas or engage them. Like speeded thoughts, we suggest labeling them as bouncy thoughts or thoughts in flight. Participants may also focus on the feeling that comes with racing thoughts: where the feeling is and what sensations come with it. Breathe acceptance into this feeling without getting tangled up in it, and just approach it with a curious, accepting observance.

Thoughts about Increased Meaningfulness and Connectedness

If these thoughts are present or voluntarily brought to mind, we would like participants to deliberately treat them as mental events, noting their occurrence in the mind. The wanting that may come with these thoughts in the body should also be noted and observed. These thoughts may be accompanied by the desire to share, and let other people be part of the insights. Note where this feeling of wanting is, bring some curious observation to it, but do not engage it, and embrace the sensations that come with the discomfort that this may cause.

Going forward, participants will continue to practice Emotion-Focused Meditation on a daily basis. Each participant's topic(s) will be specific to him or her. In the case of a participant who has only experienced a small number of manic episodes, seems to be at low risk for mania due to the presence of few or no warning signs, but experiences ongoing and intermittent depression, mania may not be the most important topic, and topics related to depression should be emphasized. On the other hand, someone who is vulnerable to mania may want to focus on topics related to mania. On a given day, however, participants are asked to notice if thoughts or feelings are present and drawing attention in a prominent way. If they are experiencing thoughts or feelings that elicit aversion or attachment, then they would want to work with these thoughts and feelings during his or her Emotion-Focused Mediation practice.

TRIGGERS

As in the previous session, participants will continue to work on trigger situations, thoughts, feelings, and behaviors associated with warning signs and when they start feeling down and/or depressed. In this session, we ask participants whether they experienced warning signs for mania during the previous week. For those warning signs of mania, participants' homework had been to initiate the Breathing Space and develop plans for how to mind-fully move forward. As in the previous sessions, we will ask participants to pair up, compare their notes, and discuss what types of trigger situations they experienced and how they handled them. Following one-on-one discussions, we open the topic up to the group, and group members share their experiences of working with trigger situations when they felt down or depressed or noticed warning signs for mood elevation. Here are some examples that pertain to mania:

"For me, this was the week of my shift," Sara announced. "Usually it sets in during April or May and I start noticing energy coming back." Like many other participants, Sara's bipolar disorder has a seasonal com-ponent. Vulnerability to mania tends to increase in the spring and summer, while depression is more common during the fall and winter. "With the increased awareness, and knowing that it would be coming, it was interest-ing to observe. I noticed myself doing more things this week, which was the first sign I started to pick up on. So, I began to implement the Breathing Space more often. Just noticing what is going on when I am about to start the next task, or when I started putting more stuff into my schedule. I had thoughts wondering whether I may be doing too much, then thoughts that I was enjoying the swing I seemed to get into. Those warning signs are what we talked about, as well as the tendency to minimize them. These thoughts and feelings feel good, like you are finally getting better! If I had not experienced this shift to optimistic thinking before, I would have gone for it." Sara implemented the action plan she had worked on. She limited her activities, and took breaks throughout the day to implement the Breath-ing Space. "This sometimes felt hard, because I could have done so much more, but allowing yourself to notice that, bring acceptance to it in those moments, was actually helpful not to engage in it too much."

Luis had begun to have frequent religious thoughts and insights. "Reli-gion is an important part of my life, but this week I noticed again that I found myself thinking about how all these different religions are inter-connected and pondering how one could unite people in their beliefs. It is exciting to think about all these connections between the different religions and how to share these ideas with other people." For Luis, this was a major warning sign. Fortunately, he detected it early. His emergency plan included contacting both his psychiatrist and the instructor. He and his psychiatrist decided to temporarily increase his antipsychotic medication. Simultane-ously, Luis would do a Breathing Space when these thoughts started. "This is such a gratifying topic to me, and it feels so important that I could make a real difference in sharing these insights. But from the past, I know that this could get out of hand quickly, so I started to accept the draw toward the thoughts without following them, just noticing them when they would come up. It was an interesting experience, as not engaging would raise tension in my body, but gradually allowing the thoughts to come in and go away, allowing the wanting, and accepting the aversion associated with not engaging, would lessen the tension after a while."

Veronica, on the other hand, experienced being more talkative than usual during the week. She found it revealing to observe the pleasure associated with the flow of talking, as well as the pressure in her body driving it. "I have a hard time stopping in those moments. If I try, the pressure to continue is really strong, and it is very uncomfortable to not keep going at that time. It even gets worse at first when I start the Breathing Space, believe it or not: I feel waves of tension in my stomach and upper chest, as if I have to get the pressure off, right now. So I keep breathing and allow myself to notice these sensations as they unfold, telling myself that this is OK. I just allow it to be there, and interestingly the tension does go down after a while, although it comes back up as I continue to go through my day—especially when I have witty thoughts and would love to turn them into a joke when I talk to others. When I notice it early enough, I have started to shorten my sentences and pause more often during those periods."

Distractibility was Justin's biggest problem. "I find myself starting something, and then remembering other things that I need to do. So I shift, because I am afraid that I will forget. But then the next thing comes to mind and so forth. This constant task shifting really makes me feel wired. So, I started to bring the Breathing Space to those moments when I have thoughts that interfere with what I am doing at the time. I may also write the thought down if it is something I should not forget, but otherwise I label those thoughts as task-interfering thoughts and allow them in, as best as I can. It's not the perfect solution, because I still get the push and the anxiety that I may forget, but as best as I can I let them be with me, breathing into them. It is still better than coming home at the end of the day not having accomplished anything, and feeling frustrated."

For Elizabeth, irritability was an issue associated with mania. "When irritability sets in, I need to be really careful. I am not always able to pinpoint why it sets in. However, when it does, I need to be careful. Often, even minor frustration can then set me off in a big way. In meetings, for example, if people have not followed up on what they said they would do, then I get the feeling that no one is doing anything, which is very frustrating. I am working my butt off, and they don't care. If I let this happen a couple of times during the day, I find myself thinking how messed up this shop is, that we need to clean house, and I get frustrated that other people are not seeing this. A few days like this, and I feel really keyed up, kind of burning on the inside, and my thoughts start to speed up and get bouncy. I have started to breathe when I notice this underlying irritability kicking in and deliberately slow down to offset it. I have also noticed the frustration that precedes the anger that follows and this is what I am trying to let in, the feeling of hurt, disappointment, and not wanting to feel this."

BREATHING SPACE

Before discussing the anger autopilot, the group practices a 3-Minute Breathing Space to reorient themselves to the present and ground themselves so that they can move forward in the session with a renewed, open, and accepting awareness.

THE ANGER AUTOPILOT

In this session, we discuss the autopilot associated with anger and irritability, broadening the view from depression and mania autopilots (use Handout 10). How do thoughts, feelings, and behaviors trigger, maintain, and intensify anger and irritability? We use the same thought/feeling autopilot from the previous sessions to keep things consistent. As in the previous sessions is drawn on the whiteboard. We begin the discussion with anger- and irritability-related thoughts, followed by feelings and mood-congruent information processing, before discussing the role of anger-related rumination and behaviors in intensifying or decreasing anger and irritability. To start, we ask participants to share thoughts they have encountered in situations where they felt angry. This sharing serves to illustrate how in the same way as depression and hypomania/mania, anger comes with a vulnerability to experiencing automatic thoughts. Anger is usually preceded by thoughts and feelings associated with frustration or feeling hurt, which the instructor should elicit as part of participants' examples. Jennifer described her recent run-in with an employee at her health club: "She is just rude to me. She ignores me when I come to the front desk if I need something, and is never friendly or accommodating. She is just so disrespectful." When the instructor asked Jennifer how she felt about getting treated that way, her first response was, "Well, just angry, of course." Upon further questioning, however, she realized that she felt hurt at being treated this way, because she felt that she did not deserve it.

As is the case with negative or hyperpositive automatic thoughts, one does not necessarily need to feel depressed or mood elevation to experience them. Rather, participants are more vulnerable to experiencing frustration- and anger-related automatic thoughts that lead to feeling hurt and angry (e.g., "People disrespect me," "People are impolite"). Handout 21 illustrates common automatic negative thoughts. After eliciting examples from the group, we share and discuss the handout. As with automatic negative and hyperpositive thoughts, it is helpful for participants to see that these thoughts follow a pattern and constitute a bias in their information processing. Common biases in anger-related automatic thoughts are listed in Handout 22 and will be shared with the group. Examples include extreme interpretations ("This is a disaster") or overgeneralizations ("He is always doing things like this to hurt me"). These biases occur automatically; participants do not need to work hard for them. They are just part of how people interpret others' behavior, as well as their own. We point out that when one becomes more aware of biases that make one prone to react with anger, it is helpful to become more mindful. Like automatic negative and hyperpositive thoughts, these angry thoughts are interpretations and mental events, not facts. This is illustrated by Scenario 1 in Handout 23:

> *Scenario 1*: "You are a guest in a hotel and would like to check out. You are the only guest at the front desk. It's a nice day and you are in a good mood. The two front desk employees are engaged in a conversation and it takes a little while before one turns toward you. While standing at the front desk waiting, what do you think?"

Together as the group, we discuss interpretations of the situation. Scenario 2 in Handout 23 illustrates that anger interpretations are facilitated by *feeling* frustrated or angry (mood-congruent information processing):

> *Scenario 2*: "You are a guest in a hotel and would like to check out. You are the only guest at the front desk. It's been a frustrating day and you are pretty irritable. The two front desk employees are engaged in a conversation and it takes a little while before one turns toward you. While standing at the front desk waiting, what do you think?"

This tends to give participants déjà vu of the mood-dependent interpretations they encountered in the previous two sessions. On a good day, thoughts or interpretations may reflect the surmise that the hotel staff is talking about something important, but when irritable, the interpretations of their behavior change to disrespect or inattention. This again demonstrates that thoughts are not facts, but interpretations of the situation. Likewise, the example illustrates mood-congruent information processing, where feeling a certain way will elicit more automatic thoughts that fit that particular theme. This vicious cycle also sets the stage for (1) rumination and (2) behaviors, which, similar to depression and mood elevation, tend to increase frustration and anger, rather than decrease it.

Anger-Related Rumination

Similar to the depression autopilot, feeling hurt and frustrated is aversive, and can trigger rumination. Thinking about what to say to someone, how to correct him or her, how to make oneself heard, or tell someone off, are ways for the brain to try to repair hurt and angry feelings. Unfortunately, as in depression, it often yields the opposite effect. Rumination increases, rather than decreases feelings of being hurt and being angry. And, likely, the process of ruminative stewing becomes more automatic and overlearned the more often someone engages in it.

Behavior

A commonly held belief is that acting on anger has a cathartic effect. That is, once one is angry, expressing it lowers one's anger level. Empirical studies suggest that the opposite may be the case: overtly expressing anger may actually increase anger rather than decreasing it. Let's return to Jennifer's example: she would show her anger to the employee who she felt was ignoring her. Then she would ask her whether she had a minute, clearly with tension in her voice. When what she requested was not immediately possible, Jennifer asked to speak with the manager and complained about the employee at the front desk. By the end of the conversation, Jennifer was visibly much angrier than she had been. She also found herself thinking about the scenario for the rest of the afternoon: how unfair the employee's behavior was, that her needs were not adequately acknowledged, that people would always walk over her, and that this needed to end. At the end of the day, she felt depressed, down, and irritable.

A study conducted at Iowa State University (Bushman, 2002) illustrates both points. We hand out the description of the study to group participants, and ask them to guess the effects on being angry (Handout 24). In the study, people were randomly assigned to one of two groups, rumination or distraction, after having been angered. Participants in the rumination group were told to hit a punching bag and think about the person who had angered them, while people in the distraction group were instructed to think about becoming physically fit. People in the rumination group felt angrier than their counterparts in the distraction and control groups, demonstrating that rumination increased, rather than decreased, anger and aggression (Bushman, 2002). Even doing nothing was more effective than venting anger. These results directly contradict the catharsis theory. We connect this back to the theme of mindfulness:

> *Instructor*: "As you find yourself thinking that you are being treated unfairly or disrespectfully, and feeling hurt, it's hard to imagine that you like this. Who wants to be treated unfairly and disrespectfully? Here is where your mind wants you to let your anger out, turn it into behavior, go into automatic fixing mode. You might think about telling someone off and expressing yourself. As you can see from your own experience, not only does this mental-fixing activity rarely make you feel less hurt or angry, but it actually maintains and likely intensifies how hurt or angry you feel. So how could you deal with this mindfully?"

Guided by the instructor and based on the previous sessions, the group now develops a game plan for dealing with situations when frustration and anger have set in. Once each participant has developed a plan (see outline below), the instructor summarizes as follows:

> *Instructor*: "As you can see, automatic, anger-related thoughts can easily lead to worsening the mood if we are not careful. The first step for dealing with them differently is recognizing automatic, anger-related thoughts for what they are: thoughts, mental events, something that the mind produces. As you have seen from the examples we have discussed, everyone has his or her own set of automatic, negative thoughts. Often they feel believable. They seem real. There always seems to be some truth in them. Nonetheless, recognizing them early for what they are before they can set the autopilot in full swing will be key. As negative, anger-related thoughts arise, they can feel quite painful and aversive, calling for fixing, leading to rumination, or prompting you to act in anger. These behaviors lead to more pain, rather than less. Therefore, from now on, as you become aware of frustration or angry thoughts, as you notice yourself feeling irritable or perhaps already fuming on the inside, fantasizing about asserting yourself, ruminating about how unfair this is, we would like you to do a 3-Minute Breathing Space right then and there. Come into the present, check in with yourself, and note what is going on in terms of feelings and sensations. Then, as you have done before in trigger situations, anchor yourself on the breath and ground yourself, before expanding your attention to include the body as a whole and bringing acceptance especially to those feelings and sensations that are particularly difficult at that moment. The Breathing Space is a means of stepping out of the

autopilot and bringing yourself back into the present and connecting with the present moment. Let's practice the Breathing Space again."

BREATHING SPACE

Before turning the attention to how to be mindful with frustration and anger, the group will do a 3-Minute Breathing Space with Acceptance (see Box 5.2) independently, without guidance from the instructor.

CHOICE POINTS: HOW TO BE MINDFUL WITH FRUSTRATION AND ANGER

As with depression and mania, the end of the Breathing Space will be a decision point for participants about how to move forward after they have completed the exercise. We guide participants to ask themselves, "Now that I feel hurt and angry, how can I best take care of myself right now?" The discussion is guided by Handout 25. The guidelines include behavioral strategies such as not acting on the feeling, excusing oneself from the situation if possible, or (despite feeling angry) acting politely even if not friendly. As participants often point out, implementing these behavioral strategies is difficult when one feels hurt and angry on the inside. On the inside, the anger wants to express itself, wants to act out, either by creating angry ruminative fantasies or by manifesting itself in one's behavior. Therefore, participants will be asked to bring an accepting awareness to the thoughts and the feelings that come with feeling hurt and angry (see Handout 25).

Thoughts

This exercise involves recognizing thoughts as thoughts, not facts. One allows oneself to see thoughts as mental events that are making one feel hurt and angry. One asks oneself whether one's mind is blowing things out of proportion, or whether one is engaging in "black-and-white thinking." This activity involves taking and maintaining the perspective of a curious observer and watching thoughts of frustration, hurt, or anger enter one's mind, in the form of images, scenes, or sentences.

Feeling Hurt and Angry

In terms of the feelings, this exercise involves noticing where the feeling of hurt or anger is located in the body. What are the raw sensations that come with it? As best as one can, bring an observant acceptance to those sensations and feelings as they are present in one's body and demanding your attention. Bring an accepting observation to the aversion, the not wanting, as best as one can. Likewise, one may experience impulses to act on the angry feelings and sensations, such as wanting to raise one's voice or even yell. As best as one can, bring acceptance to this impulse and the raw sensations that are associated with it.

Angry Rumination

Participants may find themselves ruminating: seeing images, or having interior conversations in which they express their anger and complain about how they feel they were wronged. We guide them to recognize that the mind is trying to fix the feeling hurt by having these angry fantasies, but that they are intensifying the anger rather than lessening it. We ask them, as best as they can, to redirect their attention back to the breath, focusing on breathing and reanchoring themselves whenever they notice that rumination has begun.

Every participant's experience of feeling hurt, frustrated, or angry is unique. The bodily expression may be dominant for some. Others may have prominent thoughts, and feel strongly compelled to stew and ruminate angrily. Therefore, for every participant for whom anger and irritability are relevant, we facilitate their working out their own way for how to be mindful with these experiences. This is part of the homework, and should also be part of individual sessions.

ISN'T WALKING AWAY DEFEAT?

"But walking away feels like defeat!" Daniel disagreed. "I think it is important to stand up for myself and address things when I feel I am not treated right or other people are not doing what they are supposed to." Daniel's sentiment is common. If one feels that one has been wronged or treated unfairly, and feels frustrated and angry about it, not saying anything may feel like a lack of assertiveness and may even trigger negative self-evaluations (negative automatic thoughts) such as "You let people do this to you." At first, this seems like a catch-22. Expressing anger leads to one growing more angry and worked up, while doing nothing results in having negative thoughts about oneself. The answer lies in the wise distinction between reacting and responding. Not saying anything when one feels frustration and anger burning does not mean that one cannot reflect on the situation later and problem-solve about how it could best be addressed if doing so would be worthwhile. As we will see in the next session, for Daniel this distinction became an important part of his willingness to work with his anger differently when he was triggered. We finish the session with another Emotion-Focused Meditation before reviewing the homework for the next week.

EMOTION-FOCUSED MEDITATION

After discussing how to be with frustration and anger, the group will do a second Emotion-Focused Meditation. Participants will either continue with their chosen topic or practice with whatever troublesome thoughts, feelings, or sensations are present at the time. We ask subjects to choose one of their troublesome thoughts or feelings associated with anger for practice.

HOMEWORK

For homework, we ask participants to continue with their Mood Diary and continue to pay attention to warning signs (Handout 5), They do the 3-Minute Breathing Space with Acceptance (audio track 8) when they encounter trigger situations or start feeling down, elevated, frustrated, or angry (i.e., Breathing Space for Coping). Should warning signs arise, participants are instructed to enact their action plan and if needed, contact their instructor (see Handouts 8, 15, and 20). Handout 25 provides guidance about how to move forward after the Breathing Space when feeling frustrated or angry. Trigger situations encountered during the week are recorded on the Worksheet for Trigger Situations (Handout 9). Participants are asked to do one Emotion-Focused Meditation per day (audio track 9) either with a chosen topic or with any difficult thoughts or feelings that are present at that time of the Emotion-Focused Meditation.

SESSION 8

Anxiety

OVERVIEW

- About This Session
- Welcome Back and Mood Diary Check
- Emotion-Focused Meditation: Anger
- Triggers
- Breathing Space
- The Anxiety Autopilot
- Breathing Space
- Choice Points: How to Be Mindful When Feeling Anxious
- The Breath as an Anchor
- Emotion-Focused Meditation, Habituation, and Extinction
- Why Is Giving Up So Important?
- Emotion Focused Meditation: Anxiety
- Homework
  - Mood Diary and attention to warning signs
  - Emotion-Focused Meditation: Anxiety (audio track 9)
  - Continue to work with trigger situations
  - Use 3-Minute Breathing Space with Acceptance for coping with trigger situations (audio track 8)

INSTRUCTOR MATERIAL FOR SESSION 8

- Script for the 3-Minute Breathing Space with Acceptance (Box 5.2)
- Script for Emotion-Focused Meditation (Box 5.3)

- Handout 5: Mood Diary (in case a participant forgot to bring his or hers)
- Handout 9: Worksheet for Trigger Situations
- Handout 10: The Anxiety Autopilot
- Handout 26: Automatic Catastrophic Thoughts
- Handout 27: What Can I Do When I Feel Anxious?

ABOUT THIS SESSION

Anxiety is one of the most common co-occurring issues for patients with bipolar disorder. Those with a co-occurring anxiety disorder tend to have a worse course of illness compared to those without anxiety. Finding ways to be more mindful when anxiety sets in is the topic of today's session. First, we check Mood Diaries, practice Emotion-Focused Meditation related to anger, and learn more about how participants worked with situations that made them frustrated and angry. Then, we discuss the anxiety autopilot. For formal anxiety-focused meditation home practice the Emotion-Focused Meditation (audio track 9) can be used.

WELCOME BACK AND MOOD DIARY CHECK

As usual, participants and instructors take a look at the Mood Diary before group starts. Changes in symptoms and warning signs are noted and briefly discussed individually, either at that time, after group or, as needed, in an individual phone call or meeting during the week. Additional warning signs that participants detected become the object of participants' ongoing monitoring going forward.

EMOTION-FOCUSED MEDITATION: ANGER

As in the previous week, we start the group with an Emotion-Focused Meditation (for instructions see Session 5, Box 5.3). The purpose of working with thoughts, sensations, and feelings that are associated with feeling hurt, frustrated, angry, and irritable is to increase participants' abilities to be with these feelings and disengage from or not engage in angry rumination and reactively expressing their anger. When participants encounter these situations in real life, they will hopefully be better equipped to tolerate feelings of being hurt and frustrated, and find ways to respond rather than react.

Let's consider Daniel's example from Session 7: *Isn't walking away defeat?* "Making a distinction between responding and reacting in the last session was important to me, because I realized that I am not powerless. Rather, I am choosing not to respond at the time in favor of following up later, when I am feeling less heated. I brought to mind a situation that always irks me, when I see my employees standing around and not doing anything, when there are so many things to do at any given time. How can they stand around and do nothing? This is a situation that gets me going right away. So I used this in my Emotion-Focused Meditation. I brought this moment to life in my mind, letting myself feel the frustration, the hurt, and the anger. Then I let myself notice where this was expressed in my body, and the thoughts that came with it: 'You should get going! Don't you see that there are things to do? You are wasting my time and my money.' I visualized those thoughts painted on a banner, seeing them in my mind. But, I must admit, bringing acceptance to all of this was hard, although it got easier after a while. The more often I did it, the more familiar the situation became. With practice, it felt less intense, and the less I felt that I was being dragged into it."

Described below are some common challenges that come with working with bringing acceptance to feelings of being hurt or frustrated, and thoughts of being disrespected and treated the wrong way.

"I Can't Stand This Feeling of Being Hurt."

Becoming more aware of the feelings of frustration and being hurt that elicit anger can be hard for participants to tolerate. "It's not fair that I have to work on this," Jennifer said early on. "I am the one being treated unfairly and now, in addition, I have to do all the work on this. This made me even angrier when I used the front desk situation as my practice situation during the week." When participants report this experience, the instructor has two options. He or she could point out that the "I am treated unfairly" and "This is not fair" thoughts for what they are, mental events, which should be viewed that way. In our experience, however, especially if the unfairness thought carries a high degree of believability, the instructor may choose to reframe the exercise. "Practicing with being hurt and bringing acceptance to this feeling and the sensations may put you in a better position down the road to address the situation calmer than at that moment."

On the other hand, if someone already has some recognition that the thought may be biased, treating the thought as a mental event may help to create some distance. Participants may also have difficulties with experiencing the feeling if it is intense. In our experience, it is important for participants to have the option to exercise self-compassion and respect the limits of what they can do at a given time. Therefore, we make it clear that if things become too overwhelming at any point, they may reanchor themselves around the breath or step out of the exercise altogether. Yet, after grounding and reanchoring themselves, as much as they feel capable, they may allow themselves to again approach the feeling of being hurt, the aversion it creates, and the raw bodily sensations associated with curiosity, bringing a kind acceptance to those sensations, as best as they can. We ask participants to observe and accept the bodily experience as it is unfolding in every moment. "It is OK to feel hurt, frustrated, and angry."

"I Get Really Uncomfortable Holding Back."

Especially for impulsive participants, holding back anger can be difficult. "I just get very tense if I don't let this out," Jennifer said. "It feels as if this intensifies the anger even more." Jennifer's observation is apt. Not expressing one's anger often feels aversive and thereby can intensify one's emotional experiences. We ask participants to bring attention to where the aversion is expressed in their body, and then approach it with an accepting curiosity, while acknowledging that they are engaged in a difficult task. It is particularly important to bring acceptance to the aversion and the raw sensations associated with it, as much as it is to allow oneself to feel and notice feelings of hurt and frustration. It is the aversion, the not wanting, that drives individuals to express their anger, and that is an important part of what needs to be worked with.

"I Get Drawn into Angry Rumination If I Don't Act on It."

As angry rumination, fantasies of acting out, setting things straight, and making things right are highly overlearned and ingrained (autopilot), it is not surprising that participants find themselves drifting into those kinds of thoughts during the exercise. In Daniel's first experiences with the exercise, he found himself "telling people what to do and to get going over and over and over again. It actually feels gratifying, and reduces the frustration."

When this drifting happens, we ask participants to acknowledge that angry rumination has set in. Then, we ask them to redirect themselves to the breath as their anchor, before exploring the feelings and sensations of being hurt. They may reapproach this feeling with accepting observance, again without anchoring themselves, if they feel comfortable doing so.

"It Triggers Depressive, Negative Thoughts, and Rumination."

"For me, it feels almost like being caught between a rock and a hard place," Jennifer said. "If I say anything I get angrier. If I don't say anything, my mind starts getting into ruminative mode, that things will never ever get better, and I won't ever get out of this." As with angry rumination, when depressive rumination sets in during the exercise, we simply ask participants to note its presence, labeling their thoughts as depressive rumination thoughts, perhaps writing them in the sky or on a banner in their mind, but without engaging them. As best as possible, we ask them to bring themselves back to the raw sensations of frustration and feeling hurt in their bodies, while allowing thoughts to enter the mind as they come. We instruct participants to tell themselves that it is OK to feel this way. At the same time, participants should give themselves permission to move away from that feeling at any time, reanchoring themselves on the breath, whenever they feel it would be helpful to widen their attentional window to include the whole body and the sense of the body as a whole, into the exercise to be with their experience in a more spacious way.

As with depression and mood elevation, we ask participants to continue practicing Emotion-Focused Meditation with their personal anxiety themes over the next several weeks. On any given day, distressing topics may take center stage in this exercise, but the instructors will ensure that participants continue to work with their personal themes consistently. Next, as in the previous sessions, we explore how participants handled trigger situations in their daily lives.

TRIGGERS

Participants' homework had been to initiate the 3-Minute Breathing Space as well as to begin to develop plans for how to mindfully move forward when they encounter warning signs and notice themselves feeling frustrated, hurt, or angry. As in the previous sessions, we ask participants to pair up, compare their notes, and discuss what type of trigger situations they have noticed for themselves, and how they handled those moments. Following one-on-one discussions, we open the topic up for the group members to share their experiences of working on trigger situations when they felt down or depressed, or noticed warning signs for mood elevation. Here are some examples that pertain to anger:

Since the program began, Daniel had become increasingly aware of his reactions when people, especially family members, would try to acknowledge his feelings. "I get this instant aversion," he described. "It is as if you plugged me into an outlet. I feel a surge of energy going through my body, accompanied by thoughts like, 'Don't tell me you know how I feel. You don't know how I feel. You have no idea how I feel.' Then I notice the anger. And as you have noticed in conversations with me, because we talk a lot about feelings, then I get this tense voice and my tone becomes very combative. Not only with you, with anyone who goes down that road."

As part of his homework, Daniel had started to initiate the Breathing Space in these situations, allowing himself to notice his bodily and mental reactions. "Actually, it had a paradoxically calming effect," he described, "Allowing myself to step out of being in this, taking on the role of an observer who just notices and observes whatever is going on in that moment. It's very strange." Going forward, Daniel opted to maintain this observant stance, but also reserved the right to simply change the topic of conversation or take time out when he felt that conversations might get too overwhelming for him.

Jennifer had been continuing to work with her front desk situation. In fact, she had begun to make it part of her routine to approach the front desk to ask for something, putting herself in a situation of having to wait and "be treated disrespectfully." "I would do a Breathing Space before I would approach the desk, already feeling tense about it and allowing myself to notice this, accepting this as best as I could, without doing anything about it. In a strange way, it is empowering that you can go into something and tell yourself that you will take whatever comes of it." Her practice also yielded something interesting. While she had previously focused on a single employee, she now noticed that her anger extended to others as well. This happened whenever she felt that she was not given attention quickly enough or when the employee helping her was not being friendly and accommodating enough. "It is not just limited to this one woman, it seems to be a more general theme with me," Jennifer reflected. This helped her to view these thoughts as mental events rather than hard facts. "I also started to change my behavior. When I talk to people while frustrated and angry, I have this nagging tone in my voice and don't smile. So, as much as I did not feel like it, I softened my voice, was nice and friendly, and even made a couple of jokes talking to the front desk person. Interestingly, she was much friendlier compared to how she reacts when I talk to her my usual way."

For Brian, depression had set in midway through the program. "I just felt like I had no energy, could not concentrate, and felt completely overwhelmed with my work. It was a constant battle. I felt too overwhelmed, and when I would try to get stuff done and ran into problems, I would get angry and irritable because I could not even do the simplest tasks. A lot of negative and angry thoughts were running through my head. So, I have done a lot of Breathing Spaces in the past week." For Brian, as it turned out, it was critical to recognize the automatic, negative thoughts as they entered his mind. "Ordinarily, I would have sat there in my cubicle and ruminated about how bad this all is, how unfair that I need to deal with this, and if this keeps going, how behind I will be soon. This time, I did my best to acknowledge the thoughts as 'can't get anything right' thoughts and 'this will never end' thoughts, inviting them in. This was hard. It did not make me feel good. However, compared to the alternatives of stewing and getting nothing done, it was much better. I also have begun to work with this nagging feeling of irritability that is constantly with me. I just do the Breathing Space and then keep my perspective widened as best as I can. This helps a lot, as the irritability tries to draw me in and really narrows me down which makes me feel enclosed and boxed in."

Taylor noticed that irritability sets in when she is worried. "Last week on Saturday, FedEx left a note that we had a letter, but I could not pick it up before Monday. I found myself instantly getting worried. 'What could it be? Who is sending us something via FedEx?' In those kinds of situations, my thoughts become catastrophic really fast. I assumed that it was a bill we did not pay, or something else that is going to cost us money or is going to make me feel overwhelmed. Then my husband wanted us to go grocery shopping and run a couple of other errands, and I snapped at him. It was just too much. At that point, I brought the Breathing Space in and started to watch the worry thoughts as best as I could, allowing myself to accept this nagging, anxious, irritable feeling all over my body. I found myself getting carried away in trying to figure out what it could be, but then kept redirecting myself to the breath and told myself to accept whatever may come of the letter. It took a while, but it slowly got better, and I felt less anxious and irritable." Taylor's example illustrates that the autopilots are interconnected and feelings of anxiety can trigger anger, depression, or, as we saw in the previous session, mood elevation. The anxiety autopilot is the last autopilot that we formally address as part of the group sessions, and is what we turn to next.

BREATHING SPACE

Before turning the attention to the Anxiety Autopilot, the group does a 3-Minute Breathing Space with Acceptance exercise (see Box 5.2): each participant by him- or herself without guidance by the instructor.

THE ANXIETY AUTOPILOT

The last autopilot we discuss as part of this program is the autopilot associated with anxiety. This further broadens our view of autopilots from depression, mania, and anger to include anxiety. Most participants have likely experienced panic attacks, even if they do not meet criteria for panic disorder. Therefore, to start, we ask group participants to share their experiences with panic attacks. Panic attacks often come with heart palpitations or accelerated heart rate; feeling short of breath; chest pain; and feeling shaky, dizzy, or lightheaded; they are associated with catastrophic thoughts such as fear of losing control, going crazy, having a heart attack, or fear of dying. Our discussion of panic attacks serves as a lead-in to broaden the autopilot of thoughts and feelings used in the previous sessions to anxiety (see Handout 10). The anxiety autopilot framework is largely consistent with the psychophysiological model of panic attacks that view panic as the result of the interaction of automatic catastrophic interpretations (thoughts) about bodily symptoms that trigger anxiety, which in turn intensifies catastrophic thoughts, thereby creating a vicious cycle of anxiety spiraling into panic. As in the previous sessions, we draw the anxiety autopilot on the whiteboard (see Handout 10) and write the thoughts, feelings, and physical sensations participants mention close to the respective boxes. Note that physical symptoms should be listed as part of the "Feeling" section.

Let's consider Courtney's experience as an example. "For me, it often starts with a feeling of pressure in my chest and my heart starts to beat faster. This is when I know right away that a panic attack is coming up [note her interpretation of the physical event: 'This is a panic attack']." "I do whatever I can to keep it down, but usually within a few minutes my heart is racing, I have more and more trouble getting air, and I feel like everything around me is getting unreal." Typically, automatic, catastrophic interpretations during a panic attack worsen to the point that participants fear they might be dying, losing control, or going crazy. In order to elicit these examples, the instructor may ask what would be the worst that could happen if anxiety would spiral without any way of stopping it. He or she includes those thoughts in the corresponding box on the board. After the cycle of thoughts and feelings has been developed, the instructor will summarize.

> *Instructor:* "As you can see, catastrophic thoughts and feelings create a vicious cycle that goes around and intensifies the initial feeling of anxiety into full-blown panic. Often it starts with noticing one of the physical symptoms that you might be afraid of and the thought sets

in: 'What if I am going to have a panic attack?' This triggers anxiety, which comes with physical sensations, such as a pounding heartbeat, increased breathing, and so forth. Now that these are setting in, the next thought is 'It's a panic attack.' This, in turn, increases the heart rate, the breathing, and whichever other symptoms are there even more. As you may have experienced, this happens very quickly. Now, let's take a look at some of the catastrophic thoughts that people experience when they are having or anticipating panic attacks."

We provide participants with a handout of catastrophic thoughts commonly experienced by people who have panic attacks or panic disorder (Handout 26) and ask them to rate which ones they have experienced. This provides an opportunity for the group members to see that their thoughts follow a pattern, and that they are experienced by other group members as well. Familiarizing themselves with these thoughts will facilitate the process of recognizing these thoughts as mental events. Following the discussion of these thoughts, we broaden the topic from panic attacks to social anxiety.

> *Instructor*: "One of the catastrophic thoughts that people can have in the context of panic attacks is losing control. This often has an element of social embarrassment attached to it. 'What will others think if I lose control?' If the catastrophic thoughts predominantly or exclusively center around what other people would think if one behaved inappropriately or strangely, or had symptoms that others would judge, then this would be social anxiety. Here the catastrophic thoughts center around the idea that others will think you are weird or strange if they see you turning red, sweating, trembling, or if your voice cracks or you have no voice."

The handout with catastrophic thoughts associated with panic attacks also includes examples of catastrophic thoughts associated with social situations (e.g., "People will think I am crazy," "I will embarrass myself"), which are discussed with the group. The instructor also provides information about the physical symptoms that participants may experience during panic attacks or in feared social situations. These are conceptualized as part of the anxiety response (Handout 10, Feelings box). Common symptoms include increased heart rate, palpitations, stronger heartbeat, difficulty breathing, choking, chest pressure, sweating, trembling, feeling nauseous, tingling or numbness in the extremities, difficulty concentrating, feeling that things are unreal, and feeling that one is detached from one's body.

Instructor: "Anxiety often comes with lots of associated physical symptoms. These are part of the body's built-in fight–flight reaction. By design, nature has equipped us with anxiety in order to make us fight or run away when we are in danger. This works well if there is real danger, for example, if someone is attempting to harm you. It can backfire if your anxiety system sets off a false alarm when you are not in any real danger. The physical changes you notice in your body when you are getting anxious are part of your body's fight–flight reaction."

We explain some of the processes behind some of the physical symptoms, using the list that the group has created. The emphasis is on these being processes that are part of anxiety and are in no way dangerous. Explanations for the physical symptoms are below:

• *Increased heart rate, heart palpitations.* The body prepares for starting to fight or run away. In order to fight or run, the body needs an increased blood supply in the arms and legs. Therefore, even before one starts to fight or run away, the body is already increasing the heart rate to be prepared for the moment when this happens. Therefore, even though one may not engage in any physical activity at the moment when anxiety sets in, one may notice an increase in heart rate or palpitations.

• *Not getting enough air, difficulties breathing, choking.* This is often a symptom of breathing more in anticipation of fight or flight without engaging in physical activity. Paradoxically, this may result in feeling one is not getting enough air. We point out that this is usually not dangerous. Also, heavier breathing comes with breathing against the chest wall, which can also cause the sensation of difficulty breathing.

• *Trembling and shaking* reflect an anticipatory increase in muscle tonus to prepare for fight or flight.

• *Feeling hot or cold* are expressions of the body's temperature system preparing for fight or flight.

• *Trouble concentrating, things feeling unreal, and a sensation of detachment from one's body* can be related to a change in blood distribution in the brain. Brain regions involved in anxiety (temporal lobe) receive more blood, whereas brain regions that are involved in critical thinking and planning (frontal lobes) are not needed at that time, and receive less blood and oxygen. Also, anxiety may come with a change in pupil dilation, which can make things look unreal.

Next, we bring mindfulness into the discussion about the anxiety autopilot: "So, how could being mindful make a difference when dealing with anxiety?" This questions gets at two aspects of anxiety: (1) attempts to suppress anxiety symptoms by distraction, and (2) worry as an attempt to prevent anxiety and its anticipated consequences. Both can be viewed as safety or avoidance behaviors. They are geared toward keeping anxiety under control and may create the illusion that because people are engaging in these mental strategies or behaviors, anxiety has not gotten worse, or is perhaps even slightly less intense.

Anxiety Suppression and Distraction

Let's return to Courtney's experience. Like others who experience panic attacks, she tried whatever she could to prevent the worst, namely, dying or losing control, foreshadowed by the automatic, catastrophic thoughts as anxiety increased. "I typically try to take long, deep breaths, tell myself to calm down, and to slow down my heart as best as I can. Or, I try to focus on something else other than the anxiety, just as best as I can to shift my attention away, trying not to notice it." When asked about how well this response works for her, she acknowledges, "Sometimes it works, but at other times the anxiety stays at a very high level for hours." Courtney's finding that her attempts to calm herself down are sometimes effective (i.e., anxiety or panic do not get worse), but often don't yield the desired effect, is common: when people suppress anxiety, rather than calming down, they tend to stay anxious or may get even more anxious. Thus, attempts to suppress anxiety by deliberately trying to calm oneself down may actually have the opposite effect, and prevent the process of habituation.

Worry

Courtney also found herself worrying about upcoming panic attacks, and trying to find ways to prevent them, a theme that by now will be familiar to participants: the mind, trying to find ways to fix things, devises plans that prevent uncomfortable experiences. In Courtney's case, she would experience anticipatory anxiety leading to further panic attacks. Here is where the concept of anxiety is broadened further.

> *Instructor*: "You may worry about upcoming panic attacks or situations in which you might have a panic attack. You may also worry about social situations in which you fear being anxious and people thinking negatively about you. However, worry is not limited to panic

attacks or social situations. As many of you have experienced, we can worry about a lot of things, such as losing a job, not getting a job, not having enough money, losing loved ones, and so forth. Overall, worry is related to our brains' ability to think ahead and anticipate the future. If we anticipate harm in the future, then our mind will start to think about ways to prevent this harm. Wherever there is a chance of a negative or aversive outcome for us, and it is not perfectly clear that it is not going to happen (= 100%), worry may set in as a way of the mind to make something we fear less likely. We may look for solutions, contemplate options, go over what we can do, look for *the* solution that will 100% prevent what we fear. The problem is that often this solution does not exist. There are only imperfect options, and the possibility for an aversive, feared outcome remains."

The take-home point here is that no matter how much participants may try to find solutions, there is still always the possibility that what they fear may happen. This keeps anxiety up.

Instructor: "From the perspective of mindfulness, anxiety is aversive—we do not want to lose control in front of others, go crazy, die, embarrass ourselves, lose money or loved ones. Therefore, our minds go into overdrive in order to suppress the feeling and sensations, distract ourselves, or get us to think through all of the possible scenarios for how to prevent something bad from happening, thereby keeping anxiety alive. Thus the challenge here, as you may have already anticipated, is to gradually allow yourself to observe the sensations, feelings, thoughts, and aversion that come with anxiety, and begin to bring acceptance to those experiences. Therefore, from now on, as you become aware of catastrophic thoughts or anxiety sensations or feelings, or as you notice that you have already switched into worrying, we would like you to do a 3-Minute Breathing Space right then and there. Come into the present, check in with yourself, note what is going on in terms of thoughts, feelings, and sensations. Then anchor yourself on the breath, grounding yourself, before expanding your attention to include the body as a whole and bringing acceptance especially to those feelings and sensations that are difficult at that moment. As it was for depression, mood elevation, and anger, the Breathing Space is a means of stepping out of the autopilot and bringing yourself back into the present and connecting with the present moment. Let's practice the Breathing Space again."

BREATHING SPACE

Before turning the attention to being mindful with anxiety, the group does a 3-Minute Breathing Space with Acceptance (see Box 5.2): each participant by him- or herself without guidance by the instructor.

CHOICE POINTS: HOW TO BE MINDFUL
WHEN FEELING ANXIOUS

The ending of the Breathing Space is again a point for participants to decide how to move forward after they have concluded the Breathing Space (see Handout 27). Now that I am anxious, what do I need right now? How can I best take care of myself right now? The guidelines for mindfully coping with anxiety symptoms are discussed with the group (see Handout 27).

Feelings and Physical Sensations

As participants find their attention drawn to the physical manifestations of anxiety in the body (e.g., rapid heartbeat, difficulties breathing), as best as they can, we ask them to bring acceptance to those experiences by telling themselves that it is OK to feel this way. They may continue to observe it from a wider, spacious point of view within their body, or, if they can, approach the raw sensation with curiosity, bringing acceptance to whatever may happen as they observe that sensation. As experiencing these sensations is aversive, they will likely find themselves wanting to avoid this experience. Mindfulness involves, as best as they can, allowing themselves to bring an accepting openness to experiencing this part of the anxiety, too. We remind the participants that these are natural, physiological changes in their bodies. There is nothing they need to do about them other than allowing themselves to experience them with an open, accepting stance, no matter how intense they may be.

Being with Catastrophic Thoughts

As catastrophic thoughts continue to enter participants' minds, we ask them to note them for what they are: mental events. Participants may want to label them as catastrophic thoughts or catastrophic predictions, but should not engage with them in any way. As with the sensations, when the attention is drawn to them, bring an accepting observance to their presence, without arguing with them or trying to push them out of their minds.

We ask participants not to forcefully distract themselves or think about something else. As best as they can, they should maintain an open, inviting stance, letting them into the mind, and giving the thoughts permission to stay or leave.

Being with Worry

Participants may find themselves getting caught up in worry, trying to fix things in their minds, or trying to prevent what may be foreshadowed by some catastrophic thought. We guide them to allow themselves to return to the breath for a moment, or whichever anchor they have chosen for themselves. Follow the inbreath and the outbreath for a while, grounding themselves. But then, when they feel ready, widen the field of awareness to the body and mind and again. They may ask themselves, "What are the thoughts that are making me anxious?", "What catastrophic thoughts am I having?", "Is my mind making catastrophic predictions?", or "What is my mind trying to prevent?" Then label the catastrophic thoughts that may be present at that time as mental events, and bring acceptance to their presence, no matter how scary they may be.

Behavior

We ask participants to allow themselves to gradually drop some of the things that they are doing with the intention of keeping anxiety under control. These behaviors may include holding their body in a certain position, holding onto a chair, clenching fists, or crossing one's legs. They may also find themselves avoiding situations altogether, because they are afraid that anxiety may occur and they won't be able to handle it. Going forward, once participants have more experience with Emotion-Focused Meditations for Anxiety, we encourage them to gradually approach anxiety-inducing situations. Then they may apply the mindfulness skills for thoughts, feelings, and sensations described above.

THE BREATH AS AN ANCHOR

For participants with anxiety disorders for whom shortness of breath, or the fears of not getting enough air or choking is involved, the breath may not be the best anchor or object of focus for the mindfulness practice. For many participants, the breath is a place where they can ground themselves if things feel overwhelming or if they need to collect themselves. If the breath is a trigger for anxiety, or a symptom of anxiety, focusing on the breath may increase anxiety. For such a participant, focusing on sounds or something in his or her field of vision may be a better option. In this case, the breath may be one of those anxiety-provoking physical sensations the participant may bring curiosity and an observant acceptance to, while still always having the option to return to an anchor related to sounds or sights, should the experience prove too overwhelming.

EMOTION-FOCUSED MEDITATIONS, HABITUATION, AND EXTINCTION

"But isn't this mindfulness approach the same as exposure?" a cognitive-behavioral psychologist might say. Indeed, it is. As discussed in Chapter 1, *exposure* (extinction learning) has been hypothesized to be one of the mechanisms by which mindfulness may be helpful to people. Repeatedly bringing an observant, accepting stance to feelings and sensations of anxiety over time lessens their intensity. This is called *habituation*. Over days and weeks of this practice, experiences that used to trigger anxiety, such as physical symptoms, become less scary and people grow less worried about them, a process called *extinction learning*. Being less afraid of anxiety symptoms, in turn, makes it easier for people to bring an accepting, observant stance to aversive anxiety-provoking sensations as they occur. There are different theories about the processes that underlie habituation and extinction. One hypothesis is that our body and brain assess whether something we encounter could be harmful to us. If the answer to this quick assessment is affirmative, then an alarm (anxiety) reaction is triggered. When people practice Emotion-Focused Meditation, they come to understand that being with physical symptoms in this way does not lead to them losing control, going crazy, or dying. This, in turn, may change their interpretation about these symptoms and they become less fearful about them.

WHY IS GIVING UP SO IMPORTANT?

"But allowing anxiety symptoms to happen makes me more anxious!" Michelle protested after the group had reviewed some of the options for moving forward when anxiety sets in. "It's not as if I haven't tried this before. In fact, this has been suggested to me many times. 'Let the symptoms remain.' 'Don't do anything and they will subside.' But when I try this, then it gets worse!" Michelle's observation is true. When anxious people cease their efforts to keep anxiety under control, anxiety and the intensity of its symptoms (e.g., heart rate) may briefly increase, before they start to return to normal (provided one does not try to control them again). Why is this? All behavioral and mental actions that people take to control anxiety can acquire the status of safety behaviors. That is, as long as one engages in these behaviors, and nothing bad happens and anxiety does not spiral out of control, it feels that these behaviors are working. They have acquired the status of safety behaviors (i.e., "If I do this, then the worst can be prevented"). They may not be working well (after all, one is still anxious), but subjectively they work sufficiently to prevent the worst. The downside is that not engaging in these behaviors that subjectively prevent the worst from happening often increases anxiety. This can be experienced as a temporary increase in anxiety and an increase in physical sensations when one gives up control and begins to bring acceptance to those physical sensations of anxiety. We find it helpful to ask group participants whether they have encountered the effect of rising anxiety and intensifying sensations. We acknowledge that actively giving up attempts to control what is going on in one's body can be scary, but at the same time we encourage participants to allow themselves to do so as much as they are able to.

EMOTION-FOCUSED MEDITATION II

After discussing how to be mindful with anxiety, the group will do a second Emotion-Focused Meditation. The purpose of working with anxiety thoughts, feelings, and sensations is to increase participants' abilities to be with these experiences in a way that promotes habituation rather than escalation. For the anxiety-focused meditation, we ask participants to choose a physical sensation that may trigger anxiety for them (e.g., heartbeat, tension in the stomach, pressure on the chest, or the breath). They may also choose a catastrophic thought or a feeling or situation that is anxiety-provoking. Of course, if they already feel anxious, they may choose to work with the anxiety that is already present (or any other feeling that is dominant at that time). As with the previous Emotion-Focused Meditations, we ask participants to bring an observant acceptance to the feelings, sensations, and thoughts that may arise in this context. If attention is drawn to a particular place in the body (e.g., the heart), then we ask participants to go there, with an open, curious, accepting attitude.

We ask them to allow themselves to notice aversion and the raw sensations that may come with noticing that sensation, and bring a kind, accepting welcoming to that experience in that moment. If thoughts are coming to mind, we ask them to explicitly note them as mental events, label them as "catastrophic thoughts," and give these thoughts permission to remain in their minds as long as they wish. If they find their minds wandering off, and do not want to take note of their catastrophic thoughts, then, if it feels doable at that time, gently allow themselves to go back to acknowledging catastrophic thoughts. If they find themselves feeling aversion, not wanting to notice what is on their minds, then gently, and as much as they can, they may bring acceptance to the feeling and sensations of aversion and not wanting. But at all times, participants should respect what they can do at that moment, and give themselves permission to retract and reanchor themselves on the breath or some other anchor. We conduct this exercise for about 10 minutes, but when participants practice outside of the group, we encourage them to gradually stretch the exercise to make it longer. This is because feelings of anxiety and aversion often lessen in intensity over time, and gradually lengthening the exercise will allow them to experience this effect.

HOMEWORK

For homework, we ask participants to continue with their Mood Diary and continue to pay attention to warning signs (Handout 5). They will do the 3-Minute Breathing Space with Acceptance (audio track 8) when they encounter trigger situations or start feeling down, elevated, frustrated, angry, or anxious (i.e., Breathing Space for Coping). Should warning signs arise, participants are instructed to enact their action plan and if needed contact the instructor (see Handouts 8, 15, and 20). Handout 25 provides guidance for how to move forward after completing the Breathing Space when feeling frustrated and angry. Handout 27 provides guidance for how to move forward after the Breathing Space when feeling anxious. Trigger situations encountered during the week will be recorded on the Worksheet for Trigger Situations (Handout 9). Participants are asked to do one Emotion-Focused Meditation per day (audio track 9), either with a chosen topic or with any difficult thoughts or feelings that are present at that time of the meditation.

Open Awareness
and Loving-Kindness

OVERVIEW

- About This Session
- Welcome Back and Mood Diary Check
- Emotion-Focused Meditation: Anxiety
- Triggers
- Open Awareness Meditation
- Introduction to Compassionate Coaching and Loving-Kindness
- Self-Soothing Activities
- Loving-Kindness Meditation
- Breathing Space
- Homework
  - Mood Diary and attention to warning signs
  - Alternate Open Awareness Meditation (audio track 10) and Loving-Kindness Meditation (audio track 11)
  - Continue to work with trigger situations
  - Use 3-Minute Breathing Space with Acceptance for coping with trigger situations (audio track 8)
  - Be your own compassionate coach: one self-soothing activity per day
  - Send loving-kindness to a neutral person once a day

INSTRUCTOR MATERIAL FOR SESSION 9

- Script for the 3-Minute Breathing Space with Acceptance (Box 5.2)
- Script for Open Awareness Meditation (Box 9.1)
- Script for Loving-Kindness Meditation (Box 9.2)

- Handout 5: Mood Diary (in case a participant forgot to bring his or hers)
- Handout 9: Worksheet for Trigger Situations
- Handout 28: Self-Soothing Activities

ABOUT THIS SESSION

This session represents a shift in the program. Formal Emotion-Focused Meditations as part of the group's practice are coming to an end and we now introduce the concept of open awareness. This involves practicing the ability to hold experiences such as sensations, feelings, thoughts, or sounds in a wide, open, spacious awareness without getting involved or tangled up in them. We also now explicitly introduce the concept of compassionate coaching and loving-kindness into the program. Participants begin their journey of acting as their own compassionate coaches in dealing with life issues going forward. But before we embark on this part of the program, we review participants' experiences with the anxiety-focused meditations and how they dealt with anxiety trigger situations in daily life. For home practice the Open Awareness Meditation (audio track 10) and the Loving-Kindness Meditation (audio track 11) are included as recordings.

WELCOME BACK AND MOOD DIARY CHECK

As usual, participants and instructors take a look at the Mood Diaries before group starts. Changes in symptoms and warning signs are noted and briefly discussed individually, either at that time, after group, or, as needed, in an individual phone call or meeting during the week. Additional warning signs that were not yet recognized become objects of the participants' monitoring going forward.

EMOTION-FOCUSED MEDITATION: ANXIETY

As in the previous week, we start the group with Emotion-Focused Meditation. To briefly recap, the purpose of working with anxious thoughts, feelings, and sensations is to increase participants' ability to be with these experiences in a way that promotes habituation rather than escalation. Participants choose physical sensations that may trigger anxiety for them (e.g., heartbeat) or a catastrophic thought. The following challenges may come up during anxiety-focused meditation:

"Focusing on Physical Sensations Makes Me Really Anxious"

"What if I get a panic attack?" Courtney asked anxiously when the idea of focusing on feared bodily symptoms was introduced. Especially at the beginning when participants have little or no experience with bringing mindful acceptance to anxiety, doing this exercise triggers anticipatory anxiety. The instructor may use that moment to lead right into the exercise. We asked Courtney to note what thoughts were going through her mind and to note them as mental events. Additionally, we told her to note where anticipatory anxiety was located in her body and what sensations accompany it, and to allow herself to bring an observant acceptance to the sensations that she may be noticing at that very moment. She should allow herself to experience these thoughts and sensations.

"I'm Having a Panic Attack"

During the exercise, a participant's anxiety symptoms may increase. The instructor may simply ask the participant to anchor and ground him- or herself for the time being, open the eyes, and allow the body to do whatever feels most appropriate in the moment. This gives the participant as much control as possible in that moment. For the instructor, it is important not to forget that panic attacks, while they may be uncomfortable, are not dangerous. So whenever the participant feels ready, work with the participant to readopt an allowing stance toward the feelings, sensations, and thoughts he or she is experiencing at that time. We direct him or her to allow him- or herself to be with whatever is present in the body at that moment and bring acceptance to it, as best as the participant can. The participant should continue with this exercise going forward, so that he or she may experience that eventually, anxiety symptoms will pass.

"It's Difficult Not to Distract Myself."

This is a common experience for participants who habitually distract themselves from noticing anxiety-provoking or catastrophic thoughts or sensations. Their brains are particularly well trained in finding ways to quickly distract themselves, often by thinking about something that is not anxiety-provoking and thereby shifting attention away from what would trigger or increase anxiety. We encourage such participants to bring awareness to this process as it happens. They should note that the mind has quickly wandered off to something else, and then redirect themselves as much as possible to the anxiety-provoking sensation or thought, bringing an accepting, observant stance to it.

"Allowing Makes Me More Anxious."

When participants initially try to suppress the feeling or sensation of anxiety but then attempt to loosen control and bring acceptance to that feeling, they often become more anxious. If possible, we just ask participants to continue to bring acceptance to these increased sensations, perhaps by continuing to observe them from a larger space within themselves and observing the changes that occur. We also remind participants to give themselves permission to anchor and ground themselves, to respect what they feel they can do at a given time, and to take breaks if necessary. Sometimes, it can be helpful to remind participants that the increased anxiety they feel when they give up control will be temporary; this may put some in the position to allow themselves to observe and accept what might otherwise be very difficult to tolerate.

"I Can't Stop Worrying."

Deliberately bringing concerns to mind may trigger worry. Theo, who needed to extend his visa and was running into some problems, could not help but find himself switching into "worry mode" right away when he brought the topic up during anxiety-focused exposure. He worried, "What if I can't extend it? What if I need to leave the country? What if I can't finish my degree? How can I prevent this from happening?" Quickly he found himself going over all his options as he had done so many times before. As participants become aware that worry has set in, we encourage them to gently redirect themselves to where the pain was in the first place. They want to note the catastrophic thoughts like "I may need to leave. I may not be able to finish my degree," and then also bring acceptance to the feelings and the raw sensations that come with the anxiety, allowing themselves to approach the experience with curious, accepting observance.

"It Does Get Easier."

With continued accepting observance, participants often have two experiences. First, the sensations and feelings they observe fluctuate in intensity, and second, the intensity of the sensations lessens over time. Still they may also find their mind wandering away, thinking about other things. For example, Taylor recounts that "at some point I found that I had started thinking about dinner and being home after group even though I was dealing with the anxiety minutes before." The experience that thoughts, feelings, and sensations are transient often helps participants to relate to them as events in their minds and bodies.

"It's Not Getting Easier."

Noticeably disappointed, Courtney said, "This time, I continued to find myself being anxious. It did not go down as it did all the other times." Often with continued practice, participants notice that it is easier to observe and be with anxiety-provoking bodily experiences. Participants notice this effect and begin to expect it. This can shift them away from unconditional acceptance, in which they accept anything noticed in the body, to conditional acceptance in which they are willing to accept these uncomfortable sensations only for a few minutes, but then need to have them decrease in intensity to feel more comfortable. With this conditional acceptance the anxiety intensity often remains unchanged. In those situations we simply remind participants that part of practicing mindfulness is to give up any goals or purposes attached to it.

Depersonalization and Reexperiencing Trauma

Some participants experience depersonalization during the exercise (i.e., feeling detached from one's own body). Likewise, participants who have had traumatic experiences may re-experience them during the practice. If a participant is disturbed during the practice and reports depersonalization experiences and/or re-experiencing of trauma, we focus on helping him or her to become grounded and stabilized. This can be done by advising them to open their eyes, move their body, make strong contact with the floor, such as shaking the legs against the floor, getting up, or drinking some water. It might be necessary to work one-on-one with a participant, until he or she is stable enough. Importantly, participants should be encouraged to practice self-care, to take care of themselves in the midst of the difficult experience and to not expose themselves to more than they feel they can take at that moment. We then continue to work with these participants to gradually allow anxiety-provoking images, thoughts, feelings, and sensations in during the practice.

TRIGGERS

As in the previous sessions, participants pair up in small groups and discuss what types of trigger situations they have noticed for themselves and how they handled those moments. Following the small-group discussions, we open the topic to the whole group. Here we provide some examples that pertain to anxiety.

- *Courtney*: "It was an interesting experience trying to not control the symptoms of anxiety. When I get the feeling that it is starting, there is this instant rush 'Oh my God, here we go again' and I immediately tense up and go on the defensive. It was really hard to loosen this up. It feels like you are trying to get yourself to open the floodgates fully knowing that you are drowning . . . I could only do it just a little more each time, letting it sit there, telling yourself, 'It's OK, let it be there, whatever happens happens,' while at the same time your brain is screaming, 'No, don't!' But then, you let the screaming happen, too, and then at some point, the anxiety lessens. I have also gotten better at seeing the thoughts come in and looking at them as something my mind makes up to make me feel anxious."

- *Ruth*: "I worry about schoolwork constantly. Everyday I am wondering whether I am making this class. It's a vicious cycle. I worry about the assignments, then I can't really concentrate when I try to sit down, and then what I get on papers is really not that great. As a result my grades are not that stellar and that gives me more reason to worry and I get down on myself and more depressed. I tried to do what you said with homework assignments. Breathe, be in the present, notice what is going on, and then bring acceptance to the thought that I may fail the class. I pull myself back when I find myself thinking about how bad this would be and what I could do to prevent this. But it was hard to sit with this nagging feeling and I often had to redirect myself." However, Ruth also noticed changes. Instead of worrying for a long time, she started to work on her assignments. "It's better to have something on paper than nothing" she reasoned, and interestingly she found herself increasingly focused on assignments rather than the worry. "But then it hits you again, especially at the end of a section when you try to figure out what part comes next. Then you have to do the exercise all over again."

- *Elizabeth*: Not getting all her work done was a source of worry. Worry would then make her feel keyed up, which would be a trigger for mood elevation. "I just don't like to let things hang there. When I leave work, it should all be done." In the past, this had led her to work long hours that interfered with her sleep and made her manic. Now, leaving unfinished work behind made her worried that the next day would be way too full and she would not be able to keep up. "It was an educational experience for me to watch the thoughts going through my head, deliberately leaving work behind: 'You will be overwhelmed. This will be stressful and not feel good.' So, after doing my Breathing Space, I let the thoughts in, labeled them as my catastrophic thoughts, did not argue with them, and then also let this nagging feeling in my stomach sit there, as best as I could. I would not say that I was embracing it, but I kind of told myself 'It is OK. Give it space, you don't need to like it, just be with it.' I also would try to keep myself busy. Not busy in the sense that I would try to block the thoughts out. I kind of figured from our discussion that this was not the idea, but more in a way to not overfocus on things. This also helped, but at times when the worry would creep in I would need to repeat the Breathing Space, regroup, be with it, and then keep going again. For the first few days it was hard, but interestingly, it got easier. I guess you can learn to leave stuff unfinished."

OPEN AWARENESS

"Open awareness" refers to a meditation exercise where participants no longer choose a focus for awareness, but allow experiences (e.g., sensations, feelings, thoughts, sounds) to be in the field of awareness without fixating or focusing on one thing. Over the past four sessions participants have increased their abilities to be mindful with uncomfortable sensations, feelings, and thoughts without getting drawn into mental activities geared toward fixing or suppressing them. This has set the stage for now practicing a wider, more spacious decentered way of being with experiences in any given moment.

Box 9.1. Open Awareness Meditation (10 Minutes)

(Note for the instructor: [. . .] indicates a pause.)

- Coming into a comfortable sitting position, either on a chair, or on a cushion or folded blanket on the floor. Sitting upright and relaxed at the same time. Feeling the contact points with the ground or the chair. Feeling the soles of the feet on the ground and the buttocks on the cushion or chair. Noticing how the pressure is distributed on the legs and the buttocks. Becoming aware of how the ground is holding you. Bringing awareness to the shoulders and the neck. Softening here. Bringing awareness to the face. Allowing the face muscles to relax.
- And now, tuning into the breath and being with breathing. Being with each breath as you inhale and as you exhale. Feeling the sensations of breathing at the nose, or chest or abdomen. Becoming aware of the constant flow of the breath. Not missing one single aspect of breathing. Becoming aware of the quality of the breath. And breathing the way it is naturally happening. Without modifying it in any way and without judging it in any way. Just being in contact with it as it is . . . (Longer pause).
- Sitting here, breathing, right now, right here and knowing that you are doing so. Doing this with a conscious quality, being aware of what you are doing. Being conscious of the present moment. Using the breath as an anchor that brings

you in contact with your experience of the present moment. Breathing is always happening right here and right now. And it is each single breath that is happening right now that matters. Taking each breath as an opportunity to come in contact with the present moment . . . (*Longer pause*).

- And now, opening awareness to any experience that is happening right now. Bringing attention to whatever is occurring in the field of awareness in this moment. This may be sounds, body sensations, thoughts, or the breath . . . Just being present to whatever is dominant in the field of awareness right now. Being with it without judging . . . without labeling it as pleasant or unpleasant . . . just being with it . . . and now also allowing it to pass away . . . allowing the experience to end and allowing awareness to come back to the present moment . . . (*Longer pause*)

- And now, whenever you are ready, expanding awareness to include any and all sensations in the body and mind right now: the air, the breath, hearing, thoughts, feelings or emotions, whatever it is, not separating it. Just resting in the experience of it all.

- Even bringing attention to awareness itself, the awareness that holds all of these experiences . . . (*Longer pause*).

- Allowing yourself to rest in this bigger awareness . . . and being aware that you are holding all this in a bigger, spacious awareness.

- Resting with awareness itself.

- Sitting here, in this full and complete awareness of your own complete and whole being . . . (*Longer pause*)

- And as this practice is coming to an end, slowly bringing awareness to the sitting position . . . to the body, slowly opening the eyes and as you are ready bringing movement into the body.

INTRODUCTION TO COMPASSIONATE COACHING AND LOVING-KINDNESS

Up to this point, self-compassion has been an implicit aspect of the program. Participants have been asked to respect their limits during the meditation exercises, to allow themselves to reanchor themselves around the breath when sensations, feelings, or thoughts were too overwhelming, and to be gentle and kind to themselves. Similar to the concept of thoughts, feelings, and sensations being events in and of our body, we now begin to introduce the concept of self-compassion and loving-kindness explicitly. In this session, we introduce the idea of participants becoming their own compassionate and kind coaches in dealing with the experiences of bipolar disorder. This refers both to the way they talk to themselves (inner talk) as well as the way they treat themselves. After all, depression and anxiety come with harsh, judgmental, angry, and catastrophic thoughts. Mania comes with irritability or the lure of engaging in too many or too pleasur-able activities. Who, if not the participant him- or herself, will be a kind, compassionate supporting coach in dealing with this? In this session, we ask participants to begin to take on the role of acting as their own kind and compassionate coaches and actively engage in self-soothing and pleasur-able behaviors in a mindful fashion. We also begin formal loving-kindness meditations and ask participants to practice loving-kindness in their daily lives by extending it to others, beginning with neutral people. Compassion and loving-kindness both refer to the same attitudinal stance, one that is characterized by kindness and by wishing somebody well. The difference between the two is that compassion refers to the stance when the individual receiving those good wishes is suffering. When a person does not suffer, one typically uses the term loving-kindness. Here, for simplicity, we will not make a distinction between the two terms in the following descriptions, but rather use them synonymously. In the following two sessions, partici-pants will begin to practice extending compassion and loving-kindness to themselves, particularly in situations that are difficult and distressing.

But, why, one may ask, are self-compassion and loving-kindness not explicitly introduced earlier in the program? Before the program, common ways individuals cope with feelings and thoughts include avoidance, sup-pression, distraction, reasoning, and rumination. These are all forms of mental activities that aim to either shift attention away from an experience that is distressing to a participant or to modify this experience in order to make is less distressing, although they may not work well. Therefore, we first work with participants on adopting a more observant, accepting, spacious (decentered) way of being with these difficult feelings, thoughts, or sensations without attempting to change them in any way. Participants begin to see them as mental events and temporary changes in the body. We feel that this is an important first step before gradually and actively bringing explicit self-compassion and loving-kindness to moments that are difficult or challenging. Being kind to yourself, especially if your mind likes to come up with harsh, judgmental, and catastrophic thoughts, can be extraordinarily difficult. We introduce the concept of compassionate coaching and loving-kindness through the coaching story (Otto, 2000).*

The Coaching Story

This is a story about Little League Baseball. I talk about Little League Baseball because of the amazing parents and coaches involved. And by "amazing" I don't mean good. I mean extreme. But this story doesn't start with the coaches or the parents; it starts with Johnny, who is a Little

League player in the outfield. His job is to catch fly balls and return them to the infield players. On the day of our story, Johnny is in the outfield and "crack!" One of the players on the other team hits a fly ball. The ball is coming to Johnny. Johnny raises his glove. The ball is coming to him, coming to him, and then it goes over his head. Johnny misses the ball, and the other team scores a run.

Now there are a number of ways a coach can respond to this situation. Let's take Coach A first. Coach A is the type of coach who will come out on the field and shout: "I can't believe you missed that ball! Anyone could have caught it! My dog could have caught it! You screw up like that again and you'll be sitting on the bench! That was lousy!" Coach A then storms off the field. At this point, Johnny is standing in the outfield and, if he is at all similar to me, he is tense, tight, trying not to cry, and praying that another ball will not be hit to him. If a ball does come to him, Johnny will probably miss it. After all, he is tense, tight, and may see four balls coming at him because of the tears in his eyes. If we are Johnny's parents, we may see more profound changes after the game. Johnny, who typically places his baseball glove on the mantel, now throws it under his bed. And before the next game, he may complain that his stomach hurts and that perhaps he should not go to the game. This is the scenario with Coach A.

Now, let's go back to the original event and play it differently. Johnny has just missed the ball, and now Coach B comes out on the field. Coach B says: "Well, you missed that one. Here is what I want you to remember: high balls look like they are farther away than they really are. Also, it is much easier to run forward than to back up. Because of this, I want you to prepare for the ball by taking a few extra steps backward. As the ball gets closer you can step into it if you need to. Also, try to catch it at chest level, so you can adjust your hand if you misjudge the ball. Let's see how you do next time." Coach B then leaves the field. How does Johnny feel? Well, he is not happy. After all, he missed the ball, but there are a number of important differences from the way he felt with Coach A. He is not as tense or tight, and if a fly ball does come to him again, he knows what to do differently to catch it. And because he does not have tears in his eyes, he may actually see the ball and catch it.

The instructor asks the group which coach they would choose for themselves and why. The central idea for the discussion is that as human beings we talk to, or coach, ourselves all the time. The instructor explains that if you struggle with something difficult, such as bipolar disorder, it is particularly important to be kind to yourself:

Instructor: "The idea is to treat yourself well in every respect. This will help to buffer things when difficult moments come up. It is particularly important to do this when things are difficult and you are suffering. Imagine you are going through a dark, long, cold tunnel. Isn't it easier if you have a light at the end of the tunnel? You still won't like the tunnel, but the way through is easier to bear when you encourage yourself to keep going and to make it through instead of yelling at yourself that you should not have entered the tunnel in the first place. This is at the heart of the idea of being kind and compassionate to yourself. And who else but yourself would be better suited to take on this role?"

It is important for instructors to be aware of some potential coaching pitfalls. Participants may try to replace negative feelings with positive ones. They may attempt to internally generate feeling "good" when they are feeling anxious or depressed. This is unlikely to work. When instructors learn about participants' experiences in bringing loving-kindness to difficult moments, they should be keenly aware of whether participants are trying to "patch up" feeling bad. In other words, participants are encouraged to bring mindfulness into those difficult moments, recognize maladaptive thought patterns at work as mental events, bring acceptance to those experiences, *and* now also be compassionate with themselves about their own suffering. They should extend the same warm, kind, supporting, and caring help to themselves that they would give to someone else who was in the same situation. Therefore, we encourage participants to *not* try to internally generate positive feelings if they feel anxious, angry, or depressed. Rather, they may recognize when they are in a difficult spot and nurture themselves by adopting a self-caring, self-compassionate attitude.

SELF-SOOTHING ACTIVITIES

As their own coaches, we ask participants to choose one self-soothing activity they can do for themselves. In the same way that they brought mindfulness to routine activities, we now ask them to be in the moment with this particular activity and allow themselves to notice it as they engage in this self-soothing activity. The following are examples of self-soothing/pleasurable activities that have been tried by participants:

- Going for a walk
- Taking a 5-minute break
- Having a cup of coffee
- Eating something pleasurable
- Having something pleasurable to drink
- Calling a good friend
- Calling a loved one
- Reading for a while
- Watching TV

We ask participants to brainstorm soothing activities and write them down (see Handout 28). For homework, participants do one of these self-soothing activities once a day and practice to be mindful with it, similar to bringing mindfulness to routine activities. This activity should be self-soothing and pleasurable for the participant. Awareness (i.e., observing, noticing, allowing, and accepting) should be directed to the feelings, sensations, and thoughts of engaging in this pleasurable activity.

LOVING-KINDNESS MEDITATION

Next the group practices the first Loving-Kindness Meditation. What do we include in the term "loving-kindness" in this program?

- Being compassionate with yourself
- Being empathic with yourself
- Caring for yourself
- Wishing yourself happiness; allowing yourself to feel happy
- Acknowledging suffering
- Wishing yourself good things
- Feeling safe
- Being unharmed
- Being kind to yourself in times of distress

Every participant defines this term for him- or herself. In terms of the formal practice, unlike traditional Loving-Kindness Meditations, this meditation does not start with directing loving-kindness to oneself. For participants with bipolar disorder, this may activate negative, self-critical thoughts, like "What have I done to deserve this?" Therefore, we start with a loved one, move on to a neutral person, and then slowly shift to oneself.

Box 9.2. Loving-Kindness Meditation (15 Minutes)

(Note for the instructor: [. . .] indicates a pause.)

- For this meditation please come into a comfortable, relaxed and upright position. If you wish, you can also choose a different posture, perhaps lying down. Please feel free at any time to adjust your position to enhance your comfort and ease.
- If you are comfortable, letting the eyes close and taking a moment to notice any feelings in the body. Becoming aware of any sensations that are present in the body.

- Taking a moment to become aware of any thoughts that might be occurring in the mind. And letting them be, whatever they are. Simply being with what is present.

- Taking a moment now to feel the breath moving in the body. Rising on the inhale and lowering on the exhale. Being in touch with the flow of the breath.

- And now, when you are ready, bringing to mind an image of a person who is loving and kind to you. Someone who easily evokes feelings of warmth and love in you. It doesn't have to be a person that you know personally. It could be a person that just comes to your mind, an image of someone you find inspirational. It could even be someone who is no longer alive, who has passed away. Or, if no person comes to mind, it might be a pet or animal. When you have called this person or animal to mind now beginning to send wishes for well-being to that person. Choosing phrases that help you to send him or her wishes of well-being, such as "May you be happy," "May you be healthy," "May you be safe," "May you be free from suffering" . . . "May you be free from inner and outer harm" . . . "May you live with ease."

- You can choose a few such phrases—or even just one—and silently repeat them to yourself, directing them toward this person. Choosing those phrases that resonate with you right now.

- Seeing if you can fully connect to the meaning of the phrase, choosing those phrases that seem most appropriate for you: "May you be happy," "May you be healthy," "May you be safe," "May you be free from suffering," . . . "May you be free from inner and outer harm" . . . "May you live with ease."

- And while this person may not always feel happy or at peace, you are sending them the wishes that he or she may.

- And now, as you are ready, transitioning to another person. This time choosing a neutral person. Someone you may not know very well at all . . . but might be someone you see regularly—a grocery clerk or the person at the café who makes your coffee . . . choosing someone who you do not have any strong feelings for—either positively or negatively . . . Sending this person those same wishes: "May you be happy," . . . "may you be healthy," . . . "May you be safe," . . . "May you be free from suffering," . . . "May you be free from inner and outer harm" . . . "may you live with ease."

- From time to time, you might feel that you cannot connect to the meaning of the phrase. In that case, continue repeating the phrases internally, trusting that their meaning will come back. Repeating them whether you feel them now or not: "May you be happy," . . . "May you be healthy," . . . "May you be safe," . . . "May you be free from suffering," . . . "May you be free from inner and outer harm," . . . "May you live with ease."

- Now, as you are ready, you can begin to send these same wishes to yourself. Sending these wishes of well-being directly to yourself. "May I be happy," . . . "may I be healthy" . . . may I be safe" . . . "may I be free from suffering," . . . "may I be free from inner and outer harm" . . . "may I live with ease."

- Again, feeling free to choose those words that resonate with you right now.

- It is possible that you might notice resistance toward the possibility of sending yourself wishes for well-being. Perhaps you feel you don't deserve such wishes for well-being. Or perhaps the practice feels artificial or somehow false to you. In that case, see if you can just continue the practice despite these doubts. Perhaps you can even extend the wishes for well-being toward those aspects of yourself that don't want to be gentle and kind toward yourself. Another way might be to back off a little bit. Coming back to the breath for a moment, and now trying once again: "May I be happy," . . . "May I be healthy," . . . "May I be safe," . . . "May I be free from suffering," . . . "May I be free from inner and outer harm," . . . "May I live with ease" . . . (*Longer pause*)

- And now, as we are ending this practice, as you are ready, opening your eyes, expanding awareness into the room, and gently bringing movement back into the body.

Doing a Loving-Kindness Meditation for the first time triggers a variety of reactions. The most common ones are described below.

"Sending Myself a Little Loving-Kindness Doesn't Hurt"

Michelle had a smile on her face after the exercise. "I chose to send happiness to my boyfriend. He is remarkable putting up with my mood swings all the time and this for years and years. He really deserves every bit of happiness that I could send him. And then, when it came to me, initially I figured, you know, I really do endure a lot, and I deserve the same happiness as my boyfriend. And then I allowed myself to accept the kindness I was extending to my boyfriend." As the instructor asked more about this moment when she "allowed herself to accept the kindness," Michelle described a moment of hesitation.

"Do I Deserve This?

"With all the problems I am having, all the problems that I have caused, is this something I can just take?" For Michelle, this became a moment when she exercised true self-compassion, allowing herself to accept the wishes for health and happiness that she was sending. As instructors help participants to explore their experience with the exercise, this is one of the moments when the instructor's questions about the experience will increase participants' awareness of the negative self-related thoughts, the aversion that comes with those thoughts, and the choices they may make for themselves at that moment.

"For me this did not go that easy," Veronica said. "My relationship with my boyfriend is going downhill, I am having a hard time at work because I am not getting my act together, and then sending myself happiness does not seem right." Veronica's aversive reaction is common for participants who have a self-concept with many negative aspects (e.g., not doing well in the relationship or at work, that being their fault). Instructors should be well aware of it. The instructor's curious questions about this moment—what participants experienced, how this felt, what thoughts and raw sensations were there—are geared to raise participants' awareness that sending oneself loving-kindness triggered a negative self-related thought at that moment. Participants and instructors have various options in how to work through this moment. One way is to approach the experience by labeling this thought as just another mental event or "negative self-related thinking" toward which the participant can bring active acceptance with thoughts like "Here we have negative thinking again. It is OK to feel the aversion that comes with being compassionate with yourself." This typically gets easier once participants start practicing loving-kindness on a regular basis, as they can anticipate that self-critical self-related negative thoughts might come up. This makes it easier to relate to them as mental events in their minds. However, if bringing acceptance to the self-critical negative thoughts proves too difficult or aversive at the beginning, participants may choose to stick with a neutral person or an animal until they feel ready to move on. Likewise, participants may also opt for sending themselves "little bits" of loving-kindness or just as much as they feel they can accept at the time. This may involve changing the choice of words. Instead of "happy, safe, no harm," they may chose "May you recover soon" or "May you be feeling better soon." Usually everyone can find an amount of loving-kindness they can accept.

Feeling Conflicted

Another obstacle that often comes up is when participants choose a person they love, but for whom they have conflicting feelings at the time. As Justin pointed out, "I love my girlfriend, but recently things have not been going so well and she is not sure whether she wants to continue with the relationship. I tried to send her all my love during the exercise, but then at the same time this triggered anxiety and anger." As the instructor curiously probed Justin's experience further, it turned out that he was afraid that his girlfriend may leave him. He felt that only some of the issues they were having were related to his illness, although his girlfriend thought otherwise. This made him quite angry. The simplest course of action for this exercise was to choose a different person. Another strategy was to bring observance and active acceptance to all of the feelings, thoughts, and sensations Justin was experiencing at this time (similar to "I do not deserve it") and to bring self-compassion to the experience of pain and difficulty. Justin opted for the second option and also changed the wording he was using for the exercise: "Despite all the difficulties we are having, despite all my and your shortcomings, may you be safe and protected from harm, no matter where things go and how things turn out."

Difficulty Connecting with the Phrases

Jennifer described her experience with the exercise: "I had difficulties connecting with the phrases and did not feel anything, especially when it came to myself." One reason for this problem may be the choice of words. We encourage participants to find their own phrases that convey the compassion and kindness they would like to send to others and themselves. For Jennifer, kindness to herself meant wishing that she may have the strength to continue, and find pockets of peacefulness in her "otherwise chaotic life." For Justin it meant "being able to rest in himself" going forward. For Michael, it was acknowledging his suffering. Participants should use whichever words help them to connect to kindness, caring, and self-compassion for others and themselves.

Forcing Happy Feelings

At times, participants may try to make themselves feel happy as they are sending themselves wishes of happiness. Christina acknowledged, "It did not seem to really make me happy." In this case we simply reiterate:

> *Instructor:* "The purpose of this exercise is not to make up or generate a happy feeling in yourself that you are not feeling. Rather the purpose is to allow yourself to extend the kindness you show to someone else to yourself during the exercise. No amount is too small. No amount is too large. There is no right and no wrong. On some days you may connect to lots of empathy, lots of caring and kindness, on other days, little or none. Whichever it is, this is what you can give. There is no need to generate happy feelings or try to make yourself feel happy as you are doing the exercise. Just allow yourself to give to yourself whatever drop of caring and kindness you have."

As part of their homework, we ask participants to send "happiness" to a neutral person once a day.

> *Instructor:* "For homework, we would like you to not only practice Loving-Kindness Meditation in your meditation corner, but also bring it into daily life. As a start, we would like you to send loving-kindness

to a neutral person, for whom you have no strong feelings. This can be the person who is crossing the street using the cross-walk in front of you. This can be a colleague you barely know and have barely ever talked to. Also, we would like you to choose a neutral situation, not one that contains conflict or bears strong emotions. Choose your own words for wishes of well-being and happiness. Do this once a day, or perhaps more often if you like the feel of it."

BREATHING SPACE

At the end of the session the group does a 3-Minute Breathing Space with Acceptance (see Box 5.2) without guidance from the instructor (i.e., each participant does it by him- or herself).

HOMEWORK

We ask participants to continue with their Mood Diaries and to continue to pay attention to warning signs (Handout 5). They do the 3-Minute Breathing Space with Acceptance (audio track 8) when they encounter trigger situations or start feeling down, elevated, frustrated, angry, or anxious (i.e., Breathing Space for Coping). Should warning signs arise, participants are instructed to enact their action plan and if needed contact the instructor (see Handouts 8, 15, and 20). Handout 25 provides guidance for how to move forward after the Breathing Space when frustrated and angry. Handout 27 provides guidance for how to move forward after the Breathing Space when feeling anxious. Trigger situations encountered during the week are recorded on the Worksheet for Trigger Situations (Handout 9). Participants are asked to alternate between the Open Awareness Meditation (audio track 10) and the Loving-Kindness Meditation (audio track 11): one meditation per day. They are also asked to act as their own compassionate coaches and do one self-soothing activity per day. In addition participants are asked to send loving-kindness to a neutral person or to oneself in a neutral situation once per day.

Loving-Kindness I

INSTRUCTOR MATERIAL FOR SESSION 10

- Script for the 3-Minute Breathing Space with Acceptance (Box 5.2)
- Script for Open Awareness Meditation (Box 9.1)
- Script for Loving-Kindness Meditation (Box 9.2)

PARTICIPANT HANDOUTS FOR SESSION 10

- Handout 5: Mood Diary (in case a participant forgot to bring his or hers)
- Handout 9: Worksheet for Trigger Situations

ABOUT THIS SESSION

This and most of the next session are devoted to the practice of loving-kindness using formal meditation, and implementing it in daily life. Not surprisingly, for many people with bipolar disorder, being (or becoming) a compassionate coach is not easy. Too many things have gone wrong in life to simply be kind and compassionate with oneself. Overcoming self-blame and negative self-critical thoughts that prevent oneself from becoming more compassionate is the topic of today's session. For further home practice the Loving-Kindness Meditation (audio track 11) and Open Awareness Meditation (audio track 10) and are included as recordings.

WELCOME BACK
AND MOOD DIARY CHECK

As usual, mood diaries are checked before group starts. Changes in symptoms and warning signs are noted and briefly discussed. This is done individually, as needed, before or after group, or during an individual meeting or phone call during the week.

LOVING-KINDNESS MEDITATION

We begin this session with a loving-kindness meditation (for instructions, see Session 9, Box 9.2). Following the Loving-Kindness Meditation, participants pair up and discuss their experiences with the exercise. In our experience, it is more difficult for participants with bipolar disorder to extend kindness and compassion to themselves than to people they love or to neutral people. As the participants describe their experiences, the instructors join each pair for a few minutes. After some time of paired discussions, experiences are shared with the whole group. As loving-kindness can (and often does) trigger self-critical, negative thoughts, some of our questions are geared toward raising participants' awareness of negative thoughts and the aversive feelings and sensations as they are present. We ask participants to treat them as mental events, and actively bring acceptance to those feelings, sensations, and thoughts. Depending on the capacities of the individual participant, the instructor can even encourage the participant to bring loving kindness to him- or herself while encountering those negative thoughts and self-doubts. The participant could send him- or herself warm wishes, even when experiencing self-doubts, such as "May I bring kindness and compassion to myself," "May I be able to meet myself with self-compassion and loving kindness," "May I be kind to myself," "May I love and accept myself, just as I am," or "May I learn to accept myself more and more." In that way, even the struggle of meeting oneself with compassion can be encountered with compassion.

As participants continue with their practice, they often experience less resistance and more acceptance when they send themselves loving-kindness. As Veronica described, "Over the week, I slowly noticed it getting easier. At the beginning everything in me was saying 'You don't deserve this . . . ' But then, gradually, I found that I did with this what I did with all the other unpleasant experiences that I have worked with as part of this program. I started to bring acceptance to this as well. 'Here my mind goes again, putting me down. Just the same old sayings. That's OK. Do what you are doing, but I will still be kind to myself no matter what you are saying.'" Jennifer and Justin had similar experiences. Their minds would argue that they should "Get their act[s] together first!" and "be more on the ball." They, like Veronica, brought acceptance to the self-critical thoughts and the aversion that came with them, and began to acknowledge and accept the pain, beginning to bring empathy to their suffering. As instructors we supported this process by helping them become more aware of their inner landscapes as they were sending themselves loving-kindness. At times, we may also ask them how they would feel if their children, or other loved ones, were distressed. This may help participants to relate to the idea of empathic and kind caring. Note, however, that instructors want to be careful not to reason with participants though their initial responses that might be negative, like "He ought to work harder on himself." In this case, a simple pause may help participants get past initial negative, critical, or demanding reactions, to allow themselves to realize how much compassion they would feel for a loved one in pain.

IS LOVING-KINDNESS MEANT TO BE A WAY
OF FIXING THINGS?

"Loving-kindness became a lifesaver for me last week," Michael declared. As in many other weeks, he had had a difficult time with his daughter, who was struggling in school and life in general. Often, he would feel guilty and think that it was his fault that she was not doing better. "When this comes up during meditation or otherwise," he described, "I now bring loving-kindness to this. I have accepted the fact that I can't do anything about it. Now, I don't even let myself feel bad. I immediately tell myself that I should not feel bad about this because this is not my fault. She is an adult. She has choices and I cannot live her life for her." While Michael was proud of his new way of coping, the instructor remained suspicious. This sounded like a way of avoiding the pain, rather than acknowledging, accepting, and being empathic with himself and his suffering. Yet, despite careful inquiry, Michael remained undeterred.

A couple of weeks later, things did not look so bright anymore. Michael had to bring his daughter to a psychiatric emergency room. Despite his best efforts to cope with loving-kindness, he felt utterly depressed. "I can't seem to shake it," he said, "no matter how much I try to make myself feel better, and no matter how much loving-kindness I have tried." At that time, it also became clear to Michael that loving-kindness had become a way of avoiding painful feelings for him. It had worked for a while, when "things were not as bad," but when things became more difficult with his daughter, the strategy stopped working. "So what do I do?" Michael asked, looking unhappy and disappointed. The instructor asked him to simply go back to observing and noticing what he felt. He was told to notice the thoughts, the feelings, and the sensations and, as he had done before, to bring acceptance to whatever was present at that time. Michael and the instructor also talked about what loving-kindness could mean for Michael in this challenging time: "If someone else you love had to go through what you are going through, how would you feel for them?" the instructor asked, gently helping Michael to realize that being kind and empathic with himself did not imply trying to shut off difficult feelings and thoughts. "I guess," Michael answered, "there are no shortcuts with this. But if I have to go through this, at least I can be empathic and kind with myself."

CAN LOVING-KINDNESS MAKE YOU MANIC?

Like Michael, Michelle enjoyed her first week with loving-kindness meditations. "I love this exercise," she said, "it is just making me feel good."

Compared to the weeks before, when she had mostly worked with self-critical, negative thoughts, she seemed noticeably brighter this week and her Mood Diary rating was still in the upper end of the normal range. When asked more about the experience, Michelle noted that sending herself wishes for happiness filled her with warmness and joy. "I just started to do this more and more during the day, even outside the sitting time, as this really made me feel good." This feeling also gave her more energy to do things she had procrastinated on, and made her feel even better. But she also realized that wishing herself well had become "quite addictive." "I am not sure, but I get the feeling that I am overdoing this a bit," she said, looking to the instructor for feedback. Indeed, Michelle's experience points to a fine line that participants sometimes walk, particularly if they are vulnerable for euphoric mania at the time. When Michelle discovered that sending herself wishes of happiness filled her with warmth and happiness, the purpose of doing the exercise gradually shifted toward re-creating those desired feelings. Wishing herself happiness had become a tool for generating pleasurable feelings and taking away unwanted feelings. She started to think about the warmness and joy these wishes brought her during the day, and she also more and more found herself thinking about how good it felt to be good to herself, a sign of positive rumination. Sending herself more happiness, more pleasure, and more energy encouraged partaking in more activities, some of which, Michelle acknowledged, were ones she had flagged as warning signs. But does this mean that Michelle should not or could not use loving-kindness? Not necessarily. It meant redefining loving-kindness.

For Michelle, loving-kindness had meant becoming kinder and more compassionate with herself at times when she was not feeling well, particularly when she was struggling to tolerate periods when something was not right in her relationship with her boyfriend and her daughter. She began to wish herself kindness for those times when she felt distressed and challenged, rather than sending herself unconditional happiness. In daily life, she began to direct her attention to those moments when her mind was asking for feelings of warmth and happiness. These moments became periods of noticing and kind acceptance. Michelle's example illustrates that being kind to yourself, wishing yourself to be free from harm and protected, and being empathic with yourself are different than generating positive feelings. Participants with a vulnerability to mania at the time of these exercises need to bear this distinction in mind.

> *Instructor:* "As you can see, being kind to yourself, having empathy and compassion with yourself, and wishing yourself well are not the same as trying to deliberately create the feeling of happiness or

excitement. Positive feeling may be a by-product, but if you find this becoming your primary reason of doing the exercise, then this is a departure from the original purpose. So just be aware of the attachments, the draw of 'wanting more' that may sometimes come with being kind to yourself."

COMPASSIONATE COACHING: PARTICIPANTS AS THEIR OWN COACHES

Next, we follow-up on the coaching story. Participants discuss what they have noticed about their own coaching styles during the week. Michelle pointed out that "it is amazing how much Coach A is in me. A lot of 'you got to do this, and you have to do that. And why haven't you done X yet.' This was very revealing for me to notice. No wonder that I feel tense most of the day." Other participants had similar experiences. "I still beat myself up over not writing at least one job application a day," Stephen described. "While I recognize that I am putting the pressure on myself, it is hard to step back from this, now that I have this goal to get back to work." As part of becoming more aware of their own coaching styles, or negative self-talk, we ask participants to do a Breathing Space and then to move forward by deliberately adopting a kinder, more empathic tone, resembling Coach B, in which to talk to themselves.

> *Instructor*: "From now on, whenever you become aware that Coach A is at work we ask you to pause for a moment. Do a Breathing Space, come into the present, and if you need to ground yourself, do so with the breath or whichever other anchor you have chosen. But then, however you are moving forward, deliberately adopt the style of Coach B. Move forward and be kind and gentle to yourself. Have empathy with yourself if you are suffering."

SELF-SOOTHING AND PLEASURABLE ACTIVITIES

One way to practice being a gentle and kind coach is to deliberately engage in behaviors that are self-soothing and pleasurable. In the previous session, participants had begun to identify those behaviors. They were asked to begin integrating them into their days and to bring mindful attention to the experience (i.e., feelings, sensations, and thoughts) of engaging in these behaviors. As with the initial process of becoming more mindful, the instructors curiously probe participants' experience with this exercise. The emphasis is not only on coaching themselves to engage in soothing and pleasurable behaviors, but also on allowing themselves to observe their own reactions, feelings, thoughts, and sensations as they are engaging in the chosen activity. The following experiences and obstacles commonly arise.

"I Forgot."

As with all new assignments that have not become habitual, participants may simply forget to do the exercise. They might remember at some point during the week, but then get distracted again until the day of group arrives. In this case, we simply use the reminder strategies developed when participants were beginning the process of bringing mindfulness into their days. Examples include putting reminder cues on sticky notes or using smart phone reminders. Likewise, participants may attach self-soothing activities to behaviors that are highly likely to occur. For example, Brian often felt tired after lunch and usually denied himself naps, thinking, "I have too much stuff to do." Over time, he had realized that although he tried his best he was not very productive in the afternoon. When the instructor suggested allowing himself to rest for half an hour after lunch, he was amenable to that idea: "Well, given that I don't get anything done during that time anyways, why not?" With continued practice of gentle Coach B guidance, participants will gradually find themselves relying more on internal, rather than external, reminder cues to talk to themselves in a gentler, kinder way. The same reminder strategies are also used for making time for the formal Loving-Kindness Meditation periods.

"I Didn't Find the Time."

This happens when participants are aware that they should engage in a self-soothing or pleasurable activity, but something else they feel is more important or that they ought to do always comes up. When this happens, we simply ask participants to deliberately pause in this moment, do a Breathing Space, come into the present, and ask yourself "What do I need right now to be gentle and kind to myself?" Note that it can be wise to do the soothing or pleasurable activity no matter what the mind is saying about what else might be more important. Bringing a kind, accepting awareness to the ongoing Coach A talk while engaging in Coach B behavior is something that participants must practice in order for the Coach B voice to grow stronger over time.

"I Don't Deserve It."

Negative, self-critical thoughts will continue to be an issue for many participants, as will making loving-kindness and soothing activities contingent on having achieved something else. Hence, participants often deny themselves self-soothing or pleasurable activities if the outcome of something they did was not right. We simply ask participants to pay attention to those negative thoughts and treat them as mental events.

> *Instructor*: "These thoughts are simply products of your mind designed to prevent you from treating yourself with the same gentleness, the same kindness that you would give to someone else. As they come up, as you have done before, notice them as thoughts, as mental events, bring acceptance to them, and then proceed to treat yourself with gentleness and kindness, no matter what self-critical things your mind is saying."

We also point out to participants that becoming a gentler, kinder coach to themselves needs practice, just like everything else they have learned as part of the program. The most valuable practice occurs when participants are kind and gentle to themselves, despite self-critical and negative thoughts pushing them to continue with Coach-A style thinking.

"I Didn't Have Enough Time for the Activity"

This may simply mean that participants picked self-soothing or pleasurable activities that are too time-consuming or challenging to implement. For example, visiting a friend who lives far away may not always be possible. In this case, we ask participants to pick smaller activities that can realistically fit into their days, so that they have the chance to implement them. Alternatively, it might be that the participant's mind has been generating thoughts, constraints, or contingencies to prevent Coach B from taking over. We ask participants to bring awareness to those moments, check in with themselves, and to simply treat the "I don't have the time" thought as a mental event, which they greet with acceptance. Then they should engage in whatever they decided to do as a self-soothing, pleasurable activity, like taking a break or having a cup of coffee.

"I Didn't Enjoy It."

This can be a common experience, especially if self-critical thoughts such as "I don't deserve this" or "You have to do X or Y first" are present. In fact, the lack of enjoyment may trigger additional negative thoughts such as "I cannot even enjoy the most simple things." Should this lead to participants abandoning the exercise? We don't think so. In fact, enjoyment often only increases with having done self-soothing exercises for a while. Stephen described how "when I take my coffee break, my thoughts immediately go toward thinking that I should keep working on things, otherwise I will not finish my work on time. Then I start feeling guilty for not working on it. This really made me not enjoy having the coffee and not want to keep going with the exercise." In this case, as before, we ask participants to become aware of the thoughts, feelings, and sensations that are there, treat thoughts as mental events, and recognize the old, self-critical patterns kicking in. They can also take a Breathing Space if necessary. But then they should deliberately let Coach B take the leading role and ask themselves, "Is it in my best interest to keep pushing myself, or should I grant myself some gentleness?" They may want to bring empathy to themselves, recognizing that their mind is giving them a hard time in an enjoyable moment. Then they could proceed with the self-soothing activity in a gentle and kind fashion. Participants will notice it gets easier over time, as did tolerating uncomfortable experiences, because Coach B becomes stronger with continued practice.

It is also possible that a participant chose an activity that he or she felt obligated to do. Michael described how he had scheduled running for himself as a pleasurable activity. Careful inquiry revealed he was not truly looking forward to running, that running was not his favorite thing to do—instead it was something he felt he should do for his health. Not surprisingly, he had not done any running. In this case we go back to the drawing board and help the participant to identify activities that are soothing and pleasurable and can be implemented without too much difficulty.

"I Didn't Have the Energy."

Three things can be associated with this outcome:

1. Especially if a participant is depressed, he or she may not look forward to doing things that used to be fun or enjoyable. As participants think about engaging in a self-soothing or pleasurable behavior, they may feel the lack of energy or motivation weighing on them. This is the moment we ask participants to become mindful about: come into the present; notice the thoughts, the feeling, and the sensation; be with it, notice it, but do not try to change it. In this moment, Coach B encourages doing the pleasurable activity and also bringing acceptance to the feelings of low energy, low motivation, and not wanting to do what may be pleasurable or self-soothing.

Coach B kindly and in a gentle way moves the participants to doing, rather than trying to change the underlying feeling in any way.

2. An activity may simply be too complex to execute. Going to a theater performance or to the movies may be too much. In this case, we ask participants to begin with smaller activities that are easier to implement. Give a friend a call, have something pleasurable to eat, or watch a movie at home. Choose whatever seems to be a good starting point.

3. As described before, the participant may have picked an activity that is not really enjoyable and is not really looked forward to. As described above, in this case we simply switch to self-soothing and pleasurable behaviors that are doable and that the participant is looking forward to.

"I Loved It—I Want More!"

Sometimes pleasurable activities can be a mixed bag. For participants who are vulnerable to mania, they can trigger mood elevation. "I started another experiment this week," Elizabeth announced, "and absolutely loved it. There is something very reassuring about knowing the steps, and going through them step by step. And then the anticipation about the outcome." But Elizabeth also noticed that this triggered the wish for more "successful" experiences. "I need to be careful with this," she admitted, "as I can notice that my body wants more of this. This usually comes with staying later, getting home later and then it gets into the way of sleep." Michelle had a similar experience. Trading CDs online was one of her favorite activities. But often, she had difficulties stopping and would get carried away. Her hardly being able to wait for the new CDs she traded would lead to positive rumination. Did this mean that Michelle would have to give up trading? Not necessarily, but she had to limit the number of CDs she would trade and the time she would spend trading. Some self-critical thoughts accompanied this decision. For example, "You cannot even go on the Internet without getting manic" made her feel disappointed and guilty. In those moments, she began to use Coach B, to show herself empathy, and to look at limiting her time on the Internet as an act of caring and gentleness to herself.

> *Instructor:* "Both of your experiences illustrate really important things. This is a shift toward being kind to yourself and coaching yourself to include self-soothing and pleasurable activities in your daily life. But there is the risk that your mind and body may set the autopilot in motion. Wanting more, because it is enjoyable. You have already worked on moments like these when wanting and attachment are present. Here it is particularly important to bring acceptance to whatever

wanting is present in your body, without pursuing it, whether it is wanting to do more of the same behavior or wanting to generate more pleasant thoughts or fantasies. Here, kindness to yourself means watching
out for yourself, and doing something that is not easy. Refrain from
something your body wants to do and do not beat yourself up over it.
Instead, praise yourself for having taken another step toward becoming and staying healthy."

In general, when participants and instructors choose self-soothing
activities, instructors should be aware if any of a participant's chosen pleasurable activities have been involved in their mania. Obviously, we do not
want participants to engage in high-risk or dangerous activities. Likewise,
sometimes even too much of a lower risk or nondangerous activities may
increase the risk for mood elevation. This should be carefully monitored by
participants and the instructors.

BRINGING LOVING-KINDNESS TO A NEUTRAL
PERSON AND TO YOURSELF

The next part of the discussion focuses on the practice of sending loving-
kindness to a neutral person or to oneself in a neutral situation. This is
not as easy as it sounds. As with the self-soothing activities, discussion
centers around the experience participants had with this exercise. Were
they able to complete it? What situation did they choose? Which person
did a participant opt to send loving-kindness to? How did he or she do
this? And what did participants notice in themselves as they were doing
it? For both participants and instructors, it is important to keep the basic
skills in mind: notice what feelings, thoughts, and sensations are present
as they engage in the exercise and bring acceptance to it. This basic skill,
that has been acquired, practiced, and honed since the first sessions, never
changes. For participants who forgot to do the exercise or did not find time,
we use additional reminder cues and identify times during the day when
they can do this exercise without having to make extra time for it. In fact,
this is one of those exercises that can be accomplished without changing
much in a participant's routine. Loving-kindness can be brought to the
person who is crossing the street in front of us, the person at the register
in the supermarket, or the person sitting next to us on the train to work.
In group we tend to first inquire about the experience of sending loving-
kindness to a stranger, as this can then be contrasted with the experience
that participants have when they attempt to show loving-kindness to themselves, which we inquire about second. The most common responses to

loving-kindness exercises include "This feels artificial," "I don't really feel anything toward that person," "I don't like this person," "I get jealous—I wished I could have their lives," and "Bringing this to a stranger is easy—not so much to myself."

"This Feels Artificial."

As instructors, we readily acknowledge that sending wishes for happiness to people we don't know is an unusual, likely novel, behavior for participants. So we ask another question about the experience: Is the mind coming up with self-critical judgments about doing this exercise, such that the participant is doing something odd or weird? If yes, we remind participants to bring awareness to the fact that this is a self-critical thought or judgment. The participant may acknowledge it as a mental event, give it permission to be in his or her mind, and then continue to wish that other person freedom from harm and happiness. As with all other experiences which we give permission to be present, the negativity here may be fleeting or persistent. And, as most of the participants in our groups would likely confirm, the more you begin to send out those warm wishes, the less strange it feels.

"I Don't Feel Anything toward These People—Am I Doing Something Wrong?"

Similar to the thought that this exercise is artificial, participants' lack of feeling during this exercise can quickly bring about negative and self-critical thoughts. As the experience is explored, we encourage participants to notice that this question, "Am I doing something wrong?" is masking the self-critical thought, "You are not doing this right." And as with all other experiences, they should bring acceptance to this thought. Then we simply ask them to continue with the exercise. Sometimes we may ask them to imagine that person as a really good friend, and then to imagine what they would wish for him or her. This sometimes makes it easier to relate to the loving-kindness that they are sending this person.

"I Don't Like This Person"

This thought comes up when a participant chooses a person who they thought was neutral, but ends up engendering a negative gut reaction. Or this may happen if a participant is ambitious and wants to bring loving-kindness to a difficult person. As we probe deeper, critical or negative thoughts about this person often arise like "I don't like how she looks," "He seems to be arrogant," "I don't like how he looks at people," followed by self-critical thoughts about oneself such as "I should not think this way," "I should send this person warm wishes, instead of being judgmental," and "I am such a horrible person for thinking negatively about this person, without even knowing him or her." There is no shortage of negative thoughts that this type of situation can trigger. As above, we simply use the experience to reinforce what participants have already learned and should be practicing.

> *Instructor*: "As best as you can, take this as an opportunity to again become aware of critical thoughts entering your mind. Are the judgments about the other person or actually about yourself? Is this black-and-white thinking? Are you making quick, absolute judgments? And, as you have done so many times before, you may choose to bring acceptance to the presence of these thoughts. These are events in your mind. Patterns of thinking that can be noticed and observed without getting tangled up in them. Allow yourself to let them happen and bring a kind, observant acceptance to them as you are doing this exercise. But then, with, or despite, all of this, I would like you to simply extend warmth and kindness to the person you started to think about. 'No matter what my mind is making up, may you have a life without harm. May you be happy. May you be safe . . .' "

"I Get Jealous—I Wished I Could Have Their Lives."

It is naive to assume that people do not compare themselves to others. A participant's choice to bring loving-kindness to somebody who seems to be already happy may trigger feelings of jealousy, whether those assumptions about the other person are true or not. "Why does this person seem to have nothing to deal with?" "Why is it me who has to put up with all of this?" "It's not fair that I have to deal with so much, and others with so little." As careful exploration reveals such thoughts and feelings, there is no trick or cure to employ, other than to recognize that a depression trigger has been set in motion and to recognize the thought patterns it is yielding. Acknowledge the thoughts, accept the thoughts, but then go beyond this experience and continue to extend a warm kindness to that person. Instructors should be careful not to enter into a discussion about how much or little that other person may or may not suffer in his or her life. This is not important, and would also deviate from the goal of treating self-critical thoughts and judgments as mental events. Despite having critical or self-critical thoughts, the exercise is to extend kindness and warm wishes to others.

"Bringing This to a Stranger Is Easy—Not so Much to Myself."

Even after choosing a situation where nothing in particular is going on, participants often find themselves having a difficult time extending unconditional wishes of warmth, kindness, and happiness to themselves. This is often in contrast to their ability to send those wishes to a person for whom they feel little or nothing. As we inquire about the experience, negative, self-critical thoughts typically come to light. "When I send myself these wishes," Veronica said, "my mind immediately goes into 'yes, but' mode. 'Yes, you can send yourself these wishes, but this does not mean they come true. Yes, it is nice, but if you don't get your stuff done, no matter how much love you sent yourself, your boss will still be unhappy with you.' So, why should I try?" In moments like this, instructors have choices. One could point out that Veronica may treat those thoughts as self-critical, negative judgments about herself that are present in her mind, and allow herself to observe them as they arise during the exercise. In fact, we often ask participants to explicitly invite those self-critical thoughts to become part of the exercise next time, not only to see that these are predictable occurrences, but also to realize that they can continue to practice being kind to themselves when these thoughts are present. This is what Veronica chose to do, and surprisingly, not only did she begin to look at those thoughts more and more as mental events, but also she seemed to get better at setting them aside, without pushing them out of her mind, continuing to bring a kind of caring attitude to herself. To cultivate the ability to accept negative, self-critical thoughts for what they are—mental events—we may also ask participants to change their perspective.

> *Instructor*: "Let's assume you have a really good friend, who you have been close with for a long time and who is close to your heart. If, for whatever reason, you get a glimpse into your friend's mind, and you discover all these self-critical, negative thoughts and the nasty tone they come with, what would you tell that person to express your empathy, kindness, and support?"

This change in perspective can help participants to recognize the double standard they are applying to themselves and other people. Often, we are far more forgiving with other people than we are with ourselves. Recognizing this truth can help develop a kinder, gentler, and more forgiving attitude toward ourselves. Before the discussion goes on to the relationship between acceptance and loving-kindness, the group does a Breathing Space.

RELATING ACCEPTANCE AND LOVING-KINDNESS

Up to this point, the relationship between acceptance and loving-kindness has been implicitly modeled as part of the discussion. However, we feel that it is important for participants to have a clear and explicit understanding of how these two concepts are related, especially when it comes to being mindful in moments that are distressing and difficult. We pose the question, "What is the relationship between loving-kindness and acceptance?" to the whole group. Thoughts are collected on the whiteboard based on the discussion.

> *Instructor:* "So, we have practiced mindfulness as bringing an observant, accepting awareness to whatever is happening in your mind and body at any given moment, being in the present, moment by moment. These may be moments that are pleasant and enjoyable. Often we have practiced bringing this particular way of being to uncomfortable and distressing experiences. Realize and acknowledge that these are events in our minds and temporary changes in our bodies. Actively accept whatever distressing thoughts, sensations, and feelings are present in a given moment. We have used the Breathing Space for these moments to come into the present, anchor ourselves, and then go forward with an open, accepting type of awareness, moment by moment. Now that you are becoming your own kind and compassionate coach, we would like you to be especially aware of how you coach yourself when coming into the present after using the Breathing Space. For you, as your own coach, this involves bringing empathy to yourself when things are difficult, and asking yourself at the end of the Breathing Space, 'How can I be especially kind to myself now that I am in this? How can I be most compassionate with myself going forward?' Give yourself the same kindness and empathy you wished you would receive from someone else in this moment. As you can see, the first step is always to bring an observant, accepting awareness to whatever is. Next, treat yourself with the utmost kindness and gentleness, and have empathy for yourself when things are difficult and distressing. Let's take a look at some trigger situations you have encountered in the past week and discuss how you worked with these, and reflect on this concept of being kind, compassionate, and empathic in those moments."

TRIGGERS

As in previous sessions, before opening the discussion to the whole group, participants divide into pairs or small groups and the instructor joins in when participants discuss the difficult situations they encountered in the past week. Let's consider two examples.

- *Stephen* had continued to bring an accepting awareness to those moments when discussions with his wife and daughter triggered anger. As he observed, "I now notice those thoughts coming in very clearly: 'They are being obstructive again!' It is in this moment that I sense that both of them are on the same page, and no matter what I say I am not going to make a difference. I have become much better at allowing myself to do the Breathing Space at this point, step back and let this happen, although it has not been easy, because I still think that my point is valid and that this is unfair. How should I factor loving-kindness into this? I guess this goes toward recognizing that this is a difficult situation and really patting myself on the shoulder that I am now handling it much better. After all, we don't have the big fights anymore in those moments. It's more that we have all recognized that we hit those 'moments' once in a while, and trying to push it in that moment has generally left me angry and them frustrated." As Stephen described his take on loving-kindness, the instructor picked up his point that "praising yourself for the hard work that you are doing is very important!" The instructor also gently asked about some other aspects of loving-kindness, in an open-ended fashion. "What about empathy?" This prompted Stephen to think about how this was a difficult situation for all of them. As homework, he decided to bring this empathy when they were all stuck in one of "their moments."

- Although *Veronica's* job situation (see Session 6) with her supervisor had not improved much, overall she was dealing with it much better. "I still get somewhat anxious when he is coming to me with new work assignments. When things are not clear, I still see my rumination autopilot starting up. 'Is this what he wants me to do? What if I am going about this the wrong way? Then I will get the look again.'" But Veronica had become much better at recognizing when her mind was going into this mode and reanchoring herself, bringing acceptance to those moments as best she could. She had recognized that her supervisor would not give her more guidance about the advertisement assignments. Veronica had begun to bring acceptance to the feeling of uncertainty about what she was doing with the advertisements, and less to the catastrophic thoughts foreshadowing criticism about her work and job. But treating these thoughts as mental events and acknowledging their patterns somehow incited the realization that her supervisor did not want to micromanage. He wanted her to take the lead on making the initial call, even if this meant changing things down the road. For Veronica, loving-kindness translated into "recognizing that this is difficult for me" and "being a good friend to myself who supports herself in dealing with uncertainty" rather than "putting herself down for not knowing which way she should go."

As participants continue to work on trigger situations, they are asked from now on to bring their own loving-kindness to situations after working with the Breathing Space. The goal is to develop a kinder, more empathic, and compassionate way for themselves to deal with moments or periods of depression, mood elevation, anger, irritability, or anxiety. Before ending the session, the instructor broadens the view from difficult or trigger situations to kind and loving coaching as a general way of treating oneself.

> *Instructor:* "Before we adjourn today, let's broaden the view again. Being kind to yourself is not limited to distressing situations. Every day, as you wake up, you as your own coach may want to ask yourself, "What can I do today to be kind to myself? What can I do to be good to myself?" So, for homework, we would like you to pick soothing activities that are good for you, or through which you can accomplish something."

SELF-SOOTHING ACTIVITIES AND SELF-TALK

The session ends with each participant picking another soothing activity, or an activity that is geared toward accomplishing something, in addition to the ones they have engaged in during the previous week. The purpose is to increase the frequency of these behaviors until the next session. Reminder cues can be used to help participants engage in these behaviors. Likewise, reminder cues should also be used to help participants check in with themselves at designated time points: "How am I talking to myself? Who is present right now: Coach A or Coach B?" The purpose of these scheduled check-ins is to increase participants' awareness of how they are talking to themselves at random times of the day, and give themselves the opportunity to do a Breathing Space if they discover that Coach A was present. They can then allow themselves to move forward with Coach B guiding the way. To practice loving-kindness, we ask participants once per day to bring loving-kindness to either a neutral person in a difficult situation, or to a person they find difficult. As before, we ask participants to bring loving-kindness to themselves in a neutral situation, and now also in situations that are depressing or bring about mood elevation, anger, or anxiety.

OPEN AWARENESS MEDITATION

The group ends this session by doing an Open Awareness Meditation practice exercise (for instructions, see Session 9, Box 9.1).

HOMEWORK

We ask participants to continue with their Mood Diary and continue to pay attention to warning signs (Handout 5). They do the 3-Minute Breathing Space with Acceptance when they encounter trigger situations or start feeling down, elevated, frustrated, angry, or anxious (i.e., Breathing Space for Coping). Should warning signs arise, participants are instructed to enact their action plan and, if needed, contact the instructor (see Handouts 8, 15, and 20). Handout 28 provides guidance about how to move forward after the Breathing Space when frustrated and angry. Handout 27 provides guidance about how to move forward after the Breathing Space when feeling anxious. Trigger situations encountered during the week are recorded on the Worksheet for Trigger Situations (Handout 9). Participants are asked to alternate between the Open Awareness Meditation (audio track 10) and the Loving-Kindness Meditation (audio track 11): one meditation per day. They are also asked to act as their own compassionate coaches, and add more self-soothing activities to their days. Finally, we ask participants to send loving-kindness to a neutral person in a difficult situation (or to a difficult person) once per day. We also ask them to send loving-kindness to themselves in a neutral situation.

Loving-Kindness II

OVERVIEW

- About This Session
- Welcome Back and Mood Diary Check
- Loving-Kindness Meditation
- Compassionate Coaching: Participants as Their Own Coaches
- Sending Loving-Kindness to a Neutral Person in a Difficult Situation and to One-self
- Breathing Space
- Trigger Situations: Acceptance and Loving-Kindness in Difficult Situations
- Preview: Next Week is the Last Session
- Open Awareness Meditation
- Homework
  - Mood Diary and awareness of warning signs
  - Loving-Kindness Meditation (audio track 11)
  - Continue to work with trigger situations
  - Use 3-Minute Breathing Space with Acceptance for coping with trigger situations (audio track 8)
  - Be your own compassionate coach: Self-soothing activities
  - Send loving-kindness to a neutral person in a difficult situation (or to a difficult person). Send loving-kindness to yourself even in difficult situations

INSTRUCTOR MATERIAL FOR SESSION 11

- Script for the 3-Minute Breathing Space with Acceptance (Box 5.2)
- Script for the Open Awareness Meditation (Box 9.1)
- Script for the Loving-Kindness Meditation (Box 9.2)

- Handout 5: Mood Diary (in case a participant forgot to bring his or hers)
- Handout 9: Worksheet for Trigger Situations

ABOUT THIS SESSION

In this session we continue with Loving-Kindness Meditations as we progress on participants' journey to become more compassionate with themselves in their daily lives and address common obstacles in their way. For formal home practice the Loving-Kindness Meditation (audio track 11) can be used. Because the next session is the last session of the program, we also begin the transition for participants to continue to work with themselves in order to maintain the gains they have made.

WELCOME BACK AND MOOD DIARY CHECK

As in the previous weeks, the Mood Diary is checked before group starts. As needed, changes in symptoms and warning signs are noted and briefly discussed individually with the participant.

LOVING-KINDNESS MEDITATION

The group starts with a Loving-Kindness Meditation (for instructions, see Box 9.2). Following the Loving-Kindness Meditation, the group shares the experiences participants had during the exercise. Perhaps not surprisingly, sending oneself wishes of well-being, warmth, and happiness tends to be one of the continuing challenges, especially for participants with a negative self-concept. As Jennifer pointed out, "It definitely has gotten easier to send myself those wishes. There are days where I can actually take it in. But then there are those days where my mind just fires back. I can sense the tension creeping up as I try to connect with the phrases." As before, the instructor inquires how participants work with those moments when aversion sets in. Where is it located in the body? What are the raw sensations? Have negative thoughts entered the mind?

When uncomfortable sensations, feelings, or thoughts become part of the experience, the task is to bring awareness to those experiences in that very moment and to actively accept whatever is, as it unfolds at that time. Sometimes participants try to accomplish this goal all at once, sending themselves loving-kindness and trying to accept whatever tension has arisen, getting utterly overwhelmed. "I tried this and it did not work," Daniel complained. "It was just too much. I ended up doing what you just described. Moving away from sending myself wishes of happiness and observing and accepting what was going at that time." Further exploration yielded the information that for Daniel this experience came with negative thoughts such as "You should be able to do this by now." As he had practiced it before, he used this opportunity to observe his bodily changes, noted the raw sensations in his body that were associated with the aversion, and also was able to see his thoughts as mental events in his mind. But how do you bring in loving-kindness if the mind and body are reacting this way? For Daniel and others in the group, we discovered that the answer to this question is compassion. They need to observe and accept whatever is, but then also recognize that they are suffering. Bringing the gift of compassion to themselves in those difficult moments helped them to be more compassionate with themselves as they were going through difficult times during the practice.

> *Instructor:* "Observing and bringing acceptance to whatever is never changes. It is part of everything we have worked on since the beginning of this program. Being in the moment, noticing what is going on, and accepting whatever is, no matter how unpleasant or pleasant it may be. But then, as you encounter difficult moments, either during practice or in daily life, also beginning to recognize when you are suffering and becoming more empathic with yourself that you are going through this, may be perhaps one of the biggest gifts that you can give yourself. Give yourself the same empathy you would give to a friend or a loved one who was going through a difficult time."

COMPASSIONATE COACHING: PARTICIPANTS AS THEIR OWN COACHES

Next, we discuss with the group whether participants have continued to become more aware of their own coaching style in daily life. Participants tend to encounter two obstacles: (1) awareness and (2) implementation.

Awareness

"I notice it getting better," Justin said, "But I think I still have a ways to go." As with other participants, Justin had set his phone alarm to designated times to remind him to check in with his own coaching. "It is amazing to see how wrapped up you are in what is going on, and then all of a sudden, your phone beeps, and you realize that you have been going through

your morning without paying attention to how you talk to yourself." Justin
noticed that he would pack his day full with activities, going from classes
A to B to C without having much of a break or a time to pause. "My self-
talk consists of a lot of 'Next you have got to do this, then you need to do
that.' Now that I am becoming more aware of it, I am pausing right then
and there. I got a coffee a number of times, sat down, and just sat there and
allowed myself to be where I was." Justin also started to cue himself toward
creating kinder self-talk. Whenever he became aware of "got to" or "need
to," he started to say to himself "Gentle" as a reminder to pause and to be
kind to himself. For participants whose awareness toward their own self-
coaching remains an obstacle, we tend to schedule more frequent reminders. One may also use the techniques described in the earlier phase of the
program in which participants attached cues to something they always do
in a given day, such as having breakfast or coffee in the morning or taking
medication at a given time. Attaching the reminder about becoming more
aware of a behavior that has a high likelihood of occurrence increases the
chance that a group participant may indeed pause and take a moment to
reflect on where his or her own coaching is at that time.

Implementation

"I can see what Justin is saying," Veronica said. There is always something
more important to do at that time when you become aware of it." Veronica's experience is common. If that particular task is not attended to, it
will have adverse consequences. But isn't this Coach A? Isn't this the very
coach we are trying to become aware of so that it can't keep getting in the
way of treating ourselves well? When this issue comes up—and it comes
up frequently—we ask participants to deliberately pause and listen to what
their mind is saying at this moment. Listen to the tone with which it is saying things. Is it pushing, driving, nagging, critical, or even hostile? If yes,
then Coach A is at work, and there is no easy way out, as Veronica pointed
out. She simply started coaching herself to treat herself well at work. "Your
mind is saying, 'But you need to do this!' And you know, by the end of the
day, I go home exhausted. Not only have I worried about whether what I am
doing is right or wrong, but also I didn't have enough time to really sit down.
Now, despite Coach A being present, I am slowing down. It is remarkably
simple and difficult at the same time. I just tell myself, 'Slow down, or you
are going to pay the price. Be kind to yourself. Take your break. Have lunch
outside.' I continue to notice the negative thoughts (Coach A) when I do this
and accept their presence, but I am now beginning to be kinder to myself,
just because I know that if I don't do this, then I am going to end up in the
hospital. This is taking care of me." Other participants share Veronica's
experience. Implementing Coach B, not only in the way how they *talk* to

themselves, but also in the way they *treat* themselves is often difficult at the beginning, but it gets easier with more practice.

> *Instructor:* "You have now got a taste of how surprisingly difficult it can be to be kind to yourself. Coach A often tends to be present, whispering, sneaking its way in, and making the day miserable. Becoming aware of this whispering, nagging voice that is putting you down or pushing you over the edge is critical. However, when Coach A is present, there is no magic to make it go away. It simply means deliberately making a choice to turn toward Coach B in this moment, deliberately choosing to take care of yourself, to be kind to yourself, and to act accordingly. Coach A may not like this choice and may continue to whisper negative thoughts in your ear. The challenge you are facing is recognizing this situation as just another mental event, another negative thought, and then continuing to treat yourself well. The good news is that, as with all the things we have worked on, it will get easier over time as you practice this gentler and kinder way of treating yourself."

For homework, participants will continue with the self-soothing and pleasurable activities that they have already started to implement in their daily lives and are asked to include one more item per day in order to increase the dose of practicing Coach B and self-soothing behaviors. As needed, reminder cues can be placed, and this is also further discussed in the individual sessions.

SENDING LOVING-KINDNESS TO A NEUTRAL PERSON IN A DIFFICULT SITUATION AND TO ONESELF

This aspect of the practice is again discussed in the context of becoming a gentler, more compassionate, and kinder coach for oneself. This topic can be discussed either in small groups, pairs, or within the large group. The instructor asks about participants' experiences doing this exercise. The emphasis is on learning more about participants' experiences. As for the above discussion on coaching, it is particularly important that instructors do not "prescribe" the way participants could be or should be gentle, kind, or compassionate with themselves or with other people. In our experience, only those ways that resonate with participants (e.g., gentle, kind, or compassionate moments that they have discovered for themselves) will become part of their own self-coaching. Let's consider some examples.

> • *Jennifer:* "I came across this scene at the register yesterday at the grocery store. This guy was complaining about one of the items having the wrong price, and the person at the register was not able to do anything

about it because the computer was listing it incorrectly. The longer it took, the more aggravated they both got, and the line got longer and longer, and you could see that people were not happy. I just looked at this situation and felt really sorry for all of those stuck in it. This was the first time that I could really connect to some of the phrases we had practiced. It just came to me. 'May this not ruin your day. May this not stick with you. May you be able to not take this aggravation with you into the next moments of your day.' "

- *Daniel* encountered a similar situation, but with himself involved. "I was looking for a parking spot in a very crowded lot when I saw this woman going to her parked car. I positioned myself so that I could take her spot, but it took forever. The car lights went on, and then nothing. Needless to say, I got aggravated. Why are you not moving? This is inconsiderate. Now I recognize these moments very well and did my Breathing Space. But then the car moved and slowly pulled out. The women was on the phone and she was clearly angry and aggravated at someone, trying to navigate the car out of the parking spot, holding the phone, steering and yelling. Wow, what a miserable moment for her. I really felt for her. A sunny day, perfect temperature, and here she is stuck with whatever she is dealing with, getting so angry and aggravated. . . ."

- *Veronica*, on the other hand, had begun to use loving-kindness at work when dealing with her supervisor. "I actually found myself wondering how it must be for him, having to manage all of us and making sure that the results turn out well. There are 10 employees in his group, all working on advertisement strategies. He must be under pressure too, when it comes to reporting to the one who oversees all the groups. So last week, when he did not give me clearer guidance on how to go about this ad campaign, I realized that he probably worries too, or is frustrated and angry with us at times . . . this really helped me to accept my own frustrations with how the situation is. . . ."

With respect to sending oneself loving-kindness, participants usually develop different strategies. Some just send themselves small cups full of loving-kindness distributed over the day whenever they get reminded about this. Others stick to designated times or reminder cues.

BREATHING SPACE

Before moving on to discussing trigger situations, the group does a 3-Minute Breathing Space with Acceptance exercise (see Session 5, Box 5.2), each participant by him- or herself without guidance from the instructor.

TRIGGER SITUATIONS: ACCEPTANCE
AN LOVING-KINDNESS IN DIFFICULT SITUATIONS

At this point, the emphasis is on how participants have begun to work loving-kindness into difficult moments. The instructor curiously inquires not only about participants' experiences, but also about in which way participants brought loving-kindness to themselves, how they experienced it, connected to it, and what the experience was like. This topic may first be discussed in pairs, smaller groups, or with the full group. Let's review some examples.

- For *Brian*, loving-kindness added an element that was critical for him to deal with his depression. "This was one of my more depressed weeks," he confessed. "I was very irritable and very angry at myself that I couldn't get my work done. I have learned to recognize when these kind of thoughts are coming in, and when the tension is building inside me, but despite going into observant mode, letting it in, bringing acceptance to it as best as I can, it sticks around an awful long time. This week, with this continued emphasis on self-talk, it somehow clicked how unkind I am to myself dealing with this depression situation. I was sitting in my cubicle again, noticing rumination kicking in—How in the world will I be able to get all this work done?—and I somehow realized that this is one of these moments where I really need to be kind to myself. Not yelling. Not trying to figure out how I can get everything done. Not just recognizing and accepting the negative thoughts, but being kind to me. Not to everyone else. Me. Being kind to me. . . ." In fact, that day, despite all of his work, Brian decided to leave work early. He took a long walk and had coffee in the small coffee bar at the river that he loved. "This was the best thing I have done in a long time," he said. "And you know, since then I also had a conversation with my supervisor. I told her that I simply have too much work and cannot get it done. Now my problem is out in the open, and I don't need to hide it anymore. . . ."

- For *Jennifer*, bringing loving-kindness to the moments in her health club also made a difference. Interactions with the front-desk personnel had continued to be a challenge for her, although with mindfulness she felt much more in control, and they did not ruin the rest of the day. "With all this emphasis on loving-kindness, I actually began to wonder whether to these people at the front desk I could come across as unkind. In a way, I started empathizing with them. How it must be, having to attend to all these people, often at the same time. . . . So I started to give them a smile, have a softer voice, somehow projecting low stress whenever I approached the desk in the past week. It was actually interesting to observe how this change was perceived. I even got a smile from the woman I hate so much. I still get negative thoughts that they could be more attentive, more respectful; they just occur, but now I just remind myself, 'Be kind to yourself and others, and you will receive kindness, too.' "

• For *Courtney*, loving-kindness had made a difference in dealing with her panic attacks. As she noted, "Things have got much better, since I do a good job noticing the initial signs and then allowing myself to be with whatever unfolds in my body going from there. Not fighting it has made a huge difference for me. But then, there are those moments when I would just wish it goes away completely. When I wish I would not need to deal with this. And that gets me right back into fighting mode. I know to remind myself to be gentle to myself. Not big picture. Being kind to myself, right here, right now, letting in whatever I need to let in, almost like giving myself a hug. This has helped a lot, because I don't get into my nasty mood anymore."

• For *Michelle*, loving-kindness became a critical ally for managing periods of mood elevation. "I recognize the signs, when I need to be careful, and now slow down, close accounts as necessary, no CD trading, getting away from the excitement that drives me up. And I do my Breathing Spaces, bring acceptance to the thoughts and feelings that want me to engage, talk, do, and so forth. . . . But this coaching and self-talk we did really got me to pay attention to all the self-critical negative coaching that kicks in when I am trying to be mindful with mania. There are a lot of negative thoughts I get when I slow down, such as that 'I did it again,' or 'Why I am not more successful in controlling it even after going through almost the full program?' But then I realized that this kind of thinking plays a big part in me crashing even after successfully working those mania situations. So now I not only try to recognize the negative self-critical Coach A self-talk, but then bring kindness to myself. Not in a way that I am trying to make me feel good. More along the lines of acknowledging my limitations and respecting that I may have done what I can do. In fact, it occurred to me that with all the help that I have got, and I still hit those moments once in a while, I may need to acknowledge that there is only so much I can do. Realizing this makes it much easier to be kind to myself when I am going through those periods."

• For *Elizabeth*, on the other hand, loving-kindness had translated into emphasizing quality of life. "I have those trigger moments at work," she revealed, "when new work is coming my way. Often it excites me and I get wired, wanting to work more, longer hours, and I readily willing to sacrifice my evenings and the weekend. Since we have started to talk about loving-kindness, I have found myself thinking a lot about what it means to me. What it comes down to is that loving-kindness for me means having a good life. I want to feel well. And I have realized that for me to achieve this, I will need to regiment how much work I take on, and learn to be kind and empathic with myself when I don't feel that way, no matter how much my brain wants me to be productive and engaged. . . ."

As these statements show, loving-kindness tends to take on different forms for different people. They think about kindness, compassion, a willingness to make changes in their lives they were not willing to make before, willingness to sacrifice things, and adjusting expectations in the service of well-being. In fact, this is one of the main things that is emphasized yet again by the instructor:

Instructor: "As you may have deducted at this point, well-being, feeling well, is what we have been going after in many ways. At the beginning, this meant recognizing triggers and warning signs and beginning to implement mindfulness to interrupt the autopilot that often jumps into gear in those moments. Becoming aware when it sets in, bringing an observant, nonjudgmental acceptance to things that are uncomfortable, to things that are aversive, and to things that our body wants and is pushing for. Loving kindness was our last step, bringing kindness and compassion to yourself in difficult moments or when you are making difficult decisions in the interest of your own well-being."

PREVIEW: NEXT WEEK IS THE LAST SESSION

Because the program is ending with the next session, we use the remainder of this session to set the stage for the last session. This involves emphasizing the fact that although regular sessions will come to an end, this does not mean that the mindfulness approach should end as well. To the contrary, participants should want to continue in their roles as their own coaches, bringing awareness, acceptance, and loving-kindness into their lives: recognizing warning signs, being more aware of triggers, noticing mood shifts toward depression or mania, recognizing when anger or irritability or anxiety set in, and bringing the Breathing Space to those critical moments. However, going forward, participants may develop new warning signs and encounter new trigger situations. Therefore, in the last session, we go over the elements of the model, this time with a deeper understanding on the side of the participants on how triggers, mood shifts, and coping strategies can spiral into full-blown mood episodes. In this context, we review what participants have found helpful in dealing with those situations and periods. What has been difficult? How have they implemented mindfulness and loving-kindness in their lives over the past months dealing with triggers and mood shifts? What have participants found most valuable? What would they like to continue with? For this we ask participants to bring material they have worked on as part of this program to the next session.

1. Mood Diary (Handout 5)
2. Worksheet for Warning Signs and Action Plans (Handout 8)
3. Worksheet for Trigger Situations (Handout 9)

OPEN AWARENESS MEDITATION

The group ends this session by doing an Open Awareness Meditation practice exercise (for instructions, see Session 9, Box 9.1).

HOMEWORK

We ask participants to continue with their Mood Diary and continue to pay attention to warning signs (Handout 5). They do the 3-Minute Breathing Space with Acceptance when they encounter trigger situations or start feeling down, elevated, frustrated, angry, or anxious (i.e., Breathing Space for Coping). Should warning signs arise, participants are instructed to enact their action plan and if needed contact the instructor (see Handouts 8, 15, and 20). Handout 25 provides guidance about how to move forward after the Breathing Space when frustrated and angry. Handout 27 provides guidance about how to move forward after the Breathing Space when feeling anxious. Trigger situations encountered during the week are recorded on the Worksheet for Trigger Situations (Handout 9). Participants are asked to practice the Loving-Kindness Meditation: one meditation per day (audio track 11). They are also asked to act as their own compassionate coaches and add more self-soothing activities to their days. Finally, we ask participants to send loving-kindness to a neutral person in a difficult situation (or to a difficult person) once per day. We also ask them to send loving-kindness to themselves in a difficult situation. Finally, we remind participants to bring their Mood Diaries (Handout 5), Action Plans for Mania and Depression (Handouts 8, 15, and 20), and Worksheet for Trigger Situations (Handout 9) to the final session.

Mindfulness Never Ends

- Handout 27: What Can I Do When I Feel Anxious?
- Handout 29: Mindfulness Never Ends

ABOUT THIS SESSION

This session mainly serves as a review of what participants have learned, and gives them time to reflect on what has been most helpful. Ideally, we would like participants to continue to be their own compassionate coaches, and to move forward in their lives with an increased awareness and ability to handle difficult times more mindfully. In this spirit, we review coaching strategies, triggers, warning signs, and action plans for depression and mania before saying good-bye.

WELCOME BACK AND MOOD DIARY CHECK

As in the previous weeks, the Mood Diary is checked before group starts. As needed, changes in symptoms and warning signs are noted and briefly discussed individually with the participant.

OPEN AWARENESS MEDITATION

The group starts with an Open Awareness Meditation (Session 9, Box 9.1) without guided instructions.

MINDFULNESS GOING FORWARD

In this session we review what group participants have worked on over the course of the treatment program. Much of the past 3 months have been focused on making mindfulness a part of our participants' lives. In this session, the idea of continuing with mindfulness going forward is emphasized. The different elements that have been covered as part of the program are reviewed. What has been helpful? What has not been useful? The different elements will be reviewed in reverse order. Working backward from compassionate coaching, incorporating soothing and pleasurable activities and being mindful about them, working trigger situations, warning signs, and mood monitoring, and initiating action plans. We use the example of comparing bipolar disorder to diabetes to illustrate why continued mindfulness may serve participants well.

Instructor: "In a way, bipolar disorder is a bit like diabetes. People with diabetes need to keep their blood sugar level within a zone so that their blood sugar doesn't get too low (deadly) or too high (detrimental to one's health). Thus, they are doing what people who have bipolar disorder are trying to achieve—keep the mood in the OK zone by using mood diaries. People with diabetes (if they have it from birth) take insulin (which is the hormone they are missing) on a regular basis (like people with bipolar disorder take mood stabilizers). If they wish to have a good quality of life, people with diabetes must adjust their daily routines. For example, they cannot eat a big piece of cake or numerous foods that contain a lot of sugar. This is similar to people with bipolar disorder who try to adjust their lives in a way so that they will not have too many triggers for their autopilots (difficult situations/feelings/thoughts), and adopt mindful ways of dealing with the autopilots as they arise. Hopefully mindfulness has become a useful tool or, perhaps even better, a way of being for you that has helped you to keep your 'blood sugar' in the normal range. But mindfulness is a skill. In order for this skill to remain in good shape, it needs to be honed. This is similar to other skills, many of which have become second nature so that we do not think of them as skills anymore, but as part of our lives. Mental operations would be an example. If I asked you to multiply 3 by 2, you would immediately know that the answer is 6. But if you have not done multiplication for many years, you may find yourself wondering how to do this simple calculation. This is even truer for skills that are newer, or more recently learned. New skills are even more vulnerable to lack of practice. Therefore, continuing to use those aspects of mindfulness that you have carved out for yourself will be especially important and challenging going forward. Let's review the different elements we have worked on, starting with coaching."

Participants pair up to review their experiences over the past 3 months. What are they doing different at this point? What has changed for them? What would they like to keep in their lives going forward? The instructor joins the pairs before opening the discussion to the whole group. The most common discussion points going forward are listed below.

COMPASSIONATE COACHING

The elements of mindfulness that participants have worked on are reviewed from the perspective of participants acting as their own caring coaches. Based on the individual discussions participants had, in this final session we cover:

- Awareness of coaching styles
- Self-soothing activities and mindfulness
- Awareness of trigger situations
- Compassionate coaching in trigger situations
- Stimulus control: avoidance of trigger situations

For each of these elements we briefly review the idea and ask participants to briefly share their experiences, and what they have found to be helpful.

Awareness of Coaching Styles

As emphasized from the first session onward, being aware of what is going on in the present moment puts people in a position of being able to intervene. Becoming more aware of their own coaching styles, moment by moment, was one of the skills people were working on. How did this go? As Jennifer explained, "I am noticing the shift in tone at this point when I am starting to get hard on myself. Once you become aware of it, it is still amazing how often this can slip in without noticing. So it required a conscious effort on my part for quite a while to become better at detecting it." For others, like Michael, awareness is still on the rise. "I still find myself getting caught in pushing myself and may do so for a while, before I become aware of it. I have noticed that tension in my back is a good indicator that I may have missed the occurrence of Coach A. But it is definitely getting easier to notice. . . ." The instructor emphasizes the critical point that once Coach A has been detected, participants should acknowledge whatever negative thoughts Coach A may have floated them (i.e., notice those as mental events), but then to deliberately adopt a friendlier, kinder, and gentler tone in which they talk to themselves going forward (Coach B). Based on the group discussion, the major take-home points are:

- Awareness: Check in with yourself frequently. Who is talking, Coach A or Coach B?
- Deliberately and gently adopt Coach B in favor of Coach A.

Self-Soothing Activities and Mindfulness

One way of treating oneself gentler and kinder is to deliberately engage in behaviors and activities that are self-soothing and pleasurable. This idea was first introduced in the context of trigger situations (What do I need right now?), and then carried forward as a general way of how participants want to treat themselves. Early in the program, participants were asked to bring mindfulness to routine activities. Similarly, we asked participants to bring observance to how they feel when they engage in self-soothing, enjoyable, or pleasurable behaviors. As Michelle declared, "Being mindful when I do things for myself that I enjoy was particularly important. Doing something for yourself that is good for you, but then really staying with this in the moment, enjoying it in the moment, and letting yourself feel it, this really hit home for me. Not just doing something that is soothing, but being with it." At the same time, one of the pitfalls with soothing or pleasurable behaviors is that participants may choose pleasurable behaviors that increase the risk for mania (e.g., Elizabeth—taking on more work made her feel good, but she would stay longer at work, get less sleep). Therefore, discriminating between soothing and pleasurable behaviors that participants can engage in that do not increase the risk for mania is again emphasized. As this is discussed with the group, we like to hear what kind of self-soothing and pleasurable activities participants have chosen for themselves, how they built those into their day, and how they went about succeeding (or not succeeding) in making those activities part of their daily lives. The major take-home points are:

- As Coach B, be kind to yourself by building self-soothing and pleasurable activities into your day.
- Bring mindfulness to self-soothing and pleasurable moments.
- Avoid pleasurable activities that can trigger mania.

Awareness of Trigger Situations

Becoming more aware of situations, thoughts, or feelings that increase the risk for depression or mania has been one of the cornerstones of this program. The term "trigger situations" loosely summarizes all moments and situations in which participants deal with difficult feelings, thoughts, or sensations that, if they persist, lead to more intensive mood symptoms ("warning signs") and ultimately relapse. "Learning more about my vulnerabilities has been really helpful," Elizabeth said at the end of the program. "It was interesting to learn about the variety of things that can lead back into mania, such as demands from the outside, fear of saying no, getting excited about having a chance of doing something I like and losing sleep over it." In fact, by now, after working with triggers for several weeks, participants at the end of the program should have a good sense of what their vulnerabilities are. However, they may not have encountered all their triggers. Twelve weeks of mindfulness is only a small window into a person's life. Therefore, as they become their own kind coaches, participants should continue to bring awareness to those moments that initiate feelings of depression, mood elevation, anger, and anxiety, as well as those times when they find themselves having switched into rumination. For example, for many participants with bipolar disorder, the risk for hyperpositive thoughts, positive rumination, and mania increases in the spring as compared to the winter. Based on the group discussion, participants are asked to highlight what kind of trigger situations they have become aware of and how they brought mindfulness and self-caring coaching into these moments. Overall, using the participants' experiences, the take-home point is:

- Continue to bring awareness to situations, moments, thoughts, thought patterns, and feelings that increase the risk for mood symptoms.

Coping with Trigger Situations

Two ways of dealing with trigger situations have been discussed as part of the program: (1) avoiding trigger situations, and (2) bringing mindfulness and, most recently, also loving-kindness to these moments. Why avoid trigger situations? Simply because if avoiding a situation that may cause feelings of depression, mood elevation, anger, or anxiety comes at a low cost and can be relatively easy to achieve, then this is an effective way of dealing with that situation. But often avoidance comes with personal costs or adverse long-term consequences. For example, while avoiding talking to your supervisor about the overwhelmingly high number of work assignments you receive may lessen anxiety about having that conversation, it may lead to more work assignments, feeling overwhelmed, and then ultimately getting depressed. In this situation, the outcome of avoiding the trigger (conversation) may come at a higher cost later on. But how do you deal with trigger situations?

- Universally, moments when participants start feeling depressed, notice mood elevation, feel angry or anxious, we ask participants to use the Breathing Space.
- Then, at the end of the Breathing Space, participants want to ask themselves, as their own kind Coach B, what is the best way moving forward from here? Mindfully, accept whatever is present, bring empathy and compassion to yourself as you deal with this situation.

Guidance on how to move forward mindfully may depend on what participants are experiencing at that point. Guidance for symptoms of depression, mania, anger, and anxiety is provided in Sessions 5–9 (Handouts 15, 20, 25, and 27).

MOOD MONITORING AND WARNING SIGNS

Early on, mood monitoring was introduced as a way of raising awareness about "warning signs"—mood symptoms or other thoughts and feelings that if present with a certain frequency or intensity signal the onset of depression or mania. By now, participants hopefully have a solid understanding of the warning signs of which they want to be aware. Continued mood monitoring is encouraged as part of this program. At the same time, we recognize and know from experience that many participants do not like the idea of having to monitor their mood and focus on looking out for something they don't like. As Jennifer explained, "The idea of continuously watching it is not pleasant, I need to admit this. It just keeps the idea that something is wrong with me in the forefront, especially on days where things are going well. I really don't feel like keeping a Mood Diary every day." We, as instructors, had to learn to compromise in this department. The key is that participants maintain awareness about their warning signs, no matter whether they practice this awareness using a Mood Diary, any other kind of device, or in whichever way it suits them. Some participants have made key warning signs part of their daily schedule and check off their presence or absence. Others simply tried to keep their warning signs in mind and contacted us at various points after the program when they arose for guidance. Yet others like the idea of formal monitoring and build this into their day as suggested in this program. They take-home point is:

- Continue mood monitoring and maintain awareness toward warning signs.

WHEN WARNING SIGNS ARE PRESENT: ACTION PLANS REVISITED

As most participants have learned the hard way before participating in this program, ignoring warning signs often comes at the cost of slipping into full-blown depression or mania. Therefore, having an emergency plan when warning signs are present is critical for participants' continued well-being. Action plans should be handy, well worked out, and rehearsed, so that at the time when participants need them, they don't have to come up with an emergency plan at that moment (see Handouts 15 and 20). This was done in the first half of the program. We use the last session to review those plans, discuss questions, and make modifications as needed. To review those plans, we ask participants to pair up, discuss, and rehearse their action plans and the warning signs for when these plans should be initiated. The general guidelines for how to deal with symptoms of or warning signs associated with depression, mood elevation, anger, and anxiety can be found in the session material for Session 5 (depression; Handout 15), Session 6 (mania; Handout 20), Session 7 (anger; Handout 25) and Session 8 (anxiety; Handout 27).

BREATHING SPACE

Next the group does a 3-Minute Breathing Space with Acceptance (see Session 5, Box 5.2) without guidance by the instructor (i.e., each participant does it by him- or herself).

WHEN MANIA AND DEPRESSION STRIKE

Despite participants' best efforts and hard work, depression and mania have been part of some participants' experiences as they went through this program. Is everything lost when this happens? Not at all. Present depression and/or hypomania simply means that participants will bring mindfulness (acceptance, loving-kindness) to these symptoms and make the adjustments that are described in Sessions 5–9 (see Handouts 15, 20, 25, and 27). It will be more difficult and more taxing if depression, hypomania, or mania strike early in the course of the program because at that point mindfulness skills are in the process of development and not as well established and rehearsed as in later stages of the program. Nonetheless, as long as a participant is willing and able to work with the instructors to implement these mindfulness skills, it is worthwhile to attempt to do so. However, once participants are too disorganized or their psychotic thinking has taken over, and there are concerns for their safety, that participant would need to be hospitalized. As Brian pointed out, "Being mindful with the depression, it was certainly the most peaceful period of depression I ever had in my life." Likewise, Jennifer, who continued to carry a high risk for mania, said that "for the first time, I have something that I feel gives me a tool that I know how to use with all those symptoms of mood elevation. Now, I know this does not make them go away, but with temporarily increasing my medication and then using these skills, these periods of mood elevation have been much shorter, less intense, and I have not gotten the bouncy labile mood that used to be the after-effect I had to deal with." Before saying good-bye the group does another Breathing Space. Handout 29 is distributed to the participants. It covers the most important points reviewed in this session.

BREATHING SPACE AND GOOD-BYES

Following the rehearsal of the action plan, it is time for a final Breathing Space and time to say good-bye. We ask participants for their feedback, hopes, and dreams as they go forward as their own coaches for managing bipolar disorder. Participants often wish to stay in contact. Therefore, we encourage them to exchange contact information. This last session can be very emotional for participants as they realize that for this particular group, that day is the end of the journey working together as a team. We share how much we (as instructors) have enjoyed practicing together with the group. After all, for everyone who participated, it is all about being mindful with ourselves everyday. We would like to thank all our participants for their hard work, their enthusiasm, hanging in there despite skepticism, and giving us the opportunity to learn from their experiences that have shaped this program and this book.

PART III
Reproducible Handouts

Misconceptions about Mindfulness

Everyone who considers participation in a mindfulness-based cognitive therapy program for bipolar disorder has a wish list of what they would like to accomplish, such as to have fewer mood episodes, get a quieter mind, free themselves from strong feelings, stop being pushed around by emotions, stop ruminating, have more control over thoughts, just feel normal, not feel anything, or simply find peace. False expectations can lead to disappointment. Below is a list of common misconceptions about what meditation and mindfulness can do for people with bipolar disorder

1. **With meditation, I will have no more mood episodes.** Unlikely. As part of the MBCT program, you will learn to recognize warning signs for depression and hypomania/mania, and bring mindfulness to them. This knowledge will help to prevent them from spiraling into full-blown depression, hypomania, or mania. Therefore, with this new skill there is a good chance that you may have fewer mood episodes, but likely not to the point that they can all be fully prevented.

2. **I will be able to "treat" my depression and mania with only mindfulness.** Mindfulness will become part of the treatment mix, but is unlikely to be the only component. Among other things, you will learn to bring mindfulness to the experiences that come with depression, hypomania, or mania. Hopefully this shortens periods of depression, hypomania, or mania and makes them less severe. However, especially for mania, not addressing this problem with medication is a risky course of action (see also below).

3. **Meditation will quiet my mind.** Sometimes, when people meditate, they encounter moments with few or no thoughts. However, this is not the goal or the reason why meditation is practiced. Meditation involves learning to become more aware of thoughts and paying attention to thoughts in a different way, nonjudgmentally. This helps to disengage from ruminative patterns of thinking that often worsen the mood in both depression and hypomania/mania.

4. **Meditation stops rumination.** True, although this does not mean thoughts will be blocked out. Rather, mindfulness involves learning to recognize maladaptive thought patterns and bringing a different quality of observant, nonjudgmental attention to them, rather than engaging in endless loops of rumination.

5. **Meditation stops depressive and manic thoughts.** Meditation involves learning how to disengage from these thought patterns by paying attention in a different way (nonjudgmentally) but it will not stop them per se.

(continued)

6. **Meditation relaxes, calms, and evens out strong feelings.** Sometimes, but this is not the purpose for practicing it. Rather, mindfulness involves a different way of being with thoughts and feelings, in an observant, nonjudgmental way. In fact, as many meditation teachers have pointed out, being mindful is especially important when feelings are strong and thoughts seem to take off.

7. **Meditation can help to control strong feelings.** Meditation can help to control strong feelings in a different way than most people think. Mindfulness is not about trying to relax when strong feelings are present. In this program *you* will learn to create a "wider space" within yourself from which you can observe, notice, and be with strong feelings and thoughts without getting tangled up in them.

8. **Meditation involves music and mentally going to peaceful places.** This is true for some meditation exercises, but not for those used in this program.

MBCT for Bipolar Disorder: The Roadmap

This is an overview of this mindfulness-based cognitive therapy program for bipolar disorder.

1. Overall, mindfulness is about developing skills to disengage from strong feelings and thoughts that come with depression, hypomania, and mania.

2. Although it may seem so, mood episodes (depression, hypomania, mania) usually do not occur out of the blue. Typically there are warning signs, indicating that the mood is getting worse (i.e., becoming depressed or hypomanic). For example, depression may be foreshadowed by an increased frequency of negative thoughts, more rumination, and feeling less motivated, while initial signs of hypomania/mania may involve increased energy, confidence, and motivation, or starting to feel more irritable. As part of the program you will learn to bring awareness to the presence of these warning signs and begin to implement mindfulness as they arise.

3. You will also learn to direct awareness and bring mindfulness to thoughts, feelings, behaviors, and situations that may lead to warning signs. For example, exercising before bedtime may cause lack of sleep. This may lead to speeded thoughts and increased energy (warning signs for hypomania). Likewise, not finishing a work assignment may make you feel like a failure, leading to rumination about being inadequate. The program strives to increase awareness about such situations, and the associated thoughts and feelings. The aim is to find a balance by reducing exposure to such situations (if possible), bringing mindfulness to the thoughts and feelings (if exposure is unavoidable), and apply problem-solving strategies in a mindful way (responding rather than reacting).

4. You will also learn to employ mindfulness during periods of depression or hypomania/mania. For example, if you notice increased energy and motivation, and feel more talkative, this may involve taking an observant stance toward the mind, which is producing exciting thoughts and ideas. This protective action will also involve reducing stimulation (e.g., staying home), preventing risky activities (excessive buying, gambling, etc.) limiting conversations, possibly a temporary increase in medication, and bringing mindfulness to the experience of feeling uncomfortable when you do not spend the excess energy and follow the urge to talk.

5. Finally, in the second part of the program, you will work on becoming your own kind and compassionate coach to deal most effectively with the challenges of bipolar disorder. This involves learning to take better care of your own needs, treating yourself with kindness, and also bringing in soothing and pleasurable activities that help you to buffer the stress of daily life.

(continued)

6. How is this accomplished? Over the course of the program, you will learn to observe, notice, and be with strong feelings and thoughts without getting tangled up in them. The process of learning this involves practicing mindfulness exercises. Mindfulness is a skill that can be acquired. It will be taught in 2-hour group sessions once a week. The acquisition of this skill, like any other skill, needs practice. A skill that is only practiced once a week will take a long time to grow. Therefore, practice during the week is highly encouraged. Practice will come in two forms. There are mindfulness exercises for which you are asked to set aside blocks of time to practice, on a daily basis if possible. This may involve time for movement exercises and sitting meditations. In addition, there will be informal mindfulness exercises that will be built into your day. For example, we may ask you to "check in with what is going on in a particular moment," to begin to observe more consciously which "thoughts, feelings, and bodily sensations are present in a given moment." This way you can bring a moment of mindfulness into your life. Over time, we will increase the frequency of those moments and begin to "glue" them together so that you gradually increase your dose of daily mindfulness over the course of the program. For example, one can become mindful about being in the subway, sitting in a chair, eating a meal, or in emotional situations where one feels frustrated, or angry, and so forth. Group sessions will be complemented with semiregular (once every other week) individual sessions that provide you with additional support, help tailor mindfulness to your needs, and are used for problem solving around any life issues that may interfere with participation in the MBCT program.

Mindfulness Discussion Questions

In 2010, psychologists Matthew Killingsworth and Daniel Gilbert conducted a survey to find out how much people's minds wander day to day. At random times, participants were asked to record via their smart phones what they were doing and whether they were thinking about something other than what they were currently doing. Results showed the following:

1. People's minds had wandered

   a. 34% of the time
   b. 47% of the time
   c. 63% of the time

2. For periods when people were mentally present, compared to periods when their mind had wandered, people were

   a. equally happy
   b. less happy
   c. happier

3. People were happier when the mind had wandered to happy topics compared to being present in the moment.

   a. True
   b. False

4. People were happier in the moment compared to when their mind had wandered to neutral or unpleasant topics.

   a. True
   b. False

Yoga Exercise

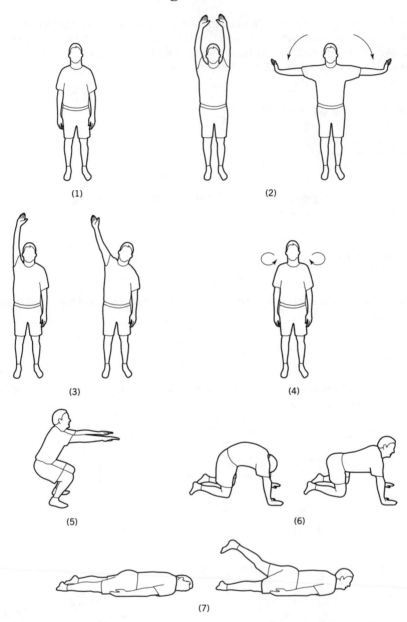

Mood Diary

Name _____   Month _____   Year _____

	DAYS	1	2	3	4	5	6	7	8	9	10	11	12	13	14	15	16	17	18	19	20	21	22	23	24	25	26	27	28	29	30	31
Elevated mood	Severe																																
	Moderate																																
	Mild																																
	Normal																																
Depressed mood	Mild																																
	Moderate																																
	Severe																																
	Anxious 0–5																																
	Irritable 0–5																																
	Hours slept last night																																
	Weight (last day of month)																																
	Notes (e.g., medication)																																

For feeling anxious or irritable: 0 = None, 5 = Severe.

293

Planning Your Mindfulness Practice

1. Choose a specific time of the day for your practice; try to find a time of the day when you have 20 minutes (or as much time as it takes) for a given exercise—for example, before or after breakfast, lunch, or dinner. Consider "attaching" the exercise to an activity that happens daily (e.g., reading the newspaper, meals).

2. Choose a specific place and prepare it. Pick a place where it is unlikely that you will be interrupted. If possible, designate a specific place solely for your practice. This can be the corner of a room, or a separate room, if that is available. It also helps to put specific things associated with your practice in this space (yoga clothes, yoga mat, candles). These objects will signal that this place is reserved for your practice and remind you about doing your exercise. This creates an atmosphere that is associated with doing the practice for the program. Prepare the place in a way so that you do not have to make long preparations before the practice. Experience shows that if people are on the fence about doing the practice, little things such as getting clothes or mats can easily derail them.

3. Try to become aware of obstacles when choosing your time and place. Conduct a mental walk-through of your exercise, including the time and activities before and after the exercise, to identify obstacles. Remember, people are always doing something, and the new activity (exercise) competes with something you used to do at this time (even if it was just resting). For example, if you decide to practice after dinner, what would you normally do after dinner? If you usually help to get the kids to bed, you may need to negotiate with your spouse to reserve this time for yourself. The kids may not agree, and ask for you to bring them to bed, which may require you to find a different time. Or you may just feel too tired to do it then, and despite your best intentions you might acknowledge that this is not the best of all times. Likewise, if you try to do your practice after lunch, incoming e-mails and smart phone hummings might derail you. Use an 80% rule: are you 80% certain that you will complete the daily exercise under the given circumstances? If not, is there a better day and time?

4. How can you remind yourself about doing the exercise?
    *   Put the exercise in your schedule book or have the phone remind you.
    *   Use colored stickers to remind you.
    *   Identify support people: have people you live with you remind you about doing the exercise.
    *   Do the exercise before or after activities you always do on a daily basis.
    *   Do the exercise before you allow yourself to do something you like (e.g., dinner with your spouse after completing the exercise).

    How many times can you practice? Set achievable goals. People typically feel good if they reach their goals, and feel they failed if they don't. So, use caution when setting your goals—how many times this week do you think you can really practice? Use the 80% rule. Do you think you can achieve you goal more than 80% of the time? If not, consider lowering the bar.

Homework Sheet

Keep this homework sheet where you do your formal practice exercises. Record after you practiced. Note anything that you experienced during the practice that you find relevant and want to talk about in group next time. Homework this week is: _____

_____

_____

_____

Day/Date	Practice: Yes/No	Comments
Monday Date:		
Tuesday Date:		
Wednesday Date:		
Thursday Date:		
Friday Date:		
Saturday Date:		
Sunday Date:		
Monday Date:		

Worksheet for Warning Signs and Action Plans

1. Warning signs for mood elevation: _____

_____

_____

_____

Plan: _____

_____

_____

2. Warning signs for depression: _____

_____

_____

Plan: _____

_____

_____

Contact Information:

Name: _____ Phone: _____ _____ E-mail: _____

Name: _____ Phone: _____ _____ E-mail: _____

Name: _____ Phone: _____ _____ E-mail: _____

Name: _____ Phone: _____ _____ E-mail: _____

Worksheet for Trigger Situations

Trigger	Thoughts	Feelings	Body sensations	How am I feeling now as I write it?

The * _____ Autopilot

*Depression, *Mania, *Anger, *Anxiety

Exercise 1 for Session 5

You work at a company, and just handed in a report to your boss. You feel you have done a really good job with this report, and look forward to discussing it with your boss. A few minutes after you handed it in, his door opens. He does not have the usual smile on his face, and asks whether you have a minute to meet.

What do you think?

_____

_____

_____

_____

_____

_____

_____

_____

_____

_____

_____

_____

_____

_____

_____

Automatic Negative Thoughts

Do you experience or have you experienced the following thoughts?

	Yes	No		Yes	No
1. I feel like I'm up against the world.			17. I hate myself.		
2. I'm no good.			18. I'm worthless.		
3. Why can't I ever succeed?			19. I wish I could just disappear.		
4. No one understands me.			20. What's the matter with me?		
5. I've let people down.			21. I'm a loser.		
6. I don't think I can go on.			22. My life is a mess.		
7. I wish I were a better person.			23. I'm a failure.		
8. I'm so weak.			24. I'll never make it.		
9. My life's not going the way I want it to.			25. I feel so helpless.		
10. I'm so disappointed in myself.			26. Something has to change.		
11. Nothing feels good anymore.			27. There must be something wrong with me.		
12. I can't stand this anymore.			28. My future is bleak.		
13. I can't get started.			29. It's just not worth it.		
14. What's wrong with me?			30. I can't finish anything.		
15. I wish I were somewhere else.					
16. I can't get things together.					

From Hollon and Kendall (1980). Reprinted with permission from Phillip C. Kendall.

Cognitive Biases in Depression

Most of us have filters and distortions in our thinking. In depression, these distortions tend to come in particular flavors. Here are some of the cognitive biases that are common to depression. As you read, consider whether you are subject to any of them.

Dichotomous Thinking (sometimes also called "All-or-Nothing Thinking"): Can you see no grey area? Do people or situations strike you as either right or wrong? This bias is evident in statements like "It's all ruined" and "I am broken, totally messed up."

Generalization: Do you see an isolated negative event as just another link in a perpetual chain of loss and failure? Generalization shows up in comments such as "Things never work out," "Things always go wrong," and "This person never understands me."

Negative Bias: Do you tend to find the negative in situations and events and focus on it to the exclusion of everything else? As an example of filtering out all but the negative, one might remark, "My garden is a wreck. There is nothing out there but weeds."

"Should" Statements: When something doesn't work out, do you assume it was supposed to have gone differently? We see this bias in statements using "should" in place of phrases expressing hopes, desires, or aspirations. For example, "I should do more to help out at my kids' school," or "I should have gone for a masters degree."

Mind Reading: Do you assume you know what people think of you? Comments like "I know she doesn't like me" and "They think I'm lazy" reflect attempts at mind reading.

Negative Forecasting: Making negative predictions (e.g., "This is not going to work out").

Magnification or Minimization: Do you notice your own mistakes more than your accomplishments, or do you notice other people's successes but not their failures? We see this bias in comments such as "After I got to work I saw the stain on my skirt, and it bugged me all day. Everyone in that office looks perfect all the time."

Inflammatory Labeling: Do you ever assign overgeneralized negative labels to yourself or to others? For example, if you don't achieve something, do you ever say things like "I am a failure"? When someone rubs you the wrong way, do you think to yourself, "He is such an idiot"?

Self-Blaming: Do you take the blame when things go wrong, even if they're not your fault? We hear self-blaming in statements like "This is all because of me" and "It's all my fault."

Exercise 2 for Session 5

Scenario 1: You are feeling happy because you and a work colleague have just been praised for good work. Shortly afterward, you see another colleague in the office and he or she rushes off quickly, saying he or she couldn't stop.

What do you think?

_____

_____

_____

_____

_____

_____

_____

_____

_____

_____

Scenario 2: You are feeling down because you have just had a quarrel with a colleague at work. Shortly afterward, you see another colleague in the office and he or she rushes off quickly, saying he or she couldn't stop.

What do you think?

_____

_____

_____

_____

_____

_____

_____

_____

_____

_____

What Can I Do
When I Start Feeling Down or Depressed?

Behavioral Strategies

- If possible, increase your activities—choose simple things, nothing complicated. Preferably, pick something that used to be fun, might be fun, or gets you involved in something. This is not the time to shoot for major accomplishments! Getting small things accomplished is key! Do things that are soothing to you.
- If it is hard to focus, do something that requires little thinking and focus (e.g., watching movies, gardening, taking a walk, listening to music, reading).
- Irritability can be part of depression. If you feel irritable, coach yourself not to express anger/irritability to others even though you may feel that your anger/irritation is justified. This does not mean that you cannot take action at a later stage, but acting on anger often increases irritability for the day.
- If your mind tends to ruminate (going over things repeatedly), choose simple activities that get you involved in something (gentle, mindful redirection coupled with engaging in tasks tends to work best for rumination).
- Remember, doing something that you may not feel like doing is difficult! Give yourself credit for trying!!

Amended Action Plan for Depression (after Session 5)

Do a 3-Minute Breathing Space, followed by one or more of the following:

1. *Activities.* Do something that is pleasurable, self-soothing, or gives you a feeling of accomplishing something. You do not have to feel like doing it. Let behavior take the leading role.

2. *Being with thoughts.* When thoughts are dominant, it may be necessary for you to spend some more time on them, going forward after the Breathing Space. Remind yourself: thoughts are mental events, not facts. Whatever thought is dominant at this time, allow it to be there, bring a welcoming stance to it without making any effort to hold on to it, just like inviting a person to stay or leave as he or she pleases. You may also write it on a sheet of paper. Or, you can imagine writing the thought in the sky, attaching it onto a cloud, and watching it from the ground.

   You may ask yourself, are the thoughts you are experiencing:
   - Confusing thoughts with facts?
   - Jumping to conclusions?
   - Painting things in black-and-white terms?
   - Condemning yourself totally because of one thing?

(continued)

- Concentrating on your weaknesses and forgetting your strengths?
- Blaming yourself for something that isn't your fault?
- Judging yourself?
- Setting unrealistically high standards for yourself so that you will fail?
- Mindreading/crystal ball gazing?
- Expecting perfection?
- Overestimating disaster?

Note, some of these questions could lead you to review evidence for or against some of these statements. This may get you back into rumination very quickly. When this happens, acknowledge the possibility that the thought might be overly negative or catastrophic.

3. *Being with feelings.* If difficult feelings and bodily sensations are dominant, allow yourself to approach these feelings and sensations with gentle curiosity. Note where the feeling is expressed in the body, note the *raw* sensations for what they are, and bring a gentle, accepting curiosity to those feelings and sensations while maintaining a sense of the body as a whole. Perhaps breathe into those sensations, and tell yourself that it is OK to feel whatever you are feeling. By the same token, respect your abilities and give yourself permission to move attention away from the sensations and feelings whenever it is becoming too overwhelming or difficult, and reanchor yourself on the breath, or any other anchor that you may have chosen for yourself. It is especially important to give yourself permission to approach or withdraw from particularly strong sensations and feelings at any time.

List of Troubling Thoughts and Feelings "Hot Topics"
(for Emotion-Focused Meditations)

1. _____

_____

2. _____

_____

3. _____

_____

4. _____

_____

5. _____

_____

6. _____

_____

7. _____

_____

8. _____

_____

9. _____

_____

10. _____

_____

Why Prevent Mania with Mindfulness?

Being hypomanic or manic can feel extremely good. What are your personal reasons for wanting to prevent the occurrence of hypomania or mania by using mindfulness?

1. _____

_____

_____

_____

_____

_____

2. _____

_____

_____

_____

_____

_____

3. _____

_____

_____

_____

_____

_____

Thoughts, Feelings, and Behaviors
Associated with Hypomania/Mania

Note: Cut the sheet into small cards

Thoughts	Feelings	Behaviors
Being more confident	More motivated	Increased activity levels
Being more hopeful	More energetic	Increased risky activities (spending money, doing drugs, etc.)
Experiencing speeded thoughts	Less sluggish	Staying up longer
Experiencing flight of ideas (jumping among topics)	Euphoric	Getting up earlier
Having lots of new ideas	Expansive	Multitasking
Being more distractible	Hyper	Doing many tasks
Being grandiose	High	Taking on new tasks
Getting paranoid	Enthusiastic	Doing things on the spur of the moment
Dismissing/minimizing adverse consequences	Being more upbeat	
Hearing voices		
Seeing colors as more intense		
Experiencing hallucinations		

Cognitive Biases in Hypomania/Mania

Most of us have biases in our thinking, and frequently we're unaware of them. Here are some of the cognitive distortions that are common to mania and hypomania (e.g., followed by exemplary statements showing those biases). As you read, consider whether you are subject to any of them, or whether you can hear yourself saying things like the statements in parentheses.

- Undue optimism about unpredictable events (e.g., "Forget the early results; I know it'll be fine").

- Counting on luck (e.g., "No, I didn't prepare, but I'm overdue for a break").

- Risk minimization (e.g., "What could go wrong? No one ever gets hurt doing this").

- Hyperconfidence (e.g., "I do better when I'm under pressure and just wing it").

- Disqualifying or ignoring problems or negative consequences (e.g., "That's all minor stuff. Basically everything at home is fine, and I am ready to do this").

- Seeking only immediate rewards (e.g., "Yes, I don't care what it costs, I'll take it").

- Inappropriate humor (e.g., "So my results were missing; I *killed* in there. They thought I was a riot").

- Misreading peoples' intentions (e.g., "She wants to sleep with me," "He wants to hurt me").

- Assigning (or inferring) special, often religious, meaning to things (e.g., "It's a sign," "That's my calling, I just know it").

- Feeling paranoid. (e.g., "Everybody is looking at me," "They are trying to ensure I screw up").

What Should I Do
When I Notice Warning Signs of Mania?

Here are some "behavioral interventions" you can do for yourself when you suspect you're heading toward a manic phase:

- Contact your group instructor; ask your psychiatrist about medication options.
- Do less; drop some activities; if you feel the urge to talk, keep quiet.
- Avoid doing things that require a lot of switching between tasks.
- No multitasking. One task at a time. Use mindfulness during routine activities to slow down and focus on one thing at a time.
- Do something that requires minimal thinking and focus (e.g., watching movies, gardening, taking a walk, listening to music, reading if you can).
- Reduce stimulation; if you need to, go into a quiet room with no people around. Stay away from people who are likely to draw you into pleasurable or risky activities.
- Decision making
    - Before acting on any plan or idea, ask two trusted support members for their opinion of it.
    - Pause for at least 2 days before taking action on the new plan.
- If needed, give up your access to pleasurable activities online.
- Have other people change your passwords.
- Surrender your credit cards and PINs to a trusted friend.

Amended Action Plan with Mindfulness (Starting in Session 6)

Do a 3-Minute Breathing Space followed by choosing one or more of the following:

1. *Behavior.* Do only one activity at a time, mindfully. In the same way that you practiced a routine activity mindfully by being in the moment, notice the activity rather than just doing it among other things. Do not switch between activities. Do not do multiple activities at the same time. Consider activities that do not require much focus, such as watching TV or resting.

2. *Thoughts.* For thoughts involving increased confidence, grandiosity, greater connectedness, understanding the meaning of things, paranoia, religious insights, exciting new plans or ideas, label thoughts as mental events being present in your mind. Bring acceptance to their presence, without engaging them or trying to refute them. Allow thoughts to exist for the time being without turning them into behaviors. Label them as hypomanic thoughts. Then reanchor yourself around the breath, or

(continued)

Behavioral interventions based on Otto et al. (2009).

another anchor of your choosing, if you find yourself getting carried away by fantasies or fearful scenarios. Repeat this process as often as you get carried away. You may find it helpful to ask yourself the following questions:

- Are these hypomanic thoughts?
- Am I getting too confident?
- Are these ideas that want me to do things on the spur of the moment?
- Am I not taking consequences into account?
- Am I overestimating the probability of a positive outcome?
- Am I taking an unnecessary risk?
- Is this a dangerous idea?
- Does this get me to do too much?
- Could this thought get me back to being manic?
- Do my insights reflect a change in the real world?
- Could this feeling of being connected be the first sign of mania?
- Could this sense of meaning and insight be the start of hypomania?

If your thoughts jump from topic to topic, let yourself observe your thoughts, allowing yourself to notice the ebbing and flowing of thoughts and ideas without trying to follow or control them. There is no need to catch all of the content. Rather, label the thoughts as bouncy, bringing acceptance to your experience of thoughts coming and going.

If your thoughts feel speeded up, allow yourself to notice the increased pace of thoughts as they enter your mind. Do not try to catch every thought or all of the content. Rather, label the rate as speedy and allow the flow of thoughts to unfold, without trying to jump in, hold on to thoughts, or slow them down. Accept the flow for now, like watching cars on a highway, the constant flow and movement.

3. *Feelings.* If you notice yourself feeling energetic and compelled to act, allow yourself to go toward the feelings of increased energy, motivation, and the impulses to talk and act. Note where these things are located in the body, and bring a curious yet accepting attention to the raw sensations that come with these bodily experiences, but do not pursue them or turn them into action. If you have the urge to talk, don't, but allow yourself to notice and observe this impulse in your body in an observant, accepting way. As best as you can, hold the impulse in your awareness without following it. Note the aversion and discomfort that may arise as you deliberately choose not to engage this urge. Bring acceptance to this, too.

Automatic Anger Thoughts

Do you experience or have you experienced the following thoughts?

Circle the items below that you can identify with. Also, add thoughts in the blanks below that would likely be relevant to you.

- Everyone pushes me around.
- People are disrespectful.
- Everyone is unfair.
- People are incompetent.
- People try to manipulate me.
- Everyone has unrealistic expectations.
- No one will take responsibility for anything.
- No one cares what I think.
- People don't care about what I need.
- No one is ever on time; I always have to wait for them.
- Everyone blames me when things go wrong.
- People exploit me.
- People take advantage of me

HANDOUT 22
Anger-Related Cognitive Biases

Black-and-White Thinking: A tendency to see/interpret things in extreme ways, usually worse than they really are; also called "catastrophic thinking" or "magnifying a situation" (e.g., "This is a disaster" instead of "This is not working out").

Personalization/Blaming: Assigning the responsibility for things that went wrong to someone else (e.g., "We could have been on time, if you hadn't procrastinated," "This could have worked out if you had just done your part right"). This involves the mistaken belief that other people are "harming" oneself intentionally.

Inflammatory Labeling: Assigning overgeneralized negative labels to events or people (e.g., if someone rubs you the wrong way, saying, "He's an idiot").

Mind Reading and Misattributions: Making inferences about someone else's intent and jumping to conclusions (e.g., "I know he was setting me up for failure").

Overgeneralization: Taking a single negative event as a pattern by using words like "never" or "always" (e.g., "He's always doing things like this to hurt me").

"Should" Statements: Thoughts that involve words such as "should," "got to," "ought to" (e.g., "They should not have done this—it was absolutely wrong").

Exercise for Session 7

Scenario 1: You are a guest in a hotel and would like to check out. You are the only guest at the front desk. It's a nice day and you are in a good mood. The two front desk employees are engaged in a conversation and it takes a little while before one turns toward you. While standing at the front desk waiting, what do you think?

_____

_____

_____

_____

_____

_____

Scenario 2: You are a guest in a hotel and would like to check out. You are the only guest at the front desk. It's been a frustrating day and you are pretty irritable. The two front desk employees are engaged in a conversation and it takes a little while before one turns toward you. While standing at the front desk waiting, what do you think?

_____

_____

_____

_____

_____

_____

_____

_____

_____

Anger Discussion Questions

Does Venting Anger Feed or Extinguish the Flame?
Catharsis, Rumination, Distraction, Anger, and Aggressive Responding

An experimental study by Brad Bushman (2002) investigated the effects of how people deal with anger. Volunteers were made angry and then randomly assigned to one of two groups. Participants in the rumination group were instructed to hit a punching bag and think about the person who had angered them. People in the distraction group were asked to think about becoming physically fit. Then, after some time, everyone was asked to report how he or she felt. Which of the following do you think that researchers found?

1. There was no difference how people felt in both groups.
2. People in the distraction group were angrier because they had to think about something else.
3. People in the rumination group were less angry because they could express their frustration.
4. People in the rumination group were angrier because they punched a bag and continued to think about what angered them.
5. People in the distraction group were less angry because they got distracted.

Solution: People in the rumination group felt angrier than did people in the distraction or control groups. Expressing anger and rumination increased rather than decreased anger and aggression. Even doing nothing at all was more effective than venting anger.

What Can I Do When I Feel Frustrated, Angry, or Irritable?

Behavioral Strategies

- When you feel hurt or angry do not act on it, as difficult as this may be.
- Act polite and perhaps even friendly, knowing that this is the opposite of how you feel.
- Take time out if you have to. If you feel that you will act angrily, remove yourself from the situation.
- If you feel compelled to approach someone and act angry, don't. Go away. Do something else.
- Do not make any decisions while you feel acutely hurt or angry.
- Do something that captures your attention without pushing the thoughts and the feelings out.

Do a 3-Minute Breathing Space followed by choosing one or more of the following:

1. *Mindfulness with angry thoughts.* Recognize thoughts as thoughts, not facts. Allow yourself to see them for what they are: mental events that are making you feel hurt and angry. What is the thought that hurt you? What is it that made you frustrated and angry?

   - When you recognize angry thoughts being present, ask yourself:
   - What is it that hurt me?
   - What is it that frustrated me?
   - Why am I hurt and frustrated?
   - Is my mind blowing things out of proportion right now?
   - Is this black-and-white thinking?
   - Is my mind making things worse than they are?
   - Is my mind telling me that this has always been this way and will never change?
   - Am I misfortune-telling?
   - Am I blaming people again?
   - Am I mind reading?
   - Did this person do this on purpose?

   Allow yourself to maintain this curious observance, and continue to watch thoughts of frustration, hurt, or anger enter your mind, whether they are in the form of images, scenes, or sentences.

2. *How to be with the feeling of being hurt or angry.* As best as you can, recognize that you have been hurt. Where is this feeling of being hurt or angry located in your body?

(continued)

What are the raw sensations that come with it? As best as you can, bring an observant acceptance to those sensations and feelings as they are present in your body and demand your attention. You don't want to be hurt, so this naturally elicits aversion. Where is this aversion? What are the sensations? Bring an accepting observation to the aversion, the not wanting, as best as you can. Likewise, your body may send you impulses to act on the angry feelings and sensations. You may wish to express your anger and dissatisfaction with your voice, and perhaps even want to yell or scream. As best as you can, bring acceptance to this impulse and the raw sensations that are associated with it as it is present in this very moment. It may be helpful to approach the impulse, the aversion, and the hurt feeling. At other times, observe it from a distance, including the body as a whole to create a wider space within yourself to maintain an accepting, observant stance.

3. *Angry rumination.* If you find yourself ruminating, having mental images or conversations in which you express your anger and how you were wronged, recognize that your mind is trying to fix the hurt feeling with angry fantasies, but that they are fueling your anger. Allow yourself to redirect your attention to the breath, focusing on breathing and reanchoring yourself whenever you notice that rumination has begun. Repeat this process as often as necessary.

Automatic Catastrophic Thoughts

Do you experience or have you experienced the following thoughts when you were anxious?

	Yes	No
1. I am going to throw up.		
2. I am going to pass out.		
3. I must have a brain tumor.		
4. I will have a heart attack.		
5. I will choke to death.		
6. I am going to act foolish.		
7. I am going blind.		
8. I will not be able to control myself.		
9. I will hurt someone.		
10. I am going to have a stroke.		
11. I am going to go crazy.		
12. I am going to scream.		
13. I am going to babble or talk funny.		
14. I will be paralyzed with fear.		
15. I am seriously ill.		
16. I am going to suffocate.		

Adapted from Chambless et al. (1984). Copyright 1984 by the American Psychological Association.

What Can I Do When I Feel Anxious?

Do a 3-Minute Breathing Space followed by choosing one or more of the following:

1. *Feelings and physical sensations.* As you find your attention drawn to the physical manifestations of anxiety in your body (e.g., faster heartbeat, difficulties breathing, trembling, shaking, feeling nauseous), as best as you can, bring acceptance to those experiences. Tell yourself that "It is OK to feel like this." Either continue to observe the sensation from a wider, spacious point of view within your body, or, if you can, approach the raw sensation with curiosity, bring acceptance to whatever may happen as you observe that sensation. Experiencing these sensations is aversive and you will find yourself wanting to turn away from this experience. As best as you can, allow yourself to also bring an accepting openness to experiencing this part of the anxiety, including it in your observance of what is unfolding at that time. These are physiological changes in your body, and there is nothing you need to do about them other than allowing yourself to experience them with an open, accepting stance, no matter how intense they may be. If you experience things that seem unreal, or you seem to be detached from your body, allow yourself to observe this experience without trying to alter it in any way. Just observe and accept it. Respect what you are able to do at any time, and feel free to return to the breath as your anchor, following the sensations of the inbreath and the outbreath. Or you may turn to any other anchor that you may have defined for yourself, for example, following sounds or visually focusing on objects.

2. *Being with catastrophic thoughts.* As catastrophic thoughts continue to enter your mind, note them for what they are: mental events. Comment on the sensations and make predictions about what catastrophe may come of them. Perhaps label them as catastrophic thoughts or catastrophic predictions, but do not engage with them in any way. As with the sensations, when your attention is drawn to them, bring an accepting observance to their presence, without arguing with them or trying to push them out of your mind. Do not attempt to distract yourself or think forcefully about something else. As best as you can, maintain an open, inviting stance, letting them into your mind, giving them permission to stay or leave.

3. *Being with worry.* When you find yourself getting caught up in worry, trying to fix things in your mind, or trying to prevent what may be foreshadowed by some catastrophic thought, allow yourself to return to the breath for a moment, or whichever anchor you have chosen for yourself. Follow the inbreath and the outbreath for a while, grounding yourself. But then, when you feel ready, widen the field of awareness to the body and mind again. You may ask yourself:
   - What are those thoughts that are making me anxious?
   - What catastrophic thoughts am I having?

(continued)

- Is my mind making catastrophic predictions?
- What is my mind trying to prevent?

Note the catastrophic thoughts that may be present at that time, label them as mental events, and bring acceptance to their presence, no matter how scary they may be.

4. *Behavior.* When you are feeling anxious and you bring mindfulness to the experience, gradually, as best as you can, allow yourself to drop some of the things that you are doing with the intention of keeping anxiety under control. These behaviors may include holding your body in a certain position, holding onto a chair, tensing your hands, or crossing your legs. You may also find yourself avoiding situations altogether, because you are afraid that anxiety may occur and you won't be able to handle it. Going forward, with more Emotion-Focused Meditations involving anxiety under your belt, we would like you to gradually approach those situations, too. Apply the mindfulness skills to thoughts, feelings, and sensations described above in those situations as well.

HANDOUT 28
Self-Soothing Activities

List activities that are pleasurable and self-soothing for you:

1. _____

_____

2. _____

_____

3. _____

_____

4. _____

_____

5. _____

_____

6. _____

_____

7. _____

_____

8. _____

_____

9. _____

_____

10. _____

_____

Mindfulness Never Ends

Coaching

- Awareness: Check in with yourself frequently. Who is talking, Coach A or Coach B?

- Deliberately and gently adopt Coach B in favor of Coach A.

- Be kind to yourself by building self-soothing and pleasurable activities into your day.

- Bring mindfulness to self-soothing and pleasurable moments.

- Avoid pleasurable activities that can trigger mania.

- Continue to bring awareness to situations, moments, thoughts, thought patterns, and feelings that increase the risk for mood symptoms.

Coping with Trigger Situations

- Universally, for all situations, in moments when you start feeling depressed, notice mood elevation, or feel angry or anxious, use the Breathing Space.

- Then at the end of the Breathing Space, ask yourself as your own, kind coach B what is the best way to move forward from here? Mindfully, accepting whatever is present, bring compassion to yourself as you are dealing with this situation.

Warning Signs

- Continue to be aware of warning signs (better to be safe than sorry).

- Initiate the rehearsed action plans whenever needed (early intervention is key).

References

Altshuler, L. L. (1993). Bipolar disorder: Are repeated episodes associated with neuroanatomic and cognitive changes? *Biol Psychiatry, 33*(8–9), 563–565.

Altshuler, L. L., Bearden, C. E., Green, M. F., van Gorp, W., & Mintz, J. (2008). A relationship between neurocognitive impairment and functional impairment in bipolar disorder: A pilot study. *Psychiatry Res, 157*(1–3), 289–293.

American Psychiatric Association. (2013). *Diagnostic and statistical manual of mental disorders* (5th ed.). Arlington, VA: Author.

Atre-Vaidya, N., Taylor, M. A., Seidenberg, M., Reed, R., Perrine, A., & Glick-Oberwise, F. (1998). Cognitive deficits, psychopathology, and psychosocial functioning in bipolar mood disorder. *Neuropsychiatry Neuropsychol Behav Neurol, 11*(3), 120–126.

Baer, R. (2003). Mindfulness training as a clinical intervention: A conceptual and empirical review. *Clinical Psychology: Science and Practice, 10*(2), 125–143.

Bauer, M. S., McBride, L., Williford, W. O., Glick, H., Kinosian, B., Altshuler, L., et al. (2006a). Collaborative care for bipolar disorder: Part I. Intervention and implementation in a randomized effectiveness trial. *Psychiatr Serv, 57*(7), 927–936.

Bauer, M. S., McBride, L., Williford, W. O., Glick, H., Kinosian, B., Altshuler, L., et al. (2006b). Collaborative care for bipolar disorder: Part II. Impact on clinical outcome, function, and costs. *Psychiatr Serv, 57*(7), 937–945.

Beck, A. T., Steer, R. A., & Brown, G. K. (1996). *Manual for the Beck Depression Inventory—II*. San Antonio, TX: Psychological Corporation.

Belmaker, R. H. (2007). Treatment of bipolar depression. *N Engl J Med, 356*(17), 1771–1773.

Bersudsky, Y., & Belmaker, R. H. (2009). "Treatment of bipolar disorder: A systematic review of available data and clinical perspectives" by Fountoulakis and Vieta. (2008). *Int J Neuropsychopharmacol, 12*(2), 285–286.

Bishop, S. R., Lau, M., Shapiro, S., Carlson, L. E., Anderson, N. D., Carmody, J., et al. (2004). Mindfulness: A proposed operational definition. *Clinical Psychology: Science and Practice, 11*, 230–241.

References

Bowen, S., Chawla, N., & Marlatt, A. (2011). *Mindfulness-based relapse prevention for addictive behaviors: A clinician's guide.* New York: Guilford Press.

Bowen, S., Witkiewitz, K., Dillworth, T. M., Chawla, N., Simpson, T. L., Ostafin, B. D., et al. (2006). Mindfulness meditation and substance use in an incarcerated population. *Psychol Addict Behav, 20*(3), 343–347.

Bushman, B. (2002). Does venting anger feed or extinguish the flame?: Catharsis, rumination, distraction, anger, and aggressive responding. *Pers Soc Psychol Bull, 28,* 724–731.

Calabrese, J. R., Bowden, C. L., Sachs, G. S., Ascher, J. A., Monaghan, E., & Rudd, G. D. (1999). A double-blind placebo-controlled study of lamotrigine monotherapy in outpatients with bipolar I depression. *J Clin Psychiatry, 60*(2), 79–88.

Carlson, G. A., & Goodwin, E. K. (1973). The stages of mania: A longitudinal analysis of the manic episode. *Arch Gen Psychiatry, 28,* 221–228.

Cavanagh, J. T., Van Beck, M., Muir, W., & Blackwood, D. H. (2002). Case-control study of neurocognitive function in euthymic patients with bipolar disorder: An association with mania. *Br J Psychiatry, 180,* 320–326.

Chambless, D. L., Caputo, G. C., Bright, P., & Gallagher, R. (1984). Assessment of fear of fear in agoraphobics: The Body Sensations Questionnaire and the Agoraphobic Cognitions Questionnaire. *J Consult Clin Psychol, 52*(6), 1090–1097.

Chambless, D. L., & Ollendick, T. H. (2001). Empirically supported psychological interventions: Controversies and evidence. *Annu Rev Psychol, 52,* 685–716.

Chan, D., & Woollacott, M. (2007). Effects of level of meditation experience on attentional focus: Is the efficiency of executive or orientation networks improved? *J Altern Complement Med, 13*(6), 651–657.

Clark, L., Iversen, S. D., & Goodwin, G. M. (2002). Sustained attention deficit in bipolar disorder. *Br J Psychiatry, 180,* 313–319.

Cochran, S. D. (1984). Preventing medical noncompliance in the outpatient treatment of bipolar affective disorders. *J Consult Clin Psychol, 52*(5), 873–878.

Colom, F., Vieta, E., Sanchez-Moreno, J., Palomino-Otiniano, R., Reinares, M., Goikolea, J. M., et al. (2009). Group psychoeducation for stabilised bipolar disorders: 5-year outcome of a randomised clinical trial. *Br J Psychiatry, 194*(3), 260–265.

Colom, F., Veita, E., Tacchi, M. J., Sanchez-Moreno, J., & Scott, J. (2005). Identifying and improving non-adherence in bipolar disorders. *Bipolar Disorders, 7*(Suppl. 5), 24–31.

Deckersbach, T., Hölzel, B. K., Eisner, L. R., Stange, J. P., Peckham, A. D., Dougherty, D. D., et al. (2012). Mindfulness-based cognitive therapy for non-remitted patients with bipolar disorder *CNS Neurosci Ther, 18*(2), 133–144.

Deckersbach, T., Nierenberg, A. A., Kessler, R., Lund, H. G., Ametrano, R. M., Sachs, G., et al. (2010). Cognitive rehabilitation for bipolar disorder: An open trial for employed patients with residual depressive symptoms. *CNS Neurosci Ther, 16*(5), 298–307.

Deckersbach, T., Savage, C. R., Reilly-Harrington, N., Clark, L., Sachs, G., & Rauch, S. L. (2004). Episodic memory impairment in bipolar disorder and obsessive-compulsive disorder: The role of memory strategies. *Bipolar Disord, 6*(3), 233–244.

Dickerson, F. B., Boronow, J. J., Stallings, C. R., Origoni, A. E., Cole, S., & Yolken, R. H. (2004). Association between cognitive functioning and employment status of persons with bipolar disorder. *Psychiatr Serv, 55*(1), 54–58.

Dittmann, S., Seemuller, F., Schwarz, M. J., Kleindienst, N., Stampfer, R., Zach, J., et al. (2007). Association of cognitive deficits with elevated homocysteine levels in euthymic bipolar patients and its impact on psychosocial functioning: Preliminary results. *Bipolar Disord, 9*(1–2), 63–70.

Duhigg, C. (2012). *The power of habit: Why do we do what we do in life and business?* New York: Random House.

Ellicott, A., Hammen, C., Gitlin, M., Brown, G., & Jamison, K. (1990). Life events and the course of bipolar disorder. *Am J Psychiatry, 147*(9), 1194–1198.

Fava, G. A., Rafanelli, C., Cazzaro, M., Conti, S., & Grandi, S. (1998). Well-being therapy: A novel psychotherapeutic approach for residual symptoms of affective disorders. *Psychol Med, 28*(2), 475–480.

Feldman, G. C., Joormann, J., & Johnson, S. L. (2008). Responses to positive affect: A self-report measure of rumination and dampening. *Cognit Ther Res, 32*(4), 507–525.

First, M. B., Spitzer, R. L., Gibbon, M., & Williams, J. B. W. (1995). *Structured Clinical Interview for DSM-IV Axis I Disorders—Patient edition* (SCID-I/D, Version 2.0). New York: Biometrics Research Department, New York Psychiatric Institute.

Frank, E. (1999). Interpersonal and social rhythm therapy prevents depressive symptomatology in bipolar 1 patients. *Bipolar Disorders, 1*, 13.

Frank, E., Hlastala, S., Ritenour, A., & Houck, P. (1997). Inducing lifestyle regularity in recovering bipolar disorder patients: Results from the maintenance therapies in bipolar disorder protocol. *Biol Psychiatry, 41*(12), 1165–1173.

Frank, E., Kupfer, D. J., Thase, M. E., Mallinger, A. G., Swartz, H. A., Fagiolini, A. M., et al. (2005). Two-year outcomes for interpersonal and social rhythm therapy in individuals with bipolar I disorder. *Arch Gen Psychiatry, 62*(9), 996–1004.

Frank, E., Swartz, H. A., & Kupfer, D. J. (2000). Interpersonal and social rhythm therapy: Managing the chaos of bipolar disorder. *Biol Psychiatry, 48*(6), 593–604.

Frye, M. A. (2011). Clinical practice: Bipolar disorder—A focus on depression. *N Engl J Med, 364*(1), 51–59.

Geddes, J. R., Calabrese, J. R., & Goodwin, G. M. (2009). Lamotrigine for treatment of bipolar depression: Independent meta-analysis and meta-regression of individual patient data from five randomised trials. *Br J Psychiatry, 194*(1), 4–9.

Germer, C. K. (2009). *The mindful path to self-compassion: Freeing yourself from destructive thoughts and emotions.* New York: Guilford Press.

Ghaemi, S. N., Hsu, D. J., Thase, M. E., Wisniewski, S. R., Nierenberg, A. A., Miyahara, S., et al. (2006). Pharmacological treatment patterns at study entry for the first 500 STEP-BD participants. *Psychiatric Services, 57*(5), 660–665.

Gildengers, A. G., Butters, M. A., Chisholm, D., Rogers, J. C., Holm, M. B., Bhalla, R. K., et al. (2007). Cognitive functioning and instrumental activities of daily living in late-life bipolar disorder. *Am J Geriatr Psychiatry, 15*(2), 174–179.

Gitlin, M. J., Swendsen, J., Heller, T. L., & Hammen, C. (1995). Relapse and impairment in bipolar disorder. *Am J Psychiatry, 152*(11), 1635–1640.

Goldberg, J. F., Perlis, R. H., Ghaemi, S. N., Calabrese, J. R., Bowden, C. L., Wisniewski, S., et al. (2007). Adjunctive antidepressant use and symptomatic recovery among bipolar depressed patients with concomitant manic symptoms: Findings from the STEP-BD. *Am J Psychiatry, 164*(9), 1348–1355.

Goleman, D. J., & Schwartz, G. E. (1976). Meditation as an intervention in stress reactivity. *J Consult Clin Psychol, 44*(3), 456–466.

Grace, J., & Malloy, P. F. (2001). *Frontal Systems Behavior Rating Scale (FrSBe) professional manual.* Lutz, FL: Psychological Assessment Resources.

Gratz, K. L., & Roemer, L. (2004). Multidimensional assessment of emotion regulation and dysregulation: Development, factor structure, and initial validation of the Difficulties in Emotion Regulation Scale. *Journal of Psychopathology and Behavioral Assessment, 26,* 41–54.

Grossman, P., Niemann, L., Schmidt, S., & Walach, H. (2004). Mindfulness-based stress reduction and health benefits: A meta-analysis. *J Psychosom Res, 57*(1), 35–43.

Hamilton, M. (1960). A rating scale for depression. *J Neurol Neurosurg Psychiatry, 23,* 56–62.

Hart, W. (1987). *The art of living: Vipassana meditation, as taught by S. N. Goenka.* New York: HarperOne.

Harvey, P. D., Twamley, E. W., Vella, L., Patterson, T., & Heaton, R. K. (2010). *Results of the Validation of Everyday Real World Outcomes (VALERO) Study: Validation of 6 real world rating scales for their relationship with neurocognitive and functional ability.* Paper presented at the 49th annual meeting of the American College of Neuropsychopharmacology, Miami, FL.

Hofmann, S. G., Sawyer, A. T., Witt, A. A., & Oh, D. (2010). The effect of mindfulness-based therapy on anxiety and depression: A meta-analytic review. *J Consult Clin Psychol, 78*(2), 169–183.

Hofmann, S. G., Sawyer, A. T., Witt, A. A., & Oh, D. (2010). The effect of mindfulness-based therapy on anxiety and depression: A meta-analytic review. *J Consult Clin Psychol, 78*(2), 169–183.

Hollon, S. D., & Kendall, P. (1980). Cognitive self statements in depression: Development of an automatic thoughts questionnaire. *Cog Ther Res, 4,* 383–395.

Isaacson, W. (2011). *Steve Jobs.* New York: Simon & Schuster.

Jaeger, J., Berns, S., Loftus, S., Gonzalez, C., & Czobor, P. (2007). Neurocognitive test performance predicts functional recovery from acute exacerbation leading to hospitalization in bipolar disorder. *Bipolar Disord, 9*(1–2), 93–102.

Jain, S., Shapiro, S. L., Swanick, S., Roesch, S. C., Mills, P. J., Bell, I., et al. (2007). A randomized controlled trial of mindfulness meditation versus relaxation training: Effects on distress, positive states of mind, rumination, and distraction. *Ann Behav Med, 33*(1), 11–21.

Jha, A. P., Krompinger, J., & Baime, M. J. (2007). Mindfulness training modifies subsystems of attention. *Cogn Affect Behav Neurosci, 7*(2), 109–119.

Jha, A. P., Stanley, E. A., Kiyonaga, A., Wong, L., & Gelfand, L. (2010). Examining the protective effects of mindfulness training on working memory capacity and affective experience. *Emotion, 10*(1), 54–64.

Johnson, R. E., & McFarland, B. H. (1996). Lithium use and discontinuation in a health maintenance organization. *Am J Psychiatry, 153*(8), 993–1000.

Johnson, S. L., McKenzie, G., & McMurrich, S. (2008). Ruminative responses to negative and positive affect among students diagnosed with bipolar disorder and major depressive disorder. *Cognit Ther Res, 32*(5), 702–713.

Judd, L. L., Akiskal, H. S., Schettler, P. J., Endicott, J., Leon, A. C., Solomon, D. A., et al. (2005). Psychosocial disability in the course of bipolar I and II disorders: A prospective, comparative, longitudinal study. *Arch Gen Psychiatry, 62*(12), 1322–1330.

Judd, L. L., Akiskal, H. S., Schettler, P. J., Endicott, J., Maser, J., Solomon, D. A., et al. (2002). The long-term natural history of the weekly symptomatic status of bipolar I disorder. *Arch Gen Psychiatry, 59*(6), 530–537.

Judd, L. L., Schettler, P. J., Solomon, D. A., Maser, J. D., Coryell, W., Endicott, J., et al. (2008). Psychosocial disability and work role function compared across the long-term course of bipolar I, bipolar II and unipolar major depressive disorders. *J Affect Disord, 108*(1–2), 49–58.

Kabat-Zinn, J. (1990). *Full catastrophe living.* New York: Bantam Dell.

Kabat-Zinn, J. (1994). *Wherever you go there you are: Mindfulness meditation in everyday life.* New York: Hyperion.

Keck, P. E. Jr., McElroy, S. L., Strakowski, S. M., West, S. A., Sax, K. W., Hawkins, J. M., et al. (1998). 12–month outcome of patients with bipolar disorder following hospitalization for a manic or mixed episode. *Am J Psychiatry, 155*(5), 646–652.

Kessler, R. C., Adler, L., Ames, M., Demler, O., Faraone, S., Hiripi, E., et al. (2005). The World Health Organization Adult ADHD Self-Report Scale (ASRS): A short screening scale for use in the general population. *Psychol Med, 35*(2), 245–256.

Kessler, R. C., Akiskal, H. S., Ames, M., Birnbaum, H., Greenberg, P., Hirschfeld, R. M., et al. (2006). Prevalence and effects of mood disorders on work performance in a nationally representative sample of U.S. workers. *Am J Psychiatry, 163*(9), 1561–1568.

Kessler, R. C., Chiu, W. T., Demler, O., Merikangas, K. R., & Walters, E. E. (2005). Prevalence, severity, and comorbidity of 12–month DSM-IV disorders in the National Comorbidity Survey Replication. *Arch Gen Psychiatry, 62*(6), 617–627.

Killingsworth, M. A., & Gilbert, D. T. (2010). A wandering mind is an unhappy mind. *Science, 330*(6006), 932.

Kim, S., Yu, B. H., Lee, D. S., & Kim, J. H. (2012). Ruminative response in clinical patients with major depressive disorder, bipolar disorder, and anxiety disorders. *J Affect Disord, 136*(1–2), e77–e81.

Kogan, J. N., Otto, M. W., Bauer, M. S., Dennehy, E. B., Miklowitz, D. J., Zhang, H. W., et al. (2004). Demographic and diagnostic characteristics of the first 1000 patients enrolled in the Systematic Treatment Enhancement Program for Bipolar Disorder (STEP-BD). *Bipolar Disord, 6*(6), 460–469.

Lam, D. H., Hayward, P., Watkins, E. R., Wright, K., & Sham, P. (2005). Relapse prevention in patients with bipolar disorder: Cognitive therapy outcome after 2 years. *Am J Psychiatry, 162*(2), 324–329.

Lam, D. H., Watkins, E. R., Hayward, P., Bright, J., Wright, K., Kerr, N., et al. (2003). A randomized controlled study of cognitive therapy for relapse prevention for bipolar affective disorder: Outcome of the first year. *Arch Gen Psychiatry, 60*(2), 145–152.

Linehan, M. M. (1993). *Skills training manual for treating borderline personality disorder.* New York: Guilford Press.

Marlatt, G. A., & Gordon, J. R. (Eds.). (2007). *Relapse prevention* (2nd ed.): *Maintenance strategies in the treatment of addictive behaviors.* New York: Guilford Press.

Martinez-Aran, A., Vieta, E., Reinares, M., Colom, F., Torrent, C., Sanchez-Moreno, J., et al. (2004). Cognitive function across manic or hypomanic, depressed, and euthymic states in bipolar disorder. *Am J Psychiatry, 161*(2), 262–270.

Martinez-Aran, A., Vieta, E., Torrent, C., Sanchez-Moreno, J., Goikolea, J. M., Salamero, M., et al. (2007). Functional outcome in bipolar disorder: The role of clinical and cognitive factors. *Bipolar Disord, 9*(1–2), 103–113.

Merikangas, K. R., Akiskal, H. S., Angst, J., Greenberg, P. E., Hirschfeld, R. M., Petukhova, M., et al. (2007). Lifetime and 12-month prevalence of bipolar spectrum disorder in the National Comorbidity Survey Replication. *Arch Gen Psychiatry, 64*(5), 543–552.

Merikangas, K. R., Ames, M., Cui, L., Stang, P. E., Ustun, T. B., Von Korff, M., et al. (2007). The impact of comorbidity of mental and physical conditions on role disability in the US adult household population. *Arch Gen Psychiatry, 64*(10), 1180–1188.

Meyer, F., & Meyer, T. D. (2009). The misdiagnosis of bipolar disorder as a psychotic disorder: Some of its causes and their influence on therapy. *J Affect Disord, 112*(1–3), 174–183.

Miklowitz, D. J. (2008a). Adjunctive psychotherapy for bipolar disorder: State of the evidence. *Am J Psychiatry, 165*(11), 1408–1419.

Miklowitz, D. J. (2008b). *Bipolar disorder: A family-focused treatment approach* (2nd ed.). New York: Guilford Press.

Miklowitz, D. J., Alatiq, Y., Goodwin, G. M., Geddes, J. R., Fennell, M. J. V., Dimidjian, S., et al. (2009). A pilot study of mindfulness-based cognitive therapy for bipolar disorder. *International Journal of Cognitive Therapy, 2*(4), 373–382.

Miklowitz, D. J., George, E. L., Richards, J. A., Simoneau, T. L., & Suddath, R. L. (2003). A randomized study of family-focused psychoeducation and pharmacotherapy in the outpatient management of bipolar disorder. *Arch Gen Psychiatry, 60*(9), 904–912.

Miklowitz, D. J., & Johnson, S. L. (2006). The psychopathology and treatment of bipolar disorder. *Annu Rev Clin Psychol, 2*, 199–235.

Miklowitz, D. J., Otto, M. W., Frank, E., Reilly-Harrington, N. A., Wisniewski, S. R., Kogan, J. N., et al. (2007). Psychosocial treatments for bipolar depression: A 1-year randomized trial from the Systematic Treatment Enhancement Program. *Arch Gen Psychiatry, 64*(4), 419–427.

Montgomery, S. A., & Asberg, M. (1979). A new depression scale designed to be sensitive to change. *Br J Psychiatry, 134*, 382–389.

Moore, A., & Malinowski, P. (2009). Meditation, mindfulness and cognitive flexibility. *Conscious Cogn, 18*(1), 176–186.

Morselli, P. L., & Elgie, R. (2003). GAMIAN-Europe/BEAM Survey I—Global analysis of a patient questionnaire circulated to 3450 members of 12 European advocacy groups operating in the field of mood disorders. *Bipolar Disord, 5*(4), 265–278.

Neacsiu, A. D., Rizvi, S. L., & Linehan, M. M. (2010). Dialectical behavior therapy skills use as a mediator and outcome of treatment for borderline personality disorder. *Behav Res Ther, 48*(9), 832–839.

Neff, K. D. (2003). Self-compassion: An alternative conceptualization of a healthy attitude towards oneself. *Self and Identity, 85*(2), 85–101.

Nierenberg, A. (2010). Evaluating the evidence for evidence-based treatment of bipolar depression. *Inter J Neuropsychoph, 13*, 28–28.

Nock, M. K., Wedig, M. M., Holmberg, E. B., & Hooley, J. M. (2008). The Emotion Reactivity Scale: Development, evaluation, and relation to self-injurious thoughts and behaviors. *Behav Ther, 39*(2), 107–116.

Nolen-Hoeksema, S. (1991). Responses to depression and their effects on the duration of depressive episodes. *J Abnorm Psychol, 100*(4), 569–582.

Orsillo, S, M., & Roemer, L. (2011). *The mindful way through anxiety: Break free]from chronic worry and reclaim your life.* New York: Guilford Press.

Ortner, C. N. M., Kilner, S. J., & Zelazo, P. D. (2007). Mindfulness meditation and reduced emotional interference on a cognitive task. *Motiv Emotion, 31*, 271–283.

Otto, M. W. (2000). Stories and metaphors in cognitive-behavior therapy. *Cognitive and Behavioral Practice, 7*(2), 166–172.

Otto, M. W., Reilly-Harrington, N., Kogan, J. N., Henin, A., Knauz, R. O., & Sachs, G. S. (2009). *Managing bipolar disorder: A cognitive-behavioral approach workbook.* New York: Oxford University Press.

Peralta, V., & Cuesta, M. J. (1998). Lack of insight in mood disorders. *J Affect Disord, 49*(1), 55–58.

Perlis, R. H., Miyahara, S., Marangell, L. B., Wisniewski, S. R., Ostacher, M., DelBello, M. P., et al. (2004). Long-term implications of early onset in bipolar disorder: Data from the first 1000 participants in the Systematic Treatment Enhancement Program for Bipolar Disorder (STEP-BD). *Biol Psychiatry, 55*(9), 875–881.

Perlis, R. H., Ostacher, M. J., Patel, J. K., Marangell, L. B., Zhang, H., Wisniewski, S. R., et al. (2006). Predictors of recurrence in bipolar disorder: Primary outcomes from the Systematic Treatment Enhancement Program for Bipolar Disorder (STEP-BD). *Am J Psychiatry, 163*(2), 217–224.

Perry, A., Tarrier, N., Morriss, R., McCarthy, E., & Limb, K. (1999). Randomised controlled trial of efficacy of teaching patients with bipolar disorder to identify early symptoms of relapse and obtain treatment. *BMJ, 318*(7177), 149–153.

Peters, A., Sylvia, L. G., Magalhaes, P. V., Miklowitz, D., Frank, E., Otto, M. W., et al. (in press). Age of onset, course of illness and response to psychotherapy in bipolar disorder: Results from STEP-BD. *Psychological Medicine.*

Peterson, R. A., & Reiss, S. (1992). *Anxiety Sensitivity Index manual* (2nd ed.). Washington, OH: International Diagnostic Systems.

Post, R. M. (1992). Transduction of psychosocial stress into the neurobiology of recurrent affective disorder. *Am J Psychiatry, 149*(8), 999–1010.

Rea, M. M., Tompson, M. C., Miklowitz, D. J., Goldstein, M. J., Hwang, S., & Mintz, J. (2003). Family-focused treatment versus individual treatment for bipolar disorder: Results of a randomized clinical trial. *J Consult Clin Psychol, 71*(3), 482–492.

Rodman, A. M., Chou, T., Peters, A. T., Ariel, A. H., Martowski, J., Peckham, A. D., et al. (2011). Bipolar disorder: How euthymic is euthymic? *Association for Behavioral and Cognitive Therapies.* San Francisco, CA.

Roemer, L., & Orsillo, S. M. (2009). *Mindfulness- and acceptance-based behavioral therapies in practice.* New York: Guilford Press.

Roemer, L., Orsillo, S. M., & Salters-Pedneault, K. (2008). Efficacy of an acceptance-based behavior therapy for generalized anxiety disorder: Evaluation in a randomized controlled trial. *J Consult Clin Psychol, 76*(6), 1083–1089.

Roth, R. M., Isquith, P. K., & Gioia, G. A. (2005). *BRIEF-A: Behavior Rating Inventory of Executive Function—Adult version.* Lutz: Psychological Assessment Resources.

Rush, A. J., Trivedi, M. H., Ibrahim, H. M., Carmody, T. J., Arnow, B., Klein, D. N., et al. (2003). The 16-Item Quick Inventory of Depressive Symptomatology (QIDS), clinician rating (QIDS-C), and self-report (QIDS-SR): A psychometric evaluation in patients with chronic major depression. *Biol Psychiatry, 54*(5), 573–583.

Ryff, C. D., & Singer, B. (1996). Psychological well-being: Meaning, measurement, and implications for psychotherapy research. *Psychother Psychosom, 65*(1), 14–23.

Sachs, G. S., Nierenberg, A. A., Calabrese, J. R., Marangell, L. B., Wisniewski, S. R., Gyulai, L., et al. (2007). Effectiveness of adjunctive antidepressant treatment for bipolar depression. *New England Journal of Medicine, 356*(17), 1711–1722.

Santorelli, S. (2000). *Heal thy self: Lessons on mindfulness in medicine.* New York: Three Rivers Press.

Scott, J., Paykel, E., Morris, R., Bentall, R., Rinderman, P., Johnson, T., et al. (2006). Cognitive-behavioural therapy for severe recurrent bipolsr disorders: Randomised controlled trial. *Br J Psychiatry, 188*, 313–320.

Scott, J., & Pope, M. (2002). Self-reported adherence to treatment with mood stabilizers, plasma levels, and psychiatric hospitalization. *Am J Psychiatry, 159*(11), 1927–1929.

Scott, J., & Tacchi, M. J. (2002). A pilot study of concordance therapy for individuals with bipolar disorders who are non-adherent with lithium prophylaxis. *Bipolar Disord, 4*(6), 386–392.

Segal, Z. V., Bieling, P., Young, T., MacQueen, G., Cooke, R., Martin, L., et al. (2010). Antidepressant monotherapy vs. sequential pharmacotherapy and mindfulness-based cognitive therapy, or placebo, for relapse prophylaxis in recurrent depression. *Arch Gen Psychiatry, 67*(12), 1256–1264.

Segal, Z. V., Williams, J. M. G., & Teasdale, J. D. (2002). *Mindfulness-based cognitive therapy for depression.* New York: Guilford.

Segal, Z. V., Williams, J. M. G., & Teasdale, J. D. (2013). *Mindfulness-based cognitive therapy for depression* (2nd ed.). New York: Guilford Press.

Sheehan, D. V., Lecrubier, Y., Sheehan, K. H., Amorim, P., Janavs, J., Weiller, E., et al. (1998). The Mini-International Neuropsychiatric Interview (M.I.N.I.): The development and validation of a structured diagnostic psychiatric interview for DSM-IV and ICD-10. *J Clin Psychiatry, 59*(Suppl. 20), 22–33; quiz 34–57.

Simon, G. E., Ludman, E. J., Bauer, M. S., Unutzer, J., & Operskalski, B. (2006). Long-term effectiveness and cost of a systematic care program for bipolar disorder. *Arch Gen Psychiatry, 63*(5), 500–508.

Simon, N. M., Otto, M. W., Wisniewski, S. R., Fossey, M., Sagduyu, K., Frank, E., et al. (2004). Anxiety disorder comorbidity in bipolar disorder patients: Data from the first 500 participants in the Systematic Treatment Enhancement Program for Bipolar Disorder (STEP-BD). *Am J Psychiatry, 161*(12), 2222–2229.

Slagter, H. A., Lutz, A., Greischar, L. L., Francis, A. D., Nieuwenhuis, S., Davis, J. M., et al. (2007). Mental training affects distribution of limited brain resources. *PLoS Biol, 5*(6), e138.

Stange, J. P., Eisner, L. R., Holzel, B. K., Peckham, A. D., Dougherty, D. D., Rauch, S. L., et al. (2011). Mindfulness-based cognitive therapy for bipolar disorder: Effects on cognitive functioning. *J Psychiatr Pract, 17*(6), 410–419.

Suppes, T., Leverich, G. S., Keck, P. E., Nolen, W. A., Denicoff, K. D., Altshuler, L. L., et al. (2001). The Stanley Foundation Bipolar Treatment Outcome Network: II. Demographics and illness characteristics of the first 261 patients. *J Affect Disord, 67*(1–3), 45–59.

Tang, Y. Y., Ma, Y., Wang, J., Fan, Y., Feng, S., Lu, Q., et al. (2007). Short-term meditation training improves attention and self-regulation. *Proc Natl Acad Sci USA, 104*(43), 17152–17156.

Teasdale, J. D., Segal, Z. V., & Williams, J. M. G. (1995). How does cognitive therapy prevent depressive relapse and why should attentional control (mindfulness) training help? *Behav Res Ther, 33*(1), 25–39.

Teasdale, J. D., Segal, Z. V., Williams, J. M., Ridgeway, V. A., Soulsby, J. M., & Lau, M. A. (2000). Prevention of relapse/recurrence in major depression by mindfulness-based cognitive therapy. *J Consult Clin Psychol, 68*(4), 615–623.

Tohen, M., Zarate, C. A. Jr., Hennen, J., Khalsa, H. K., Strakowski, S. M., GebreMedhin, P., et al. (2003). The McLean–Harvard First-Episode Mania Study: Prediction of recovery and first recurrence. *Am J Psychiatry, 160*(12), 2099–2107.

Trede, K., Salvatore, P., Baethge, C., Gerhard, A., Maggini, C., & Baldessarini, R. J. (2005). Manic–depressive illness: Evolution in Kraepelin's textbook, 1883–1926. *Harv Rev Psychiatry, 13*(3), 155–178.

U.S. Census Bureau. (2005, June 9). Population estimates by demographic characteristics. Table 2: Annual estimates of the population by selected age groups and sex for the United States: April 1, 2000 to July 1, 2004 (NC-EST2004-02). Washington, DC: Population Division, U.S. Census Bureau. Release Date: June 9, 2005. *www.census.gov/popest/national/asrh.*

Valentine, E. R., & Sweet, P. L. (1999). Meditation and attention: A comparison of the effects of concentrative and mindfulness meditation on sustained attention. *Mental Health, Religion and Culture, 2*(1), 59–70.

Van Dam, N. T., Sheppard, S. C., Forsyth, J. P., & Earleywine, M. (2011). Self-compassion is a better predictor than mindfulness of symptom severity and quality of life in mixed anxiety and depression. *J Anxiety Disord, 25*(1), 123–130.

van den Hurk, P. A., Giommi, F., Gielen, S. C., Speckens, A. E., & Barendregt, H. P. (2010). Greater efficiency in attentional processing related to mindfulness meditation. *Q J Exp Psychol* (Colchester), *63*(6), 1168–1180.

van der Loos, M. L., Mulder, P. G., Hartong, E. G., Blom, M. B., Vergouwen, A. C., de Keyzer, H. J., et al. (2009). Efficacy and safety of lamotrigine as add-on treatment to lithium in bipolar depression: A multicenter, double-blind, placebo-controlled trial. *J Clin Psychiatry, 70*(2), 223–231.

Watson, D., Clark, L. A., & Tellegen, A. (1988). Development and validation of brief measures of positive and negative affect: The PANAS scales. *J Pers Soc Psychol, 54*(6), 1063–1070.

Watson, D., & Tellegen, A. (1985). Toward a consensual structure of mood. *Psychol Bull, 98*(2), 219–235.

Wenk-Sormaz, H. (2005). Meditation can reduce habitual responding. *Alternative Therapies in Health and Medicine, 11*(2), 42–58.

Williams, J. M., Alatiq, Y., Crane, C., Barnhofer, T., Fennell, M. J., Duggan, D. S., et al. (2008). Mindfulness-based cognitive therapy (MBCT) in bipolar disorder: Preliminary evaluation of immediate effects on between-episode functioning. *J Affect Disord, 107*(1–3), 275–279.

Williams, J. M. G., Teasdale, J. D., Segal, Z. V., & Kabat-Zinn, J. (2007). *The mindful way through depression: Freeing yourself from chronic unhappiness.* New York: Guilford Press.

Young, R. C., Biggs, J. T., Ziegler, V. E., & Meyer, D. A. (1978). A rating scale for mania: Reliability, validity and sensitivity. *Br J Psychiatry, 133*, 429–435.

Zeidler, W. (2007). *Achtsamkeit und ihr Einfluss auf die Emotionsverarbeitung: Eine experimentelle Untersuchung der Wirkmechanismen [Mindfulness and its influence on emotion processing: An experimental investigation of mechanisms].* Saarbrücken, Germany: Vdm Verlag.

Index

333

List of Audio Tracks

Track	Title (size; run time)
1	**Yoga–Body Scan** (253 MB; 23:13)
2	**Introduction to the Breathing Space** (22 MB; 2:01)
3	**Body Scan** (189 MB; 17:46)
4	**Mindfulness of the Breath** (90 MB; 8:15)
5	**3-Minute Breathing Space** (37 MB; 3:23)
6	**Mindfulness of the Breath and Body** (104 MB; 9:48)
7	**Mindful Sitting with Sounds and Thoughts** (102 MB; 9:37)
8	**3-Minute Breathing Space with Acceptance** (42 MB; 3:55)
9	**Emotion-Focused Meditation** (109 MB; 10:15)
10	**Open Awareness Meditation** (111 MB; 10:29)
11	**Loving-Kindness Meditation** (140 MB; 12:48)